Osteoporosis

Fundamentals of Clinical Practice

Osteoporosis
Fundamentals of Clinical Practice

EDITOR

Murray J. Favus, M.D.
The University of Chicago
Pritzker School of Medicine
Chicago, Illinois

ASSOCIATE EDITORS

Sylvia Christakos, Ph.D.
University of Medicine and Dentistry of
New Jersey
New Jersey Medical School
Newark, New Jersey

Steven R. Goldring, M.D.
Howard Medical School
Deaconess and New England Baptist
Hospitals
Boston, Massachusetts

Geoffrey N. Hendy, B.Sc., Ph.D.
McGill University
Royal Victoria Hospital
Montreal, Quebec, Canada

Michael F. Holick, M.D., Ph.D.
Boston University School of Medicine and
Medical Center
Boston City Hospital
Boston, Massachusetts

Frederick Kaplan, M.D.
University of Pennsylvania School of
Medicine
Philadelphia, Pennsylvania

Sundeep Khosla, M.D.
Mayo Clinic and Medical School
Rochester, Minnesota

Michael Kleerekoper, M.D.,
F.A.C.E.
Wayne State University School of Medicine
Harper Hospital
Detroit, Michigan

Craig B. Langman, M.D.
Northwestern University Medical School
Children's Memorial Hospital
Chicago, Illinois

Jane B. Lian, Ph.D.
University of Massachusetts Medical School
Worcester, Massachusetts

Elizabeth Shane, M.D
Columbia University
College of Physicians and Surgeons
New York, New York

Dolores M. Shoback, M.D.
University of California, San Francisco
San Francisco Veterans Affairs Medical
Center
San Francisco, California

Andrew F. Stewart, M.D.
Yale University School of Medicine
Connecticut Veterans Affairs Medical Center
West Haven, Connecticut

Michael P. Whyte, M.D.
Washington University School of Medicine
Shriners Hospital for Crippled Children
Saint Louis, Missouri

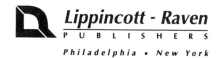

Lippincott - Raven
PUBLISHERS
Philadelphia • New York

Printed in the United States of America

9 8 7 6 5 4 3 2 1

ISBN 0-397-51823-4

WE 142
Osteoporosis

Contents

Section I. Anatomy and Biology of Bone Matrix and Cellular Elements

Section II. Calcium, Magnesium, and Phosphorus Homeostasis

Section III. Clinical Evaluation of Bone and Mineral Disorders

Section IV. Clinical Aspects of Osteoporosis

Section V. Appendix

Contributing Authors

Louis V. Avioli, M.D., F.A.C.E.
Shoenberg Professor of Medicine, and
  Professor of Orthopedic Surgery
Departments of Medicine and Orthopedic
  Surgery
Washington University Medical Center
Barnes-Jewish North Campus
216 South Kingshighway
St. Louis, Missouri 63110

Daniel T. Baran, M.D.
Professor of Medicine, Orthopedics, and Cell
  Biology
Departments of Medicine, Orthopedics, and
  Cell Biology
University of Massachusetts Medical Center
55 Lake Avenue, North
Worcester, Massachusetts 01655

Roland Baron, D.D.S., Ph.D.
Professor of Cell Biology and Orthopedics
Department of Cell Biology and Orthopedics
Yale University School of Medicine
333 Cedar Street
New Haven, Connecticut 06510

Arthur E. Broadus, M.D., Ph.D.
Professor of Medicine and Physiology
Department of Internal Medicine
Yale University
333 Cedar Street
New Haven, Connecticut 06510-8020

Sylvia Christakos, Ph.D.
Professor of Biochemisty and Molecular
  Biology
Department of Biochemistry and Molecular
  Biology
University of Medicine and Dentistry of
  New Jersey
New Jersey Medical School
185 South Orange Avenue
Newark, New Jersey 07103

Thomas A. Einhorn, M.D.
Professor of Orthopedics
Department of Orthopedics
Mount Sinai School of Medicine
Fifth Avenue and 100th Street
New York, New York 10029-6574

David R. Eyre, Ph.D.
Professor and Burgess Chairman of Orthopedic
  Research
Department of Orthopedics
University of Washington
Box 356500
1959 Northeast Pacific
Seattle, Washington 98195

Murray J. Favus, M.D.
Director, Bone Program
Director, General Clinical Research
  Center, and
Professor of Medicine
The University of Chicago
Pritzker School of Medicine
5841 South Maryland Avenue, MC5100
Chicago, Ilinois 60637

Harry K. Genant, M.D.
Skeletal Section
Radiology Department
University of California, San Francisco
Box 0628
San Francisco, California 94143-0628

Steven R. Goldring, M.D.
Associate Professor of Medicine
Harvard Medical School; and
Chief of Rheumatology
Deaconess and New England
  Baptist Hospitals
110 Francis Street
Boston, Massachusetts 02215

Robert P. Heaney, M.D.
John A. Creighton University Professor
Creighton University
2500 California Plaza
Omaha, Nebraska 68178

Geoffrey N. Hendy, B.Sc., Ph.D.
Professor of Medicine
Departments of Medicine and Physiology
McGill University; and
Calcium Research Laboratory
Royal Victoria Hospital
687 Pine Avenue West
Montreal, Quebec, Canada, H3A 1A1

Michael F. Holick, M.D., Ph.D.
Professor of Medicine, Physiology, and
*   Dermatology*
Department of Medicine
Section of Endocrinology, Diabetes, and
*   Metabolism*
Boston University School of Medicine and
*   Medical Center; and*
Boston City Hospital
80 East Concord Street, M-1013
Boston, Massachusetts 02118

Jeffrey A. Jackson, M.D.
Associate Professor of Medicine
Division of Endocrinology
Scott & White Clinic
Texas A & M University Health Science Center
2401 South 31 Street
Temple, Texas 76508

C. Conrad Johnston, Jr., M.D.
Professor of Medicine
Department of Medicine
Indiana University School of Medicine
545 North Barnhill Drive
Emerson Hall 421
Indianapolis, Indiana 46202-5124

Frederick Kaplan, M.D.
Chief, Division of Metabolic Bone Diseases
Departments of Orthopaedic Surgery and
*   Medicine*
University of Pennsylvania School of Medicine
Silverstein Pavilion
3400 Spruce Street
Philadelphia, Pennsylvania 19104

Sundeep Khosla, M.D.
Associate Professor of Medicine
Department of Endocrinology
Mayo Clinic and Medical School
200 First Street, Southwest
Rochester, Minnesota 55905

Michael Kleerekoper, M.D., F.A.C.E.
Professor of Medicine
Department of Internal Medicine
Wayne State University School of Medicine
Harper Hospital
1 Webber South
3990 John R
Detroit, Michigan 48201

Craig B. Langman, M.D.
Professor of Pediatrics
Head, Nephrology and Mineral Metabolism
Department of Pediatrics
Northwestern University Medical School; and
Children's Memorial Hospital
2300 Children's Plaza, Box 37
Chicago, Illinois 60614

Jane B. Lian, Ph.D.
Professor of Cell Biology
Department of Cell Biology
University of Massachusetts Medical School
55 Lake Avenue North
Worcester, Massachusetts 01655-0106

Robert Lindsay, Ph.D., M.B., Ch.B.,
*   **F.R.C.P.***
Professor of Clinical Medicine
Columbia University
New York, New York; and
Department of Medicine
Helen Hayes Hospital
Route 9 West
West Haverstraw, New York 10993

Barbara P. Lukert, M.D.
Professor of Medicine
Department of Medicine
University of Kansas Medical Center
3901 Cambridge
Kansas City, Kansas 66160

Robert Marcus, M.D.
Professor of Medicine
Department of Medicine
Stanford University, and
Veterans Affairs Medical Center
3801 Miranda Avenue
Palo Alto, California 94304

L. Joseph Melton III, M.D.
Eisenberg Professor of Epidemiology
Department of Health Sciences Research
Mayo Clinic and Foundation
200 First Street, Southwest
Rochester, Minnesota 55905

Gregory R. Mundy, M.D.
Department of Medicine, Endocrinology and
*   Metabolism*
University of Texas Health Science Center
7703 Floyd Curl Drive
San Antonio, Texas 78284-7877

Michael E. Norman, M.D.
Clinical Professor of Pediatrics
Department of Pediatrics
University of North Carolina School of
*   Medicine*
Chapel Hill, North Carolina 27599

Eric S. Orwoll, M.D.
Chief, Department of Endocrinology and
*   Metabolism*
Portland Veterans Affairs Medical Center; and
Associate Professor of Medicine
Oregon Health Sciences University
3181 Southwest Sam Jackson Park
Portland, Oregon 97201

Socrates E. Papapoulos, M.D., Ph.D.
Associate Professor of Medicine
Department of Endocrinology and Metabolic
*   Diseases*
University Hospital Leiden
Rijnsburgerweg 10
2333 AA Leiden, The Netherlands

J. Edward Puzas, Ph.D.
Donald and Mary Clark Professor of
*   Orthopedics*
Department of Orthopaedics
University of Rochester School of Medicine
575 Elmwood Avenue
Rochester, New York 14642

Pamela Gehron Robey, Ph.D.
Chief, Bone Research Branch
National Insititutes of Health
9000 Rockville Pike MSC 4320
Bethesda, Maryland 20892

Elizabeth Shane, M.D.
Associate Professor of Clinical Medicine
Department of Medicine
Columbia University
College of Physicians and Surgeons
630 West 168th Street
New York, New York 10032

Dolores M. Shoback, M.D.
Associate Professor of Medicine
Department of Medicine
University of California, San Francisco, and
San Francisco Veterans Affairs Medical Center
4150 Clement Street
San Francisco, California 94121

Charles W. Slemenda, M.P.H., Dr. P.H.
Associate Professor of Medicine
Department of Medicine
Indiana University School of Medicine, and
Riley Hospital
702 Barnhill Drive
Indianapolis, Indiana 46202

Andrew F. Stewart, M.D.
Professor of Medicine
Department of Endocrinology
Yale University School of Medicine; and
Chief, Department of Endocrinology
Connecticut Veterans Affairs Medical Center
950 Campbell Avenue, 151C
West Haven, Connecticut 06516

John D. Termine, Ph.D.
Executive Director
Lilly Research Labs
Eli Lilly and Company
Lilly Corporate Center
Indianapolis, Indiana 46285

Richard D. Wasnich, M.D., F.A.C.P.
Hawaii Osteoporosis Center
401 Kamakee Street, Second Floor
Honolulu, Hawaii 96814

Michael P. Whyte, M.D.
Professor of Medicine and Pediatrics
Division of Bone and Mineral Diseases
Washington University School of Medicine; and
Medical Director, Metabolic Research Unit
Shriners Hospital for Crippled Children
2001 South Lindbergh Boulevard
St. Louis, Missouri 63131-3597

The American Society for Bone and Mineral Research

The diseases of bone are growing not just in prevalence but also in importance. Osteoporosis is one of the most talked-about conditions of the 1990s, and new diagnostic tests and medications are changing the face of this common disease. However, other diseases of the bone, such as osteolytic bone disease and Paget's disease, are increasingly common in our patient population, and therapeutic approaches are changing as our knowledge of these conditions increase.

In the 20 years of its existence, The American Society for Bone and Mineral Research (ASBMR) has become the primary forum for the presentation of new knowledge in the field of bone and mineral metabolism. This is accomplished mainly through its Annual Scientific Meeting and the *Journal of Bone and Mineral Research* (JBMR). Both the Annual Meeting and the JBMR attempt to cover this entire field, from the most basic mechanisms to practical aspects of the clinical management of patients with common diseases of bone. The Education Committee of the ASBMR launched *The Primer* in 1990 as a comprehensive account of the field for all those interested, including not only society members but also students, residents, and fellows who might eventually be attracted to this rapidly growing field. Now in its third edition, *The Primer* has been extremely popular as an authoritative, educational, and up-to-date account of this field compiled by workers at the very forefront. We anticipate that this abridged version will provide a user-friendly window to this field for busy practitioners. We hope you like it.

Gregory R. Mundy, M.D.
President, American Society for Bone
and Mineral Research
June 1997

Preface

The rapid growth of interest in osteoporosis and related disorders has attracted basic scientists of diverse backgrounds to the study of bone biology, who have gathered important new information to facilitate the treatment of bone disease. Clinical investigators from many disciplines have applied this new basic knowledge to improve diagnosis and treatment of osteoporosis. To disseminate this new information on the causes, diagnoses, and treatments of osteoporosis to a wider audience, the Education Committee of the American Society for Bone and Mineral Research has selected 22 chapters and portions of the Appendix from the third edition of its publication titled *Primer of Metabolic Bone Diseases and Disorders of Mineral Metabolism* to create *Osteoporosis: Fundamentals of Clinical Practice*. The Editors of *The Primer* believe that primary care physicians will find this concise but informative format their first choice of information on osteoporosis. We hope that this publication will foster timely, effective, and cost-efficient patient care, and we welcome your comments and suggestions for future editions.

Murray J. Favus. M.D.
The University of Chicago
Pritzker School of Medicine
June 1997

Preface to the Third Edition

As with the first two editions of the *Primer*, the *Third Edition* is written for those clinicians, basic scientists, students, residents, and fellows who seek a concise yet thorough description of basic bone biology, mineral metabolism, and the diseases that affect these systems. While the basic organization of the *Primer* has been retained the large volume of important new information in both the basic sciences and clinical realms has resulted in the extensive revision of nine chapters and the addition of 30 new chapters.

Over the past several years, the scientific contributions of a relatively small group of investigators have attracted increasing numbers of basic scientists and clinical investigators into the field of bone and mineral metabolism. The broad array of scientists entering the bone field also reflects the movement away from the traditional separation of disciplines, as research turns from descriptive science to the understanding of molecular processes. This general evolution of science is reflected in the basic science chapters, whose authors have backgrounds in cellular and molecular biology, physiology, biochemistry, embryology, and molecular genetics. The clinical chapters also show the breadth of interest in the field, with contributions from authors with backgrounds in internal medicine, endocrinology, genetics, nephrology, pediatrics, rheumatology, radiology, nuclear medicine, nutrition, and orthopedic surgery. The breadth and depth of the current expanding research effort has created an anticipation for further advances, making this an exciting time to be in this field.

Murray J. Favus. M.D.
Bone Program
University of Chicago Medical Center
June 1996

Acknowledgments

Credit for any success the *Primer* may enjoy is due to the contributing authors' devotion to their areas of interest, and their commitment to present their material in the most comprehensible manner. The high standards set by the authors of the first two editions are greatly appreciated and are responsible for the excellent chapters prepared for the Third Edition. Yet, the greatest asset continues to be the Associate Editors and members of the ASBMR Task Force for *Primer, Third Edition,* including Sylvia Christakos, Steven R. Goldring, Geoffrey N. Hendy, Michael F. Holick, Sundeep Khosla, Frederick Kaplan, Michael Kleerekoper, Craig B. Langman, Jane B. Lian, Elizabeth Shane, Dolores M. Shoback, Andrew F. Stewart, and Michael P. Whyte. I am deeply grateful for their hard work, creativity, dedication, and thoughtful criticism. I also wish to acknowledge the strong support we have received from our publisher, Lippincott-Raven. My deep appreciation is extended to Judy Hummel for her diligence and good spirit in coordinating the day-to-day communications between the authors, Associate Editors, and Lippincott–Raven Publishers.

Murray J. Favus, M.D.
June 1996

Osteoporosis

Fundamentals of Clinical Practice

SECTION I

Anatomy and Biology of Bone Matrix and Cellular Elements

1. Anatomy and Ultrastructure of Bone

Roland E. Baron, D.D.S., Ph.D.

Departments of Orthopedics and Cell Biology, Yale University, School of Medicine, New Haven, Connecticut

Bone is a specialized connective tissue that makes up, together with cartilage, the skeletal system. These tissues serve three functions: (i) mechanical: support and site of muscle attachment for locomotion; (ii) protective: for vital organs and bone marrow; and (iii) metabolic: as a reserve of ions, especially calcium and phosphate, for the maintenance of serum homeostasis, which is essential to life.

In bone, as in all connective tissues, the fundamental constituents are the cells and the extracellular matrix. The latter is particularly abundant in this tissue and is composed of collagen fibers and noncollagenous proteins. In bone, cartilage, and the tissues forming the teeth, however, unlike in other connective tissues, the matrices have the unique ability to become calcified.

BONE AS AN ORGAN: MACROSCOPIC ORGANIZATION

Anatomically, two types of bones can be distinguished in the skeleton: flat bones (skull bones, scapula, mandible, and ileum) and long bones (tibia, femur, and humerus). These two types are derived by two distinct types of histogenesis, intramembranous and endochondral, respectively (see later section, Bone Histogenesis and Growth), although the development and growth of long bones actually involve both types of histogenesis.

External examination of a long bone (Fig. 1) shows two wider extremities (the epiphyses), a more or less cylindrical tube in the middle (the midshaft or diaphysis), and a developmental zone between them (the metaphysis). In a growing long bone, the epiphysis and the metaphysis, which originate from two independent ossification centers, are separated by a layer of cartilage, the *epiphyseal cartilage* (also called growth plate). This layer of proliferative cells and expanding cartilage matrix is responsible for the longitudinal growth of bones; it becomes entirely calcified and remodeled by the end of the growth period (see later section, Bone Histogenesis and Growth). The external part of the bones is formed by a thick and dense layer of calcified tissue, the *cortex* (compact bone) which, in the diaphysis, encloses the medullary cavity where the hematopoietic bone marrow is housed. Toward the metaphysis and the epiphysis, the cortex becomes progressively thinner and the internal space is filled with a network of thin, calcified trabeculae; this is the *cancellous bone,* also named spongy or *trabecular bone.* The spaces enclosed by these thin trabeculae are also filled with hematopoietic bone marrow and are in continuity with the medullary cavity of the diaphysis. The bone surfaces at the epiphyses that take part in the joint are covered with a layer of articular cartilage that does not calcify.

There are consequently two bone surfaces at which the bone is in contact with the soft tissues (Fig. 1): an external

surface (the periosteal surface) and an internal surface (the endosteal surface). These surfaces, the *periosteum* and the *endosteum,* are lined with osteogenic cells organized in layers. Cortical and trabecular bone are constituted of the same cells and the same matrix elements, but there are structural and functional differences. The primary structural difference is quantitative: 80% to 90% of the volume of compact bone is calcified, whereas 15% to 25% of the trabecular bone is calcified (the remainder being occupied by bone

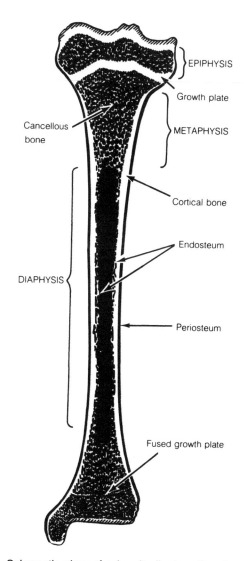

FIG. 1. Schematic view of a longitudinal section through a growing long bone. (From: Jee WSS. The skeletal tissues. In: Weiss L (ed) *Histology, Cell and Tissue Biology.* Elsevier Biomedical, New York, 200–255, 1983.)

marrow, blood vessels, and connective tissue). The result is that 70% to 85% of the interface with soft tissues is at the endosteal bone surface, which leads to the functional difference: the cortical bone fulfills mainly a mechanical and protective function and the trabecular bone a metabolic function.

BONE AS A TISSUE

Microscopic Organization

Bone Matrix and Mineral

Bone is formed by *collagen fibers* (type I, 90% of the total protein), usually oriented in a preferential direction, and noncollagenous proteins. Spindle- or plate-shaped crystals of hydroxyapatite $[3Ca_3(PO_4)_2 \cdot (OH)_2]$ are found on the collagen fibers, within them, and in the ground substance. They tend to be oriented in the same direction as the collagen fibers. The ground substance is primarily composed of glycoproteins and proteoglycans. These highly anionic complexes have a high ion-binding capacity and are thought to play an important part in the calcification process and the fixation of hydroxyapatite crystals to the collagen fibers.

Numerous noncollagenous proteins present in bone matrix have recently been purified and sequenced (see Chapter 4), but their role has been only partially characterized. Most of these proteins are synthesized by bone-forming cells, but not all: a number of plasma proteins are preferentially absorbed by the bone matrix, such as α_2-HS-glycoprotein, which is synthesized in the liver.

The preferential orientation of the collagen fibers alternates in adult bone from layer to layer, giving to this bone a typical *lamellar* structure, best seen under polarized light or by electron microscopy. This fiber organization allows the highest density of collagen per unit volume of tissue. The

lamellae can be parallel to each other if deposited along a flat surface (trabecular bone and periosteum), or concentric if deposited on a surface surrounding a channel centered on a blood vessel (haversian system, Fig. 2). However, when bone is being formed very rapidly (during histogenesis and fracture healing, or in tumors and some metabolic bone diseases), there is no preferential organization of the collagen fibers. They are then found in somewhat randomly oriented bundles: this type of bone is called *woven bone* (see later section, Bone Histogenesis and Growth), as opposed to lamellar bone.

Cellular Organizations Within the Bone Matrix: Osteocytes

The calcified bone matrix is not metabolically inert, and cells (osteocytes) are found embedded deep within the bone in small osteocytic lacunae ($25,000/mm^3$ of bone) (Figs. 2,3). They were originally bone-forming cells (osteoblasts), and they were trapped in the bone matrix that they produced and which later became calcified. These cells have numerous and long cell processes rich in microfilaments, which are in contact with cell processes from other osteocytes (i.e., there are frequent *gap junctions*), or with processes from the cells lining the bone surface (osteoblasts or flat lining cells in the endosteum or periosteum). These processes are organized during the formation of the matrix and before its calcification; they form a network of thin canaliculi permeating the entire bone matrix (Fig. 2).

Between the osteocyte's plasma membrane and the bone matrix itself is the *periosteocytic space.* This space exists both in the lacunae and in the canaliculi, and it is filled with extracellular fluid (ECF).

The physiological significance of this system is readily demonstrated by some numbers. The total bone surface area of the canaliculae and lacunae is 1000 to 5000 m^2 in an adult (compared to a surface area of 140 m^2 for lung capillaries); the volume of bone ECF is 1.0 to 1.5 L; and the surface calcium contained on bone mineral crystals is approximately 5 to 20 g, which accounts for a significant percentage of the total exchangeable bone calcium. The fact that the calcium concentration in the bone ECF (0.5 mmol/L) is lower than in plasma (1.5 mmol/L) suggests that there is a constant flow of calcium ions out of the bone.

The morphology of the osteocytes varies according to their age and functional activity. A young osteocyte has most of the ultrastructural characteristics of the osteoblast from which it was derived, except that there has been a decrease in cell volume and in the importance of the organelles involved in protein synthesis (rough endoplasmic reticulum, Golgi). An older osteocyte, located deeper within the calcified bone, shows these decreases further accentuated, and, in addition, there is an accumulation of glycogen in the cytoplasm. These cells have been shown to be able to synthesize new bone matrix at the surface of the osteocytic lacunae, which can subsequently calcify. Although historically they have been considered able to resorb calcified bone from the same surface, this point has recently been dis-

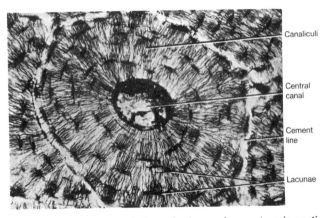

FIG. 2. Cross-sectional view of a haversian system in cortical bone, showing the lamellar organization of collagen in mature bone matrix, and the morphology and canalicular organization of osteocytes. (From: Jee WSS. The skeletal tissues. In: Weiss L (ed) *Histology, Cell and Tissue Biology.* Elsevier Biomedical, New York, 200–255, 1983.)

Canaliculi

Central canal

Cement line

Lacunae

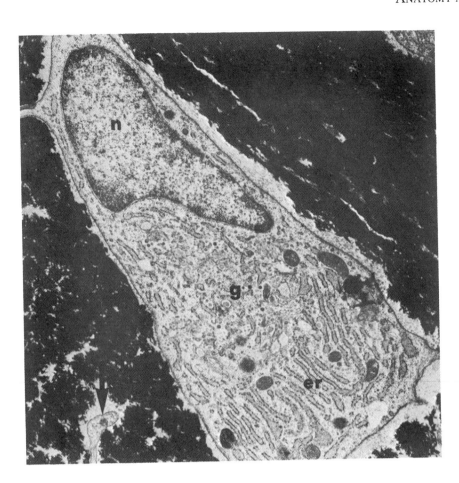

FIG. 3. Osteocyte. Electron micrograph of an osteocyte embedded in calcified bone matrix (black, hydroxyapatite crystals). The cell has a basal nucleus (n), a large Golgi complex (g), and a relatively well-developed endoplasmic reticulum (er). Cytoplasmic extensions can be seen in the matrix *(arrow)* in their canaliculi. Approximate magnification, ×5000.

puted. The fate of the osteocytes is to be phagocytized and digested, together with the other components of bone, during osteoclastic bone resorption. These cells may also play a role in local activation of bone turnover.

The Bone Surface

Most of the bone tissue turnover occurs at the bone surfaces, mainly at the endosteal surface where it interfaces with bone marrow. This surface is morphologically heterogeneous, reflecting the various specific cellular activities involved in remodeling and turnover.

The Osteoblast and Bone Formation

The osteoblast is the bone lining cell responsible for the production of the matrix constituents (collagen and ground substance) (Fig. 4). It originates from a local mesenchymal stem cell (bone marrow stromal stem cell or connective tissue mesenchymal stem cell). These precursors, with the right stimulation, undergo proliferation and differentiate into preosteoblasts and then into mature osteoblasts. Osteoblasts never appear or function individually but are always found in clusters of cuboidal cells along the bone surface (~100–400 cells per bone-forming site). At the light microscope level, the osteoblast is characterized by a round

nucleus at the base of the cell (opposite to the bone surface), a strongly basophilic cytoplasm, and a prominent Golgi complex located between the nucleus and the apex of the cell. Osteoblasts are always found lining the layer of bone matrix that they are producing, before it is calcified (called, at this point, *osteoid tissue*). Osteoid tissue exists because of a time lag between matrix formation and its subsequent calcification (the osteoid maturation period), which is approximately 10 days. Behind the osteoblast can usually be found one or two layers of cells: activated mesenchymal cells and preosteoblasts. At the ultrastructural level, the osteoblast is characterized by (i) the presence of an extremely well-developed rough endoplasmic reticulum with dilated cisternae and a dense granular content, and (ii) the presence of a large circular Golgi complex comprising multiple Golgi stacks. Cytoplasmic processes on the secreting side of the cell extend deep into the osteoid matrix and are in contact with the osteocyte processes in their canaliculi. Junctional complexes (gap junctions) are often found between the osteoblasts. The plasma membrane of the osteoblast is characteristically rich in alkaline phosphatase (whose concentration in the serum is used as an index of bone formation) and has been shown to have receptors for parathyroid hormone, but not for calcitonin. Osteoblasts also express receptors for estrogens and vitamin D_3 in their nuclei. Toward the end of the secreting period, the osteoblast becomes either a flat lining cell or an osteocyte.

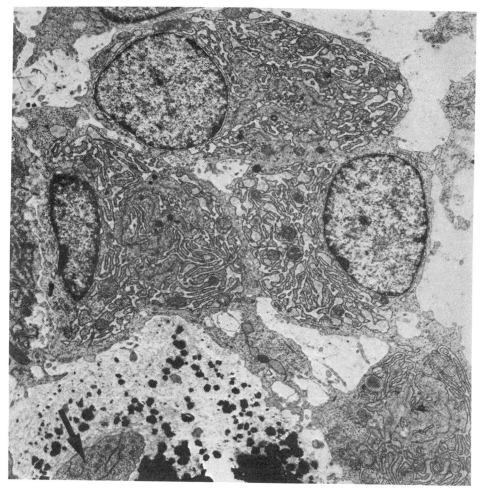

FIG. 4. Osteoblasts and osteoid tissue. Electron micrograph of a group of osteoblasts *(top)* covering a layer of mineralizing osteoid tissue *(bottom)* with a newly embedded osteocyte *(arrow)*. Basal nuclei, prominent Golgi, and endoplasmic reticulum, and characteristics of active osteoblasts. Approximate magnification, ×3000.

The Osteoclast and Bone Resorption

The osteoclast is the bone lining cell responsible for bone resorption (Fig. 5).

Morphology. The osteoclast is a giant multinucleated cell, containing four to 20 nuclei. It is usually found in contact with a calcified bone surface and within a lacuna (Howship's lacunae) that is the result of its own resorptive activity. It is possible to find up to four or five osteoclasts in the same resorptive site, but there usually are only one or two. Under the light microscope, the nuclei appear to vary within the same cell: some are round and euchromatic, and some are irregular in contour and heterochromatic, possibly reflecting the asynchronous fusion of mononuclear precursors. The cytoplasm is "foamy" with many vacuoles. The zone of contact with the bone (the sealing zone) is characterized by the presence of a ruffled border with dense patches on each side.

Characteristic ultrastructural features of this cell are the abundant Golgi complexes characteristically disposed around each nucleus, the mitochondria, and the transport vesicles loaded with lysosomal enzymes. The most prominent features of the osteoclast are, however, the deep foldings of the plasma membrane in the area facing the bone matrix, which form the sealing zone: the ruffled border surrounded by a ring of contractile proteins that serve to attach the cell to the bone surface, thus sealing off the subosteoclastic bone-resorbing compartment. The attachment of the cell to the matrix is performed via integrin receptors, which bind to specific sequences in matrix proteins. The plasma membrane in the ruffled border area contains proteins that are also found at the limiting membrane of lysosomes and related organelles, and a specific type of electrogenic proton ATPase involved in acidification. The basolateral plasma membrane of the osteoclast is highly and specifically enriched in (Na^+, K^+) ATPase (sodium-potassium pumps), HCO_3^-/Cl^- exchangers, and Na^+/H^+ exchangers.

Mechanisms of Bone Resorption. *Lysosomal enzymes* are actively synthesized by the osteoclast and are found in the

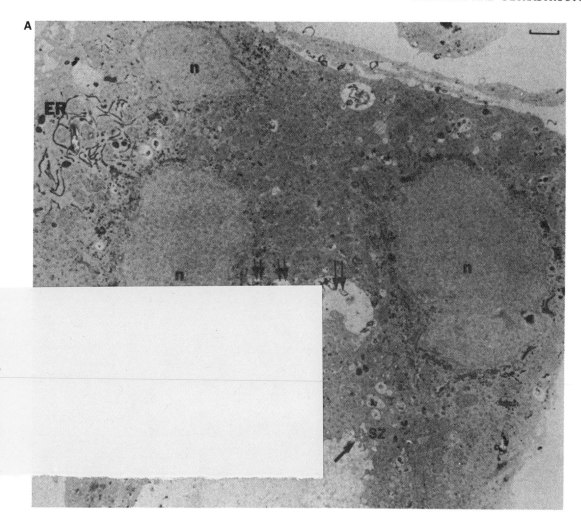

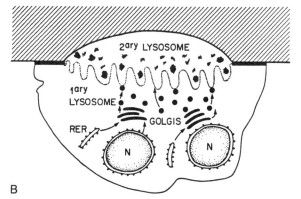

OSTEOCLAST

FIG. 5. Osteoclast. **A:** Section of an osteoclast stained for the lysosomal enzyme arylsulfatase. The osteoclast contains multiple nuclei (n), an endoplasmic reticulum where lysosomal enzymes are synthesized (ER), and prominent Golgi stacks around each nucleus. The cell is attached to bone matrix *(bottom)* and forms a separate compartment underneath itself, limited by the sealing zone (SZ) *(single arrows)*. The plasma membrane of the cell facing this compartment is extensively folded and forms the ruffled border, with pockets of extracellular space between the folds *(double arrows)*. Multiple small vesicles for transporting enzymes toward the bone matrix can be seen in the cytoplasm. Approximate magnification, ×9000. **B:** Schematic representation of enzyme secretion polarity in osteoclasts. (From: Baron R, Neff L, Louvard D, Courtoy PJ. *J Cell Biol* 101:2210–2222, 1985.)

endoplasmic reticulum, Golgi, and many transport vesicles. The enzymes are secreted, via the ruffled border, into the extracellular bone-resorbing compartment; they reach a sufficiently high extracellular concentration because this compartment is sealed off. The transport and targeting of these enzymes for secretion at the apical pole of the osteoclast involves mannose-6-phosphate receptors. Furthermore, the cell secretes nonlysosomal enzymes such as collagenase.

The acidifies the extracellular compartment by secreting protons across the ruffled-border membrane (by proton pumps). Recent evidence suggests the presence of an electrogenic proton-pump ATPase, related to but different from that of the kidney-tubule-acidifying cells. The protons are provided to the pumps by the enzyme carbonic anhydrase, and they are highly concentrated in the cytosol of the osteoclast; ATP and CO_2 are provided by the mitochondria. The basolat-

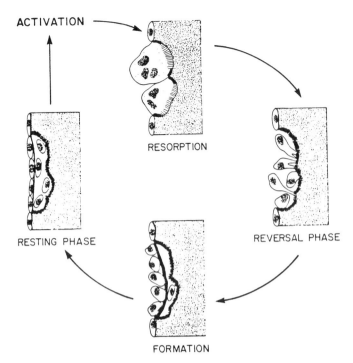

ACTIVATION

RESORPTION

RESTING PHASE

REVERSAL PHASE

FORMATION

FIG. 6. Bone remodeling. The bone remodeling sequence as it occurs in trabecular bone. (The same principles apply to haversian remodeling; see text.)

eral membrane activity exchanges bicarbonate for chloride, thereby avoiding an alkalinization of the cytosol. The basolateral sodium pumps might be involved in secondary active transport of calcium and/or protons in association with a Na^+/Ca^{2+} exchanger and/or a Na^+/H^+ antiport. This cell could therefore function in a manner similar to that of kidney tubule or gastric parietal cells, which also acidify lumens.

The extracellular bone-resorbing compartment is therefore the functional equivalent of a secondary lysosome, with (i) a low pH, (ii) lysosomal enzymes, and (iii) the substrate. The low pH dissolves the crystals, exposing the matrix. The enzymes, now at optimal pH, degrade the matrix components; the residues from this extracellular digestion are either internalized, or they are transported across the cell (by transcytosis) and released at the basolateral domain, or they are released during periods of relapse of the sealing zone,

possibly induced by a calcium sensor responding to the rise of extracellular calcium in the bone-resorbing compartment.

First, the hydroxyapatite crystals are mobilized by digestion of their link to collagen (the noncollagenous proteins) and dissolved by the acid environment. Then, the residual collagen fibers are digested either by the activation of latent collagenase or by the action of cathepsins at low pH.

Clinically, this explains why (i) bone resorption helps to maintain calcium and inorganic phosphate levels in the plasma, and (ii) the concentrations of hydroxyproline and N-terminal collagen peptides in the urine are used as indirect measurements of bone resorption in humans (collagen type I is highly enriched in hydroxyproline and pyridoxiline links).

Origin and Fate of the Osteoclast. It is the work of Walker on osteopetrotic mice that established the hematogenous origin of the osteoclast. Cells of the mononuclear/phagocytic lineage are the most likely candidates for differentiation into osteoclasts. Although this differentiation may occur at the promonocyte stage, monocytes and macrophages, already committed to their own lineage, might still be able to form osteoclasts under the right circumstances.

Recent work has suggested that, despite its mononuclear/phagocytic origin, the osteoclast membrane is devoid of Fc and C_3 receptors, as well as of several other macrophage markers; it is, however, rich in nonspecific esterases, it synthesizes lysozyme, and it expresses colony-stimulating factor 1 (CSF-1) receptors, as do mononuclear phagocytes. Monoclonal antibodies have been produced that recognize osteoclasts but not macrophages. Receptors for calcitonin, but not for parathyroid hormone, are present on the osteoclast membrane, and estrogen, but not vitamin D receptors, have been found in these cells.

BONE REMODELING

The previously described activity of bone cells is performed along the surfaces of bone, mainly the endosteal surface, and it results in bone remodeling, which is the process of bone growth and turnover. Bone formation and bone resorption do not, however, occur along the bone surface at random: they are part of the turnover mechanism by which old bone is replaced by new bone. In the normal adult skeleton, bone formation occurs only where bone resorption has previously occurred. The sequence of events at the remodeling site (Figs. 6,7) is the

Remodeling Sequence

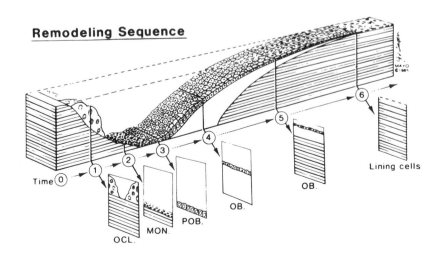

Time ⓪ ① ② ③ ④ ⑤ ⑥

OCL. MON. POB. OB. OB. Lining cells

FIG. 7. Bone remodeling in cancellous bone as seen in longitudinal sequence and cross sections. Five different phases can be distinguished over time: (1) osteoclastic resorption, (2) reversal, (3) preosteoblastic migration and differentiation into osteoblasts, (4) osteoblastic matrix (osteoid) formation, and (5) mineralization. The end-product of remodeling in cancellous bone is the completed cancellous bone structural unit (BSU) covered by lining cells (6). (From: Eriksen EF, Axelrod DW, Melsen F. *Bone Histomorphometry*. Raven Press, New York, 3–12, 1994.)

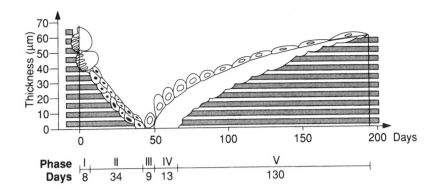

FIG. 8. Duration and depth of the various phases of the normal cancellous-bone-remodeling sequence, calculated from histomorphometric analysis of bone biopsy samples obtained from young individuals. Note the balance between the erosion depth and the mean wall thickness. (From: Eriksen EF, Axelrod DW, Melsen F. *Bone Histomorphometry*. Raven Press, New York, 13–20, 1994.)

activation-resorption-formation (ARF) sequence. During the intermediate phase between resorption and formation (the reversal phase), some macrophage-like, uncharacterized mononuclear cells are observed at the site of the remodeling, and a cement line is formed, which marks the limit of resorption and acts to cement together the old and the new bone. The duration of these various phases has been measured (Fig. 8): the complete remodeling cycle takes about 3 to 6 months.

Although cortical bone is anatomically different, its remodeling follows the same biological principles (Fig. 9). Lamellar bone being formed within such a system gives the characteristic structure of an haversian system when seen in cross section (see Fig. 2).

BONE HISTOGENESIS AND GROWTH

There are two types of histogenesis of bone: intramembranous ossification (flat bones) and endochondral ossification (long bones). The main difference between them is the presence of a cartilaginous phase in the latter.

Intramembranous Ossification

In intramembranous ossification, a group of mesenchymal cells within a highly vascularized area of the embryonic connective tissue undergoes division and differentiates directly into preosteoblasts and then into osteoblasts. These cells synthesize a bone matrix with the following characteristics: (i) the collagen fibers are not preferentially oriented but appear as irregular bundles, (ii) the osteocytes are large and extremely numerous, and (iii) calcification is delayed and does not proceed in an orderly fashion but in irregularly distributed patches. This type of bone is called woven bone.

At the periphery, mesenchymal cells continue to differentiate, following the same steps. Blood vessels incorporated between the woven bone trabeculae will form the hematopoietic bone marrow. Later, this woven bone is remodeled following the ARF sequence, and it is progressively replaced by mature lamellar bone.

Endochondral Ossification

Formation of a Cartilage Model

Mesenchymal cells undergo division and differentiate into prechondroblasts and then into chondroblasts. These cells secrete the cartilaginous matrix. Like the osteoblasts, the chondroblasts become progressively embedded within their own matrix, where they lie within lacunae, and they are then called chondrocytes. But, unlike the osteocytes, they continue to proliferate for some time, this being allowed in part by the gel-like consistency of cartilage. At the periphery of this cartilage (the perichondrium), the mesenchymal cells continue to proliferate and differentiate. This is called appositional growth. Another type of growth is observed in the cartilage by synthesis of new matrix between the chondrocytes (interstitial growth). In the growth plate, the cells appear in regular columns called isogenous groups. Later on, the chondrocytes enlarge progressively, become hypertrophic, and die.

Vascular Invasion and Longitudinal Growth (Remodeling)

The embryonic cartilage is avascular. During its early development, a ring of woven bone is formed by intramem-

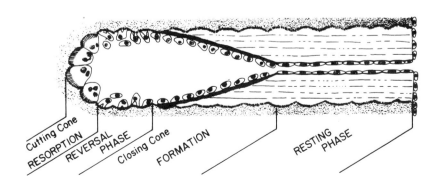

FIG. 9. The bone-remodeling activity in cortical bone as seen in longitudinal sequence. Osteoclasts dig out a tunnel, creating a "cutting cone." Subsequently, new bone is formed in the area of the "closing cone," leading to the creation of a new BSU (i.e., the haversian system).

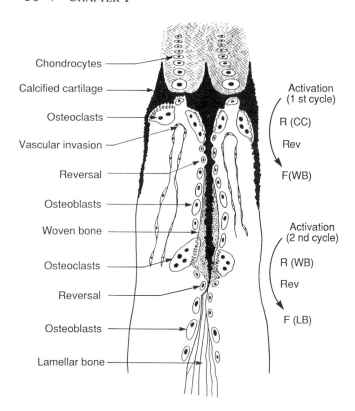

Chondrocytes

Calcified cartilage

Osteoclasts

Vascular invasion

Reversal

Osteoblasts

Woven bone

Osteoclasts

Reversal

Osteoblasts

Lamellar bone

Activation
(1 st cycle)

R (CC)

Rev

F(WB)

Activation
(2 nd cycle)

R (WB)

Rev

F (LB)

FIG. 10. Bone growth and remodeling at the epiphyseal plate. Schematic representation of the cellular events occurring at the growth plate in long bones. R, resorption; Rev, reversal; F, formation; CC, calcified cartilage; WB, woven bone; LB, lamellar bone.

branous ossification in the future midshaft area under the perichondrium (which is then a periosteum). Just after the calcification of this woven bone, blood vessels (preceded by osteoclasts) penetrate it and the cartilage, bringing the blood supply that will form the hematopoietic bone marrow.

The growth plate in a growing long bone shows, from the epiphyseal area to the diaphyseal area, the following cellular events (Fig. 10). In a proliferative zone, chondroblasts divide actively, forming isogenous groups and actively synthesizing the matrix. These cells become progressively larger, enlarging their lacunae in the hypertrophic zone, and then they undergo programmed cell death (apoptosis). At this level of the epiphyseal plate, the matrix of the longitudinal cartilage septa selectively calcifies (zone of provisional calcification). Once calcified, the cartilage matrix is resorbed, but only partially, by osteoclasts, and then blood vessels appear in the zone of invasion. After resorption, osteoblasts differentiate and form a layer of woven bone on top of the cartilaginous remnants of the longitudinal septa.

Thus, the first ARF sequence is complete: the cartilage has been remodeled and replaced by woven bone. The resulting trabeculae are called the primary spongiosum. Still lower in the growth plate, this woven bone is subjected to further remodeling (a second ARF sequence), in which the woven bone and the cartilaginous remnants are replaced with lamellar bone, resulting in the mature state of trabecular bone called secondary spongiosum (Fig. 11).

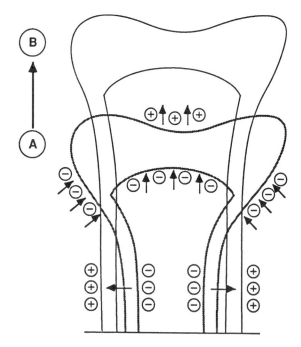

FIG. 11. Resorption (–) and formation (+) activities during the longitudinal growth of bones. During growth from A to B, the cortex in the diaphysis must be resorbed inside and reformed outside *(bottom)*. The growth plate moves upward (see Fig. 10), and the wider parts of the bone must be reshaped into a diaphysis. (From: Jee WSS. The skeletal tissues. In: Weiss L (ed) *Histology, Cell and Tissue Biology.* Elsevier Biomedical, New York, 200–255, 1983.)

Growth in Diameter, and Shape Modification (Modeling)

Growth in the diameter of the shaft is the result of a deposition of new membranous bone beneath the periosteum that will continue throughout life. In this case, resorption does not immediately precede formation. The midshaft is narrower than the metaphysis, and the growth of a long bone progressively destroys the lower part of the metaphysis and transforms it into a diaphysis, accomplished by continuous resorption by osteoclasts beneath the periosteum (Fig. 10).

SUGGESTED READINGS

1. Baron R, Chakraborty M, Chatterjee D, Horne W, Lomri A, Ravesloot J-H: Biology of the osteoclast. In: Mundy GR, Martin TJ (eds) *Physiology and Pharmacology of Bone.* Springer-Verlag, New York, 111–147; 1993
2. Eriksen EF, Axelrod DW, Melsen F: *Bone Histomorphometry.* Raven Press, New York, 1994
3. Jee WSS: The skeletal tissues. In: Weiss L (ed) *Histology, Cell and Tissue Biology.* Elsevier Biomedical, New York, 200–255, 1983
4. Nijweide P, Burger EH, Feyen JHM: Cells of bone: Proliferation, differentiation and hormonal regulation. *Physiol Rev* 66:855–886, 1986
5. Suda T, Takahashi N, Martin TJ: Modulation of osteoclast differentiation. *Endocr Rev* 13:66–80, 1992

2. Osteoblast Cell Biology—Lineage and Functions

J. Edward Puzas, Ph.D.

Department of Orthopedics, University of Rochester School of Medicine, Rochester, New York

Bone-forming cells are, by definition, the cells responsible for the production of authentic bone. For the purposes of this discussion, bone is defined as the tissue that is formed by the deposition of mineral ions within a collagenous framework. The mineral must be in the form of carbonated hydroxyapatite and the collagen must be predominantly type I collagen. Although this definition seems self-evident, it does exclude a number of mineralized tissues that, through the years, have been grouped with authentic bone. Some examples of such mineralizing nonbone tissues are dentin and enamel in teeth, calcifying cartilage in the developing growth plate of long bones, virtually any organ undergoing pathologic calcification (e.g., arterial and aortic walls), and renal stones. There are, however, some forms of ectopic or heterotopic bone which do fit the criteria of authentic bone. These forms of bone frequently occur after orthopedic surgery or in rare metabolic disease states. A discussion of this type of pathologic bone or related calcification syndromes is found elsewhere (1). The reader is also referred to review articles on the topic (2,3).

The term *bone-forming cell* can be equated with the term *osteoblast*. That is, wherever there is authentic bone being formed, there must be present a population of osteoblasts. This dissertation is organized into four categories: (i) the ultrastructural and functional properties of osteoblasts, including specific characteristics and biochemical markers of the cells, (ii) the osteoblast lineage, (iii) key processes involved in bone formation, and (iv) unique regulatory mechanisms related to these cells.

ULTRASTRUCTURE AND PROPERTIES OF BONE-FORMING CELLS

The ultrastructural and histologic features of osteoblasts underscore the fact that these are very metabolically active cells. They have an extensive rough endoplasmic reticulum composed of polysomal structures that stain intensely basophilic. The predominant genes that are transcribed and translated in these cells are those dealing with the synthesis of an extracellular matrix, i.e., collagenous and noncollagen matrix proteins. Fully 20% of the total protein produced by osteoblasts is type I collagen. When one considers the number of genes that need to be expressed to maintain function, for a cell to devote one fifth of its activity to a single gene product is extraordinary. The predominant noncollagen protein secreted by osteoblasts is osteocalcin [bone gla-protein (BGP)], making up approximately 1% of extracellular matrix protein. Moreover, a host of regulatory factors are produced and deposited in bone by osteoblasts. These include the family of bone morphogenetic proteins (BMPs), the beta transforming growth factors (TGF-βs), the insulin-like growth factors (IGFs), platelet-derived growth factors

(PDGFs), and basic fibroblast growth factor (bFGF), among others. Though these proteins represent a minor component of the extracellular matrix, they play a critical role in bone remodeling (see later).

A well-developed Golgi apparatus is also present in osteoblasts. This cellular structure is responsible for the secretion of collagen and noncollagen proteins. It is usually found near the center of the cell as a negatively stained organelle. The negative staining results from the high lipid composition of the Golgi lamellae.

All osteoblasts are mononuclear. The nucleus is usually positioned eccentrically in the cell opposite the rough endoplasmic reticulum. The nuclear material is similar to that of other eukaryotic cells and remains in a diffuse, uncondensed state during interphase. There are usually present one to three nucleoli. A mature, functioning osteoblast does not divide. That is, the mitotic forms of prophase, metaphase, anaphase, and telophase do not appear in osteoblasts. If ever such structures are observed, the cell must be considered, by convention, a progenitor form of an osteoblast or a pre-osteoblast.

Figure 1, an electron micrograph of five osteoblasts and one osteoprogenitor cell, shows examples of osteoblasts with well-developed rough endoplasmic reticulum, Golgi apparatus, and nuclei with nucleoli.

A characteristic of osteoblasts that can be demonstrated histochemically is the presence of a substantial amount of the enzyme alkaline phosphatase. Bone-specific alkaline phosphatase has been localized to the plasma membrane of osteoblasts, and, although it is known to be present in large amounts, its true function has not yet been determined. Speculations as to its role in mineralization have been published since 1923 (3); it is clear that alkaline phosphatase activity correlates with bone formation, but its exact mechanism of action is not yet known. Elevated levels of bone-specific alkaline phosphatase in the blood indicate excessive osteoblast activity, or bone formation. Normal levels in an adult would be 20 to 70 international units (IU); in a growing child, 100 to 150 IU; and, in pathologic high-bone-turnover states such as Paget's disease, 350 to 700 IU.

The osteoblast also plays a key role in bone resorption. Recent evidence has shown that osteoblasts possess receptors for a number of bone-resorbing stimulatory factors, such as parathyroid hormone, vitamin D, prostaglandins, interleukins, and TGF-β, and that the primary target for these agents in the modulation of osteoclast activity is the osteoblast (or stromal lining cells) (5–8). The hypothesis under which most investigators are working is that the systemic signal to resorb bone is received and processed by osteoblasts, which then elaborate a molecule (or molecules) that recruits and stimulates the activity of osteoclasts. Also, because osteoclasts do not resorb bone that is lined by intact osteoblasts or stromal cells (9), the presence

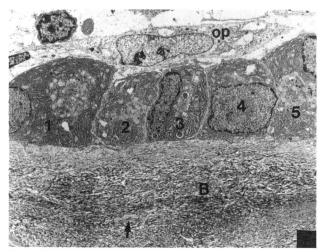

FIG. 1. Electron micrograph of osteoblasts and a pre-osteoblast; five osteoblasts line the bone surface. A well-developed rough endoplasmic reticulum and Golgi apparatus can be seen in most of the cells. The elongated cell with an elongated nucleus immediately above the osteoblasts is an osteoprogenitor cell, or pre-osteoblast. This cell still has the capacity for division, and it will take the place of one of the osteoblasts when the latter becomes encased in the bone matrix as an osteocyte. The *arrow* indicates the presence of a canaliculus from an osteocyte deeper within the bone. (From: Marks SC, Popoff SN. *Am J Anat* 183:1–44, 1988.)

or absence of these cells can determine what bony sites are to be resorbed. Thus, it is clear that the osteoblast plays a pivotal role in directing both when and where bone resorption will occur.

THE OSTEOBLAST LINEAGE

Three forms of the osteoblast cell lineage are recognized. They are progenitor osteoblasts (pre-osteoblasts), mature osteoblasts, and osteocytes. From a phylogenetic point of view, it is known that osteoblasts arise from cells in the con-

densing mesenchyme, and as such they are one form of connective tissue. Because mesenchymal cells can give rise to a number of tissue types, it is not until a cell is committed to the osteoblast lineage that it can be classified as a bone-forming cell.

Figure 2 summarizes the osteoblast lineage pathways.

The Pre-osteoblast

A committed progenitor cell destined to become an osteoblast has a number of distinguishing features. First, these cells are physically near bone-forming surfaces. That is, they are usually present where active mature osteoblasts are synthesizing bone. They are elongated cells, each with an elongated nucleus (Fig. 1). Most often, they are found in a stratum type of configuration, a few cell layers distant from the active osteoblasts. Second, they have the capacity to divide. Frequently, mitotic characters can be found in these cells. Third, these cells usually stain less intensely for alkaline phosphatase and there is no evidence of a developed rough endoplasmic reticulum. That is, they have not yet acquired many of the protein-synthesizing characteristics of mature osteoblasts.

Pre-osteoblasts give rise to osteoblasts at two distinctly different sites: the endosteum and the periosteum. Endosteal pre-osteoblasts are those bone-forming cells that are active on trabecular and endocortical bone surfaces. They are derived from the stromal group of cells that, along with the hemopoietic group, populate marrow spaces. These stromal cells are self-renewing (10), and with each cell division they have the capacity to create a determined osteoprogenitor cell (DOPC) that will ultimately become a mature osteoblast, and an inducible osteoprogenitor stem cell (IOPC) that will retain stem cell potentiality. The nomenclature of DOPC and IOPC was coined by Friedenstein et al. (11).

The periosteal pre-osteoblast is one of the cells that form the fibrous periosteum surrounding all bones. These cells give rise to osteoblasts on the bone surfaces and may also provide progenitor cells for the fibroblasts in the fibrous layers. They

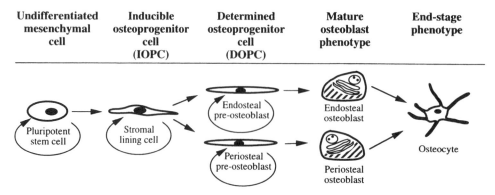

FIG. 2. Diagrammatic representation of the osteoblast lineage. This figure indicates that osteoblasts have their origin from undifferentiated mesenchymal stem cells that have the potential for differentiation into many connective tissue cell types. The first stage of differentiation is into a noncommitted osteoprogenitor cell (IOPC) and then to a committed osteoprogenitor cell (DOPC). All three of these cell phenotypes have the capacity for proliferation and self-renewal. Mature osteoblasts are found on both endosteal and periosteal surfaces. Eventually, osteoblasts may encase themselves in a bony matrix, at which point they become osteocytes.

are derived from a pool of cells that more closely resemble DOPCs than IOPCs. That is, there is no evidence for the presence of a stromal stem cell such as those in the marrow space. Nevertheless, the periosteal cell layers are also a self-renewing population (12).

Differentiation of an osteoprogenitor cell into an osteoblast is not a quantal process. Osteoblasts express all of the genes necessary for bone formation, but they are not all expressed simultaneously. A number of cell models (both *in vivo* and *in vitro*) have been used to investigate this, but perhaps the most information has come from the molecular models of Stein et al. (13). Although their model is an *in vitro* one, it does provide a framework for studying the differentiation process. It is clear that in the early stages of bone development there is extensive proliferation of progenitor cells with expression of growth-related genes (such as c-*myc* and c-*fos*). Also during the proliferative phase, a number of matrix genes begin to be expressed (i.e., type I collagen, fibronectin, and some growth factors such as TGF-β). These genes remain active for a number of days and are joined by gene products that are associated with a mature matrix, such as alkaline phosphatase and matrix gla-protein. As the matrix and matrix-maturing proteins are suppressed, new gene products associated with the mineralization phase begin to be expressed (i.e., osteocalcin and osteopontin), thus leading to hydroxyapatite accumulation and complete mineralization.

When viewed as a continuum, the maturation of a pre-osteoblast into a mature osteoblast is quite a complex process. Gene products are expressed and repressed at specified stages, and unless all of the actions are in concert, a normal bone matrix will not be formed.

Osteoblast

A mature osteoblast is derived from a pre-osteoblast and expresses all of the differentiated functions required to synthesize bone. As discussed above, there is a gradient of differentiation which becomes fully expressed when the mature form of the cell reaches the bone surface. Once the osteoblast has reached the surface, its function is to synthesize and secrete collagen, noncollagen matrix proteins, and regulatory factors into a structured array, and to ultimately mineralize it. Usually, active osteoblasts are found within a matrix that they themselves have synthesized. It is within this matrix at the mineralization front that the process of hydroxyapatite crystal growth occurs. The mineralization front is the advancing edge of calcification and is usually 5 to 50 microns away from the osteoblast surface. The area between the osteoblast and the mineralizing front is often referred to as an osteoid seam. The depth and character of the osteoid seam can be diagnostic for some forms of bone disease, such as osteomalacia and rickets. (14–16).

Osteocyte

An osteocyte is an osteoblast which has become encased in calcified bone. During the process of bone formation, the osteoblast determines its own fate by calcifying itself into a lacunae. Approximately 15% of osteoblasts eventually become osteocytes, and, although it can be said that not all osteoblasts survive as osteocytes, it is true that all osteocytes had their origin from osteoblasts. At the point of total encasement, the metabolic activity of the cell dramatically decreases as a result of the lack of nutrient diffusion. The

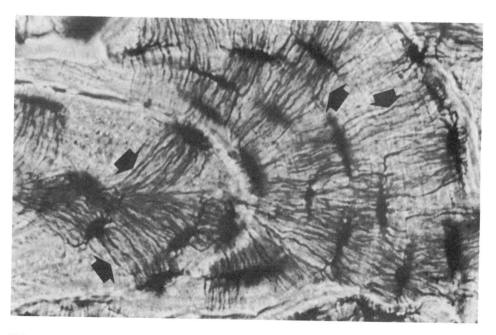

FIG. 3. Photomicrograph of mature bone. This unstained section of bone was prepared by hand grinding a fragment of adult bone until it became translucent. The osteocytes form concentric layers around a central nutrient vessel. The canaliculi of the osteocytes *(arrows)* form a fine network of tubules through which diffusion of solutes and gases can occur. The canaliculi may also form a communication network between the cells.

only source of nutrients and gas exchange to which the osteocyte has access is that which can occur through small canals known as canaliculi. These channels are actually the remnants of cellular processes which extended from the osteoblast during bone mineralization. The canaliculi form an extensive array of connecting tubules, and it has been speculated that these tubules form a communication as well as a nutrient network. Figure 3 is a photomicrograph of mature bone in which a number of osteocytes and the numerous canaliculi between them are visible.

Progression Through the Osteoblast Lineage

Many very enlightening studies demonstrating the origin and fate of pre-osteoblasts, osteoblasts, and osteocytes were performed a number of years ago (17,18). These works utilized timed radiolabeled-thymidine exposure to monitor the progression of a cell through the osteoblast lineage. Because thymidine is incorporated only into newly forming DNA, the bone cells that were labeled immediately after the injection were pre-osteoblasts in the process of cell division. There was no label in osteoblasts or osteocytes. A few days after the injection, the cells that contained the radioactive label were the osteoblasts, and after a few weeks the cells with the label were the osteocytes. Because it is known that osteoblasts and osteocytes do not divide, it was evident that the label that appeared in these cells originated in the pre-osteoblasts. In fact, the lifetime and differentiation time for osteoblasts could be calculated with these and other techniques, and it was shown that mature osteoblast appearance required not more than a few days and that they were active for up to 12 weeks before progressing into osteocytes (19,20).

KEY PROCESSES IN BONE FORMATION

Matrix Maturation

One of the major and yet poorly understood areas of collagen metabolism in bone formation is the so-called maturation of the osteoid matrix. This alteration of collagen fibers must occur before the matrix is competent to support mineralization. The best way to illustrate this is to describe the process of bone formation at a remodeling site, which involves three distinct stages of collagen synthesis and its mineralization. In the first stage, collagen is deposited at a rapid rate, and an ever-thickening osteoid seam is produced. In the second stage, the rate of mineralization increases to match the rate of collagen synthesis, and the osteoid seam width remains constant. In the third stage, the rate of collagen synthesis decreases and mineralization continues until

the osteoid seam disappears. The maturation of the collagen matrix is expressed as the ratio of the mineralization rate (in microns per day) to the osteoid seam width (in microns). Thus, the maturation of the collagen has a unit of time (days). This ratio has become known as the mineralization lag time: the length of time it takes for the osteoid matrix to acquire the characteristics necessary to support mineralization. The mineralization lag time is roughly 5 to 15 days in adults, and its magnitude can sometimes be diagnostic for metabolic bone diseases. Biochemically, the mineralization lag time remains undefined. Some theories support a role for crosslinking of collagen in the osteoid, others support the removal of a mineralization inhibitor (see later). Whatever the actual mechanism of osteoid maturation, it is apparent that newly deposited collagen cannot provide a substrate for normal mineralization until it has matured.

Mineralization

Mineralization of the collagen substructure is another unique function of the osteoblast. Although not all the details of this process are known, many important pieces of data have been collected. For example, the mineral in mature, fully calcified bone is mostly in the form of carbonated hydroxyapatite crystals. These crystals are needle-shaped and rodlike, with a diameter of 30 to 50Å and a length of up to 600Å. They lie linearly along the collagen fibrils and in some instances may penetrate some of the larger fibers. The actual process of mineral precipitation, however, remains obscure. In fact, a number of paradoxical observations have been made in trying to experimentally examine the process of calcification. For example, it appears that once the hydroxyapatite has been formed, further growth of the crystal can occur in the absence of cell activity. In other words, under physiologic conditions, the extracellular fluid is supersaturated with calcium and phosphate in the presence of hydroxyapatite. If crystal growth were not somehow mediated, the extracellular fluid would be depleted of calcium and phosphate at the expense of hydroxyapatite formation. This finding was one of the major pieces of evidence for proposing an ionic barrier between bone and blood, and it is the reason that devitalized bone will support mineralization if implanted in tissue fluids or bathed in physiologic solutions of calcium and phosphate. Therefore, the continuing processes of mineralization appear to be controlled at both the initiation stages and the deposition stages of hydroxyapatite formation.

Measurements of Bone Formation

Although we may not understand all the physical and chemical processes of osteoid maturation and mineraliza-

Table 1. *Parameters of bone formation under the control of osteoblasts*

Bone volume (microscopic area that is cancellous bone)	22.8%
Osteoid volume (volume of uncalcified osteoid, compared to bone)	4.4 mm³/cm³ bone
Osteoid surface (bone surface covered by osteoid)	7.5%
Osteoid seam width	10.0 µ
Mineral apposition rate	0.65 µ/day
Trabecular diameter (mean diameter of trabeculae in cancellous bone)	283.0 µ
Bone–osteoblast interface (bone surface in direct contact with osteoblasts)	3.8%

Table 2. *Endocrine, paracrine, and autocrine factors affecting osteoblasts*

Endocrine hormones	Paracrine factors	Autocrine factors
Parathyroid hormone	Parathyroid–hormone–related protein	
Vitamin D	TGF-β1, -β2, and -β3	TGF-β1, -β2, and -β3
Glucocorticoid hormones	Fibroblast growth factors (1 and 2)	Fibroblast growth factors (1 and 2)
Calcitonin	Insulin-like growth factors	Insulin-like growth factors
Gonadal steroids (estrogen and testosterone)	Platelet-derived growth factors	Platelet-derived growth factors
Insulin	BMPs 2–7	BMPs 2–7
	Interleukin-6	

tion, it has been possible to define and measure many parameters of bone formation. An entire histologic discipline has grown up around the methods needed to make these accurate measurements of skeletal activity. Variables such as sampling sites, embedding and sectioning techniques, and staining and quantification techniques must be considered when measuring formation (and resorption) rates. Table 1 is a brief list of some of the normal values that have been obtained from human bone. Typically, over 50 different measurements (or calculations from measurements) can be made from a bone section, and with these measurements an accurate picture of the metabolic activity of osteoblasts can be obtained. A detailed discussion of bone histomorphometry with excellent histologic and morphometric examples has recently been published (14,21).

UNIQUE REGULATORY MECHANISMS RELATED TO OSTEOBLASTS

This area is one of the most active and important topics being investigated in bone research today. It is in this arena that molecular biologic, immunologic, and biochemical techniques have been merged in an attempt to understand not only the disease processes but the normal processes of bone metabolism. It is probably from these lines of research that new therapies will emerge for diseases such as osteoporosis.

Control of osteoblast function occurs at three levels: endocrine, paracrine, and autocrine (Table 2). Endocrine control is exerted through the action of hormones such as parathyroid hormone (PTH), 1,25-dihydroxyvitamin D_3, growth hormone, glucocorticoid hormones, and gonadal steroids. These agents are secreted into the circulation by endocrine glands, and they ultimately affect all bone, no matter how distant from the site of hormone synthesis. Of these agents, PTH and 1,25-dihydroxyvitamin D_3 have been the most widely studied with regard to bone formation. Although both of these hormones are known to be responsible for increasing the level of calcium in the blood, PTH by stimulating bone resorption and 1,25-dihydroxyvitamin D_3 by stimulating intestinal calcium transport, they have also been shown to have important effects on bone formation. For example, in osteoblasts, PTH mediates ion and amino acid transport, stimulates cyclic adenosine monophosphate, regulates collagen synthesis, and binds to a specific receptor (22–26). 1,25-dihydroxyvitamin D_3 also stimulates matrix and alkaline phosphatase synthesis, production of bone-specific proteins, and binds to a receptor. In fact, we now have direct evidence that under certain conditions both PTH and 1,25-dihydroxyvitamin D_3 are direct anabolic agents for skeletal mass (27–30).

Paracrine control of osteoblast activity occurs when cells adjacent to the osteoblasts produce and release locally acting factors that influence bone formation. There are many examples of this in the skeleton, ranging from (i) the initial developmental stages in the embryo, (ii) long-bone growth and fracture healing, and (iii) the basal remodeling that occurs throughout life. Specific examples include the role of bFGF (or FGF-2) in development and expression of the limb rudiments, the production of the TGF-βs and BMP-2 by chondrogenic cells in the growth plate and fracture callus, and the production of interleukins by osteoclasts at sites of bone remodeling. These examples demonstrate the synthesis of a key factor by a nonosteoblast cell type that influences the activity of a nearby osteoblast.

Last, autocrine regulation of osteoblasts also occurs: factors produced by osteoblasts are eventually used to regulate their own activity. In the bone remodeling process, this pathway is best represented by the growth factors embedded in bone by osteoblasts, which are released to influence these cells at a later time. Some of the best studied of these factors are the insulin-like growth factors, IGF-I and IGF-II. These molecules can be extracted from bone and have been shown to have proliferation- and differentiation-stimulating activity for osteoblasts.

SUMMARY

Osteoblasts are complex and pivotal cells that participate in all aspects of bone metabolism. They serve two main functions: they form the structural components of bone (i.e., matrix and mineral) and they produce regulatory factors that influence both bone formation and bone resorption. Osteoblasts are derived from a progenitor mesenchymal cell through the expression of a series of genes that are coordinately regulated. These cells ultimately develop receptors that recognize endocrine hormones, and they translate these hormonal signals to control both bone formation and bone resorption at locally specific sites. The end-stage phenotype of an osteoblast is an osteocyte. Although viable, osteocytes are completely encased in bone and have a very much reduced metabolic activity. A clear-cut regulatory action for osteocytes has not been identified.

REFERENCES

1. Section IX: Extraskeletal (ectopic) calcification and ossification. In: Favus MJ, Christakos S, Goldring SR, et al. (eds) *Primer on the Metabolic Bone Diseases and Disorders of Mineral Metabo-*

lism, Third edition. Lippincott-Raven Publishers, Philadelphia, 421–430, 1996

2. Sawyer JR, Myers MA, Rosier RN, Puzas JE: Heterotopic ossification: Clinical and cellular aspects. *Calcif Tissue Int* 49: 208–215, 1991

3. O'Conner JM: *Soft Tissue Ossification.* Springer-Verlag, New York, 1983

4. Robison R: The possible significance of hexosephosphoric esters in ossification. *Biochem J* 17:286–293, 1923

5. Rodan GA, Martin TJ: Role of osteoclasts in hormonal control of bone resorption—a hypothesis. *Calcif Tissue Int* 33:349–351, 1981

6. Burger EH, Van der Meer JWM, Nijweide PJ: Osteoclast formation from mononuclear phagocytes: Role of bone forming cells. *J Cell Biol* 99:1901–1905, 1984

7. Chambers TJ, McSheehy PMJ, Thomson BM, Fuller K: The effect of calcium–regulating hormones and prostaglandins on bone resorption by osteoclasts disaggregated from neonatal rabbit bones. *Endocrinology* 116:234–239, 1985

8. Martin TJ, Ng KW: Mechanism by which cells of the osteoblast lineage control osteoclast formation and activity. *J Cell Biochem* 56:357–366, 1994

9. Zambonin-Zallone A, Teti A, Primavera MV: Resorption of vital or devitalized bone by isolated osteoclasts in vitro: The role of lining cells. *Cell Tissue Res* 235:561–564, 1984

10. Owen ME: Bone growth at the cellular level: A perspective. In: Dixon AD, Sarnat BG (eds) *Factors and Mechanisms Influencing Bone Growth.* Alan R Liss, New York, 1982, 19–28

11. Friedenstein AY, Chailakhyan RK, Latsinik NY, Panasyuk AF, Keiliss-Borok IV: Stromal cells responsible for transferring the microenvironment of the hemopoietic tissues. *Transplantation* 17:331–340, 1974

12. Nijweide PJ, van der Plas A: Embryonic chick periosteum in tissue culture: osteoid formation and calcium uptake. *Proc K Ned Akad Wet C* 78:410–417, 1975

13. Stein GS, Lian JB, Own TA: Relationship of cell growth to the regulation of tissue-specific gene expression during osteoblast differentiation. *FASEB J* 4:3111–3123, 1990

14. Recker RR: Bone biopsy and histomorphometry in clinical practice. In: Favus MJ, Christakos S, Goldring SR, et al. (eds) *Primer on the Metabolic Bone Diseases and Disorders of Mineral Metabolism, Third edition.* Lippincott-Raven Publishers, Philadelphia, 164–167, 1996

15. Klein GL: Nutritional rickets and osteomalacia. In: Favus MJ, Christakos S, Goldring SR, et al. (eds) *Primer on the Metabolic Bone Diseases and Disorders of Mineral Metabolism, Third edition.* Lippincott-Raven Publishers, Philadelphia, 301–305, 1996

16. Bikle DD: Drug-induced osteomalacia. In: Favus MJ, Christakos S, Goldring SR, et al. (eds) *Primer on the Metabolic Bone Diseases and Disorders of Mineral Metabolism, Third edition.* Lippincott-Raven Publishers, Philadelphia, 333–337, 1996

16. Bikle DD: Drug-induced osteomalacia. In: Favus MJ, Christakos S, Goldring SR, et al. (eds) *Primer on the Metabolic Bone Diseases and Disorders of Mineral Metabolism, Third edition.* Lippincott-Raven Publishers, Philadelphia, 333–337, 1996

17. Tonna EA, Cronkite EP: The periosteum: Autoradiographic studies on cellular proliferation and transformation utilizing tritiated thymidine. *Clin Orthop* 30:218–232, 1963

18. Tonna EA, Cronkite EP: An autoradiographic study of periosteal cell proliferation with tritiated thymidine. *Lab Invest* 11:455–461, 1962

19. Kimmel DB, Jee WSS: Bone cell kinetics during longitudinal bone growth in the rat. *Calcif Tissue Int* 32: 123–133, 1980

20. Tran VPT, Vignery A, Baron R: Cellular kinetics of the bone remodeling sequence in the rat. *Anat Rec* 202:445–451, 1982

21. Malluche HH, Faugere M-C: *Atlas of Mineralized Bone Histology.* Karger, New York, 1986

22. Donahue HJ, Fryer MJ, Eriksen EF, Heath H: Differential effects of parathyroid hormone and its analogs on cytosolic calcium ion and cAMP levels in cultured rat osteoblast-like cells. *J Biol Chem* 263:13522–13527, 1988

23. Rosenbusch JP, Nichols G Jr: Parathyroid hormone effects on amino acid transport into bone cells. *Endocrinology* 81:553–557, 1967

24. Lomri A, Marie PJ: Effect of parathyroid hormone and forskolin on cytoskeletal protein synthesis in cultured mouse osteoblastic cells. *Biochim Biophys Acta* 970:333–42, 1988

25. Kream BE, Rowe D, Smith MD, Maher V, Majeska R: Hormonal regulation of collagen synthesis in a clonal rat osteosarcoma cell line. *Endocrinology* 119:1922–1928, 1986

26. Hesch RD, Brabant G, Rittinghaus EF, Atkinson MJ, Harms H: Pulsatile secretion of parathyroid hormone and its action on a type I and type II PTH receptor: A hypothesis for understanding osteoporosis. *Calcif Tissue Int* 42:341–344, 1988

27. Harrison JR, Clark NB: Avian medullary bone in organ culture: Effects of vitamin D metabolites on collagen synthesis. *Calcif Tissue Int* 39:35–43, 1986

28. Fritsch J, Grosse B, Lieberherr M, Balsan S: 1,25-dihydroxyvitamin D is required for growth-independent expression of alkaline phosphatase in cultured rat osteoblasts. *Calcif Tissue Int* 37: 639–645, 1985

29. Price PA, Baukol SA: 1,25-dihydroxyvitamin D increases synthesis of the vitamin K dependent bone protein by osteosarcoma cells. *J Biol Chem* 255:11660–11663, 1980

30. McDonnell DP, Pike JW, O'Malley BW: The vitamin D receptor: A primitive steroid receptor related to thyroid hormone receptor. *J Steroid Biochem* 30:41–46, 1988

3. Bone-Resorbing Cells

Gregory R. Mundy, M.D.

Department of Medicine, Endocrinology and Metabolism, University of Texas Health Science Center, San Antonio, Texas

The major and possibly sole bone-resorbing cell is the osteoclast, and this cell will be the focus of attention in this chapter. Other cells, however, have been linked to bone resorption. These include osteocytes, monocytes, tumor cells, and osteoblasts. Osteocytic bone resorption, also called osteocytic osteolysis, was first described over 30 years ago by histologists examining light microscopy sections. It was thought that osteocytic osteolysis resulted from expansion of the osteocyte lacunae, in which osteocytes are embedded in bone. However, more recent observations with scanning electron microscopy make it unlikely that osteolysis by osteocytes occurs (1). Using this technique, it is apparent that bone resorption is characterized by easily discernible degradative changes in the bone matrix, which are not observed around osteocytes. Jones and coworkers (1) consider apparent osteolysis by osteocytes an artifact of observations made in bone that is rapidly turning over (fetal or woven bone). From time to time, other cells have also been linked to bone resorption. Monocytes and macrophages have been shown to degrade devitalized bone (2,3). These observations strengthen the notion that monocytes and osteoclasts have a common precursor, a concept that, in light of subsequent data, appears likely to be true. However, there are no resorption pits associated with monocytes or macrophages when they lie against bone surfaces, and it is unlikely that they have a major role in bone degradation. Similarly, tumor cells have also been shown to resorb devitalized bone by causing release of previously incorporated calcium (4), but resorption pits are not found around tumor cells, even *in vivo* (5). It has been suggested that osteoblasts may act as helper cells in the process of osteoclastic resorption by preparing the bone surface for later attack by osteoclastic enzymes, although there is still little direct evidence to support this interesting concept.

Although osteoclasts are clearly the major bone-resorbing cells, osteoclast activity may be modulated by other cells such as osteoblasts and immune cells.

OSTEOCLAST MORPHOLOGY

Osteoclasts have been studied extensively using light microscopy, transmission electron microscopy, and scanning electron microscopy. They are unique and highly specialized cells. They are localized on endosteal bone surfaces, in haversian systems, and also occasionally on periosteal surfaces. They are not commonly seen on normal bone surfaces but are found frequently at sites of actively remodeling bones, such as the metaphyses of growing bones or in pathologic circumstances, such as adjacent to collections of tumor cells. They are large, multinucleated cells, varying in size up to 100 μ in diameter in pathologic states and containing, on average, 10 to 20 nuclei. The number of nuclei in osteoclasts is related to the species, more being

seen in the cat and fewer in the mouse. The nuclei are centrally placed and usually contain 1 to 2 nucleoli. Osteoclasts have primary lysosomes, numerous and pleomorphic mitochondria, and a specific area of the cell membrane, known as the ruffled border, which abuts against the bone surface. This area of the cell membrane is composed of folds and invaginations that allow intimate contact with the bone surface. This is the site at which resorption of bone occurs and the resorption bay (also known as the Howship's lacuna) is formed. Some workers have considered the confined and circumscribed space between the ruffled border and the bone surface to be equivalent to a secondary lysosome (6). The ruffled border is surrounded by a clear zone which appears free of organelles but in fact contains actin filaments and appears to anchor the ruffled border area to the bone surface undergoing resorption.

CRITERIA FOR DEFINITION OF THE OSTEOCLAST

Some of the morphologic features of the osteoclast have been used as criteria for identification. These include multinuclearity, pleomorphic mitochondria, and presence of the ruffled border adjacent to areas of resorbed bone. These criteria have received much attention in recent years as investigators have attempted to isolate osteoclasts *in vitro* and distinguish them from other cells. Osteoclasts are difficult to distinguish from macrophage polykaryons, which are related cells with a similar lineage. Some of the features of the osteoclast that aid in the distinction from macrophage polykaryons include the capacity to resorb bone, capacity to form a ruffled border, contraction of the cytoplasm on exposure to calcitonin, presence of calcitonin receptors, crossreactivity with osteoclast-specific monoclonal antibodies (although it has not been convincingly shown that any antibody is absolutely specific for the osteoclast), appropriate responses to calciotropic hormones, and absence of the Fc receptor. The presence of tartrate-resistant acid phosphatase is a helpful marker, but it is not useful for distinguishing human osteoclasts from macrophage polykaryons. Responsivity to osteotropic hormones also has been used as a criterion for identification of osteoclasts. Osteoclast-stimulating agents, including parathyroid hormone, interleukin-1, tumor necrosis factor, transforming growth factor α, and 1,25-dihydroxyvitamin D, activate osteoclasts. Inhibitors of osteoclast activity include calcitonin, gamma interferon, and transforming growth factor. However, the effects of some of these factors are not specific for osteoclasts. For example, 1,25-dihydroxyvitamin D promotes not only the fusion of osteoclasts but also enhances the fusion of macrophages to form polykaryons (7). Moreover, some of these factors are species specific. For example, calcitonin may not cause contraction of avian osteoclast cytoplasmic membranes. The evidence suggests that macrophages can be induced to form multinucleated cells, form resorption pits, and respond to calcitonin. A reasonable compromise is to denote cells as functional osteoclasts if they form resorption pits, are multinucleated, and respond to calcitonin, while recognizing that some authentic osteoclasts are not multinucleated, do not form resorption pits, and do not respond to calcitonin.

MOLECULAR MECHANISMS OF BONE RESORPTION

Osteoclasts resorb bone by the production of proteolytic enzymes and hydrogen ions in the localized environment under the ruffled border of the cell. Hydrogen ions are generated in the cell by the enzyme carbonic anhydrase type II. They are then pumped across the ruffled border by a proton pump, apparently similar, but not identical, to the complex vacuolar ATPase in the intercalated cells of the kidney (8). Lysosomal enzymes are also released by the osteoclast, and the hydrogen ions produced by the proton pump ATPase provide an optimal environment for these proteolytic enzymes to degrade the bone matrix.

The extrusion of protons across the ruffled border of the cell (apical surface) requires the presence of a number of ion exchanges, pumps, and channels in the basolateral membrane of the cell to maintain electrochemical balance of the osteoclast. These include an Na^+/H^+ antiporter, an Na^+/K^+ ATPase, an HCO_3^-/Cl^- exchanger, a Ca^{2+} ATPase, and a K^+ channel.

The osteoclast is a motile cell. It resorbs bone to form a lacuna and then moves across the bone surface to resorb a separate area of bone. The tracks of its path can often be followed (1). Periods of locomotion are not associated with resorption. When the cell stops moving, it usually starts resorbing bone.

Some diseases are caused by disturbances in the molecular mechanisms responsible for bone resorption. For example, it has been shown that there is an unusual form of inherited osteopetrosis in children, in which there is a deficiency of the carbonic anhydrase type II isoenzyme (9). The osteoclasts in this disease are incompetent, bone is not resorbed, and the bone marrow cavity is not formed. Children with this disease also have renal tubular acidosis, caused by a similar enzyme defect in renal tubular cells, leading to impairment of hydrogen ion secretion.

Several other processes may be involved in the complex process of osteoclastic bone resorption. Some workers have suggested that the surface of the bone is prepared for the osteoclast by the actions of collagenase released by bone lining cells or osteoblasts. The osteoclasts then produce acid and lysosomal enzymes that complete the process. Because osteoblasts have the capacity to produce enzymes that could activate latent collagenase, such as plasminogen activator, such a mechanism is possible. However, it has already been shown that osteoclasts also secrete cysteine proteinases that are capable of degrading collagen in the acid environment under the ruffled border.

Recent data have suggested that oxygen-derived free radicals are involved in the resorption of bone by osteoclasts

(10). Many degradative processes of phagocytic cells are associated with free radical production, and bone resorption seems another. The use of radical-generating systems *in vivo* and *in vitro* shows that enzymes that deplete tissues of radicals, such as superoxide dismutase, block osteoclastic bone resorption stimulated by parathyroid hormone or interleukin-1. Staining reactions with nitroblue tetrazolium show that radical generation occurs within osteoclasts. Radicals could be involved in the degradation of bone under the ruffled border. However, the demonstration that radical generation is associated with new osteoclast formation suggests that radicals also have a cellular effect on the formation of osteoclasts.

The active resorbing osteoclast is a highly polarized cell. The ruffled border is the highly specialized area of the osteoclast cell membrane that lies adjacent to the bone surface. The attachment of the osteoclast to the bone surface has been shown to be an essential requirement for resorption to occur. This attachment process involves, at least in part, cell-membrane-bound proteins called integrins. Integrins attach to specific proteins in the bone matrix. One of the integrins important for osteoclast function is the vitronectin receptor (11), also known as the α_{v3} integrin. Antibodies to this receptor preferentially recognize osteoclasts. Attachment to bone matrix proteins involves specific Arg-Gly-Asp (RGD) amino acid sequences in the bone matrix proteins, and synthetic peptides are being developed that compete with osteoclast integrins for binding to these proteins, preventing osteoclast attachment to the bone surface and thereby inhibiting bone resorption. The snake venom *Echistatin* binds to this integrin and inhibits bone resorption *in vitro* and *in vivo* (12).

Recent observations have shown that the 60-kilodalton non receptor tyrosine kinase that is the product of the c-*src* proto-oncogene is required for osteoclasts to form resorption pits. This proto-oncogene is a ubiquitous intracellular tyrosine kinase which is membrane bound and has been linked to function of the cytoskeleton. In experiments in which the c-*src* gene was deleted from mice by targeted disruption in embryonic stem cells, it has been possible to breed mice that do not have the capacity to express *src*. In these mice, it was found unexpectedly that the mice have osteopetrosis, the bone disease characterized by nonfunctioning osteoclasts (13). More detailed examination of these mice has shown that multinucleated cells form on bone surfaces in *src*-deficient animals, but these multinucleated cells cannot form ruffled borders and resorb bone (14). These results indicate that this intracellular tyrosine kinase is essential for normal bone resorption, and they suggest a potential therapeutic target for the development of new inhibitors of bone resorption. Even more recently, gene knockout of the proto-oncogene c-*fos* has also been shown to cause osteopetrosis (15).

FORMATION AND ACTIVATION OF OSTEOCLASTS

Osteoclasts arise from hematopoietic mononuclear cells in the bone marrow (7). Mononuclear osteoclast precursors can circulate in the blood. At endosteal bone surfaces, the precursors proliferate, fuse to form multinucleated cells, form ruffled borders, and resorb bone. The cell of origin for the osteoclast in the bone marrow is still debated. The weight of evidence suggests it is a pluripotent stem cell that has the capacity, in response to appropriate stimuli, to differentiate into a granulocyte, monocyte, or osteoclast. The most likely stem cell is a CFU-GM (colony-forming unit for the granulocyte-macrophage series).

It was shown over 20 years ago that osteoclasts formed by fusion of precursors at the bone surface. These precursors circulated in the blood as mononuclear cells (16,17).

OSTEOCLAST APOPTOSIS

The disappearance of osteoclasts from bone remodeling sites may be as important as their formation for the control of bone resorption. Recent observations have suggested that osteoclasts undergo apoptosis at the conclusion of the resorbing phase of the bone remodeling process (18). Osteoclast apoptosis can be recognized by characteristic morphologic appearances of the osteoclast, including condensation of the nuclear chromatin. Another characteristic feature is loss of the ruffled border and detachment of the osteoclast from the surfaces of mineralized bone matrix. Apoptosis is modulated by drugs which regulate osteoclast function (but in an inverse manner). Drugs that inhibit bone resorption, such as bisphosphonates and estrogen, induce osteoclast apoptosis both *in vitro* and *in vivo* (18).

LESSONS FROM OSTEOPETROSIS

Osteopetrosis is the bone disorder characterized by impaired osteoclast function. It is clearly a heterogeneous disorder. There are a number of different variants in rodents that have now been well described, as well as a number of different forms that occur in humans. Although a rare disease, this is a very informative condition for osteoclast biologists. Because specific molecular and genetic defects have been found in some types of osteopetrosis, studies of variants of this disorder have characterized some of the molecular mechanisms responsible for osteoclastic bone resorption. For example, in one rare variant seen in humans, there is deficient expression of the osteoclast enzyme carbonic anhydrase type II, which is responsible for proton production in osteoclasts (9). Because proton production is necessary for normal bone resorption, patients with abnormalities in expression of this enzyme have impaired bone resorption and subsequent osteopetrosis. In several of the murine models of osteopetrosis, it has been possible to identify genes that are essential for osteoclast function. For example, in one naturally occurring animal model of osteopetrosis, the op/op murine variant, there is impaired production of colony-stimulating factor 1 (CSF-1) by stromal cells in the osteoclast microenvironment (19). As a consequence, osteoclasts fail to form and bone is not resorbed. This model shows that during the neonatal period in mice, production of normal CSF-1 is required for normal osteoclast formation. In another murine variant, tumor biologists experimenting with specific disruption of the *src* proto-oncogene have shown that this proto-oncogene, which encodes an intracellular tyrosine kinase, is

required for normal osteoclastic bone resorption (13). However, the defect is different from that seen in the op/op variant of osteopetrosis. In *src*-deficient mice, osteoclasts form, but they do not become polarized and are incapable of forming ruffled borders and resorbing bone. Unlike the op/op variant, the defect in *src* deficiency is not in the microenvironment of the osteoclast, but rather in the mature osteoclast itself. More recently, similar gene knockout experiments in mice with the c-*fos* proto-oncogene have also led unexpectedly to osteopetrosis (15). The precise mechanism is not known.

TECHNIQUES FOR STUDYING OSTEOCLASTS

Osteoclasts are very inaccessible cells, and so direct studies on these cells have been difficult to perform. Detailed information on their behavior was therefore not available until isolation techniques were developed for studying them *in vitro*. Techniques are now available for studying isolated preformed osteoclasts obtained from chicks, rodents, and baboons, as well as from human giant-cell tumors, and for studying the formation of osteoclasts from marrow precursors (7,20). These techniques are providing a tremendous boon to advances in this area of bone cell biology, for they allow the determination of the modes of actions of factors that stimulate and inhibit bone resorption.

REGULATION OF OSTEOCLAST ACTIVITY

Osteoclasts lie on bone surfaces in a bed of elliptical or fusiform, spindle-shaped cells called lining cells, which are probably members of the osteoblast lineage. When exposed to a bone-resorbing agent, the first response is that these lining cells retract and the osteoclasts insinuate an arm into the retracted area; then a ruffled border forms, and bone is resorbed at the exposed surface (1). The molecular mechanisms by which these complicated processes are controlled are unknown. Why lining cells retract at specific sites and how the osteoclast is activated is still not clear. It appears most likely that the osteoclast is activated by a soluble signal released from the lining cell (21,22).

Many hormones and factors have now been shown to stimulate osteoclast activity. Their mechanisms of action differ. Osteoclastic resorption may be stimulated by factors that enhance proliferation of osteoclast progenitors, which cause differentiation of committed precursors into mature cells or activation of the mature multinucleated cell to resorb bone (23). Similarly, osteoclasts could be inhibited by agents that block proliferation of precursors, that inhibit differentiation or fusion, or that inactivate the mature multinucleated resorbing cell. Current evidence indicates that most factors that stimulate or inhibit osteoclasts act on at least two of these steps (Fig. 1).

Systemic Hormones

The systemic hormones parathyroid hormone (PTH), 1,25-dihydroxyvitamin D, and calcitonin all influence osteoclast activity.

Parathyroid Hormone

PTH stimulates differentiation of committed progenitors to fuse, forming mature multinucleated osteoclasts. It also activates preformed osteoclasts to resorb bone. However, it does not increase CFU-GM, the earliest detectable cells in the osteoclast lineage. The activation of osteoclasts is probably indirect, probably mediated through cells in the osteoblast lineage such as the lining cells (22). The mechanisms by which osteoblasts send the second signal to the multinucleated osteoclasts in response to PTH is not known.

Parathyroid–hormone–related protein (PTH-rP) has effects on osteoclasts identical to those of PTH.

1,25-Dihydroxyvitamin D

1,25-Dihydroxyvitamin D is a potent stimulator of osteoclastic bone resorption. Like PTH, it stimulates osteoclast progenitors to differentiate and fuse (7). It has a similar effect on macrophage polykaryons, which are not osteoclasts. It also activates mature preformed osteoclasts, possibly by a similar mechanism to that of PTH. 1,25-Dihydroxyvitamin D also has other effects on bone resorption, which are indirect. It is a potent immunoregulatory molecule (24). It inhibits T cell proliferation and the production of the cytokine interleukin-2. Under some circumstances, it can enhance interleukin-1 production in cells with monocyte characteristics. Thus, the overall effects of 1,25-dihydroxyvitamin D on bone resorption are multiple and complex.

Calcitonin

Calcitonin is a polypeptide hormone that is a potent inhibitor of osteoclastic bone resorption, but its effects are only transient. Osteoclasts escape from the inhibitory effects of calcitonin following continued exposure (25). Thus, patients treated for hypercalcemia with calcitonin will respond for only a limited period of time (usually 48 to 72 hours) before hypercalcemia recurs. Even in patients with Paget's disease, the beneficial effects of calcitonin may eventually be lost with continued treatment. The "escape" phenomenon is likely a result of down-regulation of mRNA for the receptor (26). Calcitonin causes cytoplasmic contraction of the osteoclast cell membrane, which has been correlated with its capacity to inhibit bone resorption (27). It also causes the dissolution of mature osteoclasts into mononuclear cells. However, it also inhibits osteoclast formation, both inhibiting proliferation of the progenitors and inhibiting differentiation of the committed precursors. The effects of calcitonin on osteoclasts are mediated by cyclic adenosine monophosphate.

Local Hormones

Local hormones may be more important than systemic hormones for the initiation of physiologic bone resorption

Osteoclast Life Cycle

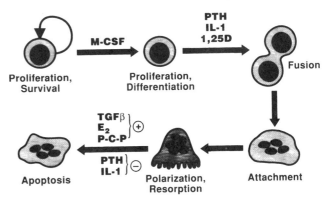

FIG. 1. Events involved in osteoclastic bone resorption. Osteoclasts develop from pluripotent mononuclear precursors (CFU-GM) present in the bone marrow. Early cells in the osteoclast lineage can differentiate along the granulocyte-macrophage lineage or the osteoclast lineage and have high proliferative capacity. As these cells become further committed to the osteoclast lineage, they gradually lose proliferative potential. Monocyte–macrophage colony-stimulating factor (M-CSF) is an important cytokine required for survival of these precursors. As the mononuclear cells proceed down the osteoclast lineage, they become further differentiated and eventually fuse to form immature osteoclasts. This process may involve cell attachment molecules such as E-cadherin. It is enhanced by systemic factors such as parathyroid hormone, 1,25-dihydroxyvitamin D, and cytokines such as interleukin-1. In the presence of bone, the mature osteoclast becomes polarized, forms a ruffled border, and, with appropriate stimulation, begins to resorb bone. A number of the molecular mechanisms that are required in the osteoclast for polarization include the expression of the *src* proto-oncogene, a nonreceptor tyrosine kinase. The osteoclast also utilizes other specialized molecules to resorb bone, including a vacuolar ATPase which is responsible for pumping protons across the ruffled border. The osteoclast undergoes apoptosis (programmed cell death) during bone remodeling and in response to agents such as transforming growth factor-β (TGF-β), estrogens, and bisphosphonates.

and for the normal bone remodeling sequence. Because bone remodeling occurs in discrete and distinct packets throughout the skeleton, it seems probable that the cellular events are controlled by factors generated in the microenvironment of bone. A number of potent local stimulators and inhibitors of osteoclast activity have been identified.

Interleukin-1

There are two interleukin-1 molecules, interleukin-1α and β. Their effects on bone appear to be the same and are mediated through the same receptor. Interleukin-1 is released by activated monocytes, but also by other types of cells including osteoblasts and tumor cells. It is a potent stimulator of osteoclasts. It works at all phases in the formation and activation of osteoclasts. It stimulates proliferation of the progenitors and differentiation of committed precursors into mature cells (28). It also activates the mature multinucleated osteoclast indirectly through another cell (possibly a bone lining cell) (29).

Interleukin-1 also stimulates osteoclastic bone resorption when infused *in vivo,* and it causes a substantial increase in the plasma calcium (30,31). At least part of its effects may be mediated via prostaglandin generation. It has been implicated as a potential mediator of bone resorption and increased bone turnover in osteoporosis (32). It may be responsible for the increase in bone resorption seen in some malignancies, as well as the localized bone resorption associated with collections of chronic inflammatory cells in diseases such as rheumatoid arthritis.

Lymphotoxin and Tumor Necrosis Factor

Lymphotoxin and tumor necrosis factor (TNF) are molecules that are related functionally to interleukin-1. Many of their biologic properties overlap with those of interleukin-1. They share the same receptor with each other, which is distinct from that of interleukin-1. They are synergistic with interleukin-1 in their effects on bone. Lymphotoxin is released by activated T-lymphocytes, and TNF by activated macrophages. TNF is one of the mediators of the systemic effects of endotoxic shock. It also causes wasting (cachexia) and suppresses erythropoiesis (red blood cell formation). Lymphotoxin and TNF stimulate proliferation of osteoclast progenitors, cause fusion of committed precursors to form multinucleated cells, and activate multinucleated cells (through cells in the osteoblast lineage) to resorb bone (33–35). Lymphotoxin may be an important mediator of bone resorption in myeloma (36). Lymphotoxin and TNF cause osteoclastic bone resorption and hypercalcemia when infused or injected *in vivo* (34,36,37).

Colony-Stimulating Factor-1

The growth regulatory factor CSF-1, which was once thought to be specific for the monocyte-macrophage lineage, has been shown to be required for normal osteoclast formation in rodents during the neonatal period. In the op/op variant of osteopetrosis, there is impaired production of CSF-1, and the consequence is osteopetrosis because of decreased normal osteoclast formation (see earlier). The disease can be cured by treatment with CSF-1 (38). CSF-1 is produced by stromal cells in the osteoclast microenvironment. Presumably, cells in the osteoclast lineage contain the CSF-1 receptor (a receptor tyrosine kinase), and this is the mechanism by which CSF-1 mediates osteoclast formation.

Osteoclastpoietic Factor

Since the osteoclast shares a common precursor with the formed elements of the blood, and CFU-GM are precursors for the osteoclast, it has long been wondered if there is a lineage-specific growth-regulatory factor for osteoclast forma-

tion. Two reports have suggested that such a factor may exist (39,40). Tumors that are associated with hypercalcemia often also cause leukocytosis due to production of various colony-stimulating factors. In human and murine tumors associated with the hypercalcemia–leukocytosis syndrome, in addition to colony-stimulating factors, these tumors have been shown to produce a 17-kDa peptide that stimulates osteoclast formation. Complete purification and cloning of this factor are awaited with interest.

Interleukin-6

Interleukin-6 is a pleiotropic cytokine that has important effects on bone. It is expressed and secreted by normal bone cells in response to osteotropic hormones such as PTH, 1,25-dihydroxyvitamin D, and interleukin-1 (41). The osteoclast is the most prodigious cell source of interleukin-6 so far described. Interleukin-6 is a fairly weak stimulator of osteoclast formation, and less powerful than other cytokines such as interleukin-1, TNF, and lymphotoxin (42,43). It has recently been implicated in the bone loss associated with estrogen withdrawal (ovariectomy) in the mouse (44).

Gamma Interferon

Gamma interferon is a multifunctional lymphokine produced by activated T-lymphocytes. In contrast to the other immune cell products, it inhibits osteoclastic bone resorption (45,46). Its major effect appears to be to inhibit differentiation of committed precursors to mature cells (47). It also has less potent effects on osteoclast precursor proliferation. Unlike calcitonin, it does not cause cytoplasmic contraction of isolated osteoclasts.

Transforming Growth Factor-β

TGF-β is a multifunctional polypeptide that is produced by immune cells but is also released from the bone matrix during resorption. TGF-β has unique effects on osteoclasts. In most systems, it inhibits osteoclast formation by inhibiting both proliferation and differentiation of osteoclast precursors (28,48). In addition, it directly inhibits the activity of mature osteoclasts by decreasing superoxide production, and it inhibits accumulation of tartrate-resistant acid phosphatase in osteoclasts. Because TGF-β has a powerful effect on osteoblasts (it stimulates proliferation and synthesis of differentiated proteins and increases mineralized bone formation) (49), it may be a pivotal factor in the bone-remodeling process. For example, it could be released during this resorption process and then be available as a natural endogenous inhibitor of continued osteoclast activity. At the same time, working in conjunction with other bone factors, it may lead to osteoblast stimulation and the eventual formation of new bone. However, the effects of TGF-β are complex and may differ in different species. In one system, neonatal mouse calvariae, it stimulates prostaglandin generation, which in turn leads to bone resorption, which is the opposite effect to that seen in the rat or human systems (50).

Other Factors

A number of other factors whose precise role in physiologic and pathologic bone resorption are still to be delineated.

Retinoids

Vitamin A is the only fully characterized factor that has a direct stimulatory effect on osteoclasts (51). Vitamin A excess eventually leads to increased bone resorption *in vivo* and hypercalcemia. It is unknown if the effects of vitamin A on osteoclasts have physiologic significance.

Transforming Growth Factor-α

TGF-α, like the related compound epidermal growth factor (EGF), is a powerful stimulator of osteoclastic bone resorption (50,52–54). TGF-α is produced by many tumors and is likely involved in increased bone resorption associated with cancer. It is probably produced normally during embryonic life. It stimulates the proliferation of osteoclast progenitors and probably also acts on immature multinucleated cells. Its actions on osteoclasts are comparable to those of the CSFs on other hematopoietic cells (55). The effects of TGF-α on bone cells are mediated through the EGF receptor, although it is more potent than EGF for bone resorption. Injections or infusions of TGF-α increase the plasma calcium levels *in vivo* (37).

Neutral Phosphate and Calcium

Neutral phosphate inhibits osteoclast activity in organ cultures (56). The precise mode of action is not clear. Phosphate is a useful form of therapy in patients with increased bone resorption, diseases such as cancer, or primary hyperparathyroidism, although it may have other effects in addition to those of inhibiting bone resorption, such as impairment of calcium absorption from the gut.

High extracellular calcium concentrations also lead to decreased osteoclast activity, associated with an increase in intracellular calcium concentrations. This suggests that increased local calcium concentrations may be another mechanism by which osteoclast activity to resorb bone may be regulated.

Prostaglandins

Prostaglandins have complex and multiple effects on osteoclasts, depending on the species. Prostaglandins have been linked to the hypercalcemia and increased bone resorption associated with malignancy and chronic inflammation (57). However, the effects of prostaglandins are confusing. Prostaglandins of the E series stimulate osteoclastic bone resorption in organ culture. Moreover, some bone-resorbing factors, and particularly growth factors, appear to mediate their effects through the production of prostaglandins in mouse bones. Prostaglandins inhibit the formation of human osteoclasts and cause cytoplasmic contraction of isolated osteoclasts in much the same way as calcitonin. However, prostaglandins stimulate the formation of mouse multinucleated osteoclasts from marrow progenitors. The overall significance of prostaglandins depends on the species studied. Their overall effects on bone resorption in humans are still a mystery.

Leukotrienes

Leukotrienes, like prostaglandins, are arachidonic acid metabolites that have been linked to osteoclastic bone resorption (58). They are produced by the metabolism of arachidonic acid by a 5-lipoxygenase enzyme. Several of these leukotrienes have been shown to activate osteoclasts *in vitro,* and they may be related to the bone resorption seen in giant cell tumors of bone. These arachidonic acid metabolites have effects on osteoclasts that are different from those of the E series prostaglandins, which stimulate osteoclastic bone resorption in organ culture and cause transient inhibition of the activity of isolated osteoclasts. In contrast, the leukotrienes stimulate osteoclastic bone resorption in organ culture, but they also enhance the capacity of isolated osteoclasts to form resorption pits.

Thyroid Hormones

The thyroid hormones thyroxine and triiodothyronine stimulate osteoclastic bone resorption in organ cultures (59). Some patients with hyperthyroidism have increased bone loss, increased osteoclast activity, and hypercalcemia. Thyroid hormones act directly on osteoclastic bone resorption, but their precise mode of action is unknown.

Glucocorticoids

Glucocorticoids inhibit osteoclast formation *in vitro* and inhibit osteoclastic bone resorption in organ cultures. Their efficacy depends on the stimulus to bone resorption. They are less effective in inhibiting bone resorption stimulated by parathyroid hormone than they are in inhibiting bone resorption stimulated by cytokines such as interleukin-1 (60).

In vivo, glucocorticoid administration is associated with increased bone resorption. This is an indirect effect that results from the effects of glucocorticoids to inhibit calcium absorption from the gut. As a consequence, parathyroid gland activity is stimulated and secondary hyperparathyroidism leads to a generalized increase in osteoclastic bone resorption.

Estrogens and Androgens

Estrogen lack is associated with increased osteoclastic bone resorption in the 10 years following the menopause (61). The mechanisms are not clear. It has been suggested that estrogens may affect osteoclasts directly (62), but, in addition, estrogens may mediate their effects on osteoclasts indirectly by suppressing the production of bone-resorbing cytokines such as interleukin-1 and interleukin-6 (32,44,63). These notions suggested that estrogen withdrawal, for example at the menopause, leads to enhanced bone resorption.

Pharmacologic Agents

A number of pharmacologic agents have been used as inhibitors of bone resorption and are useful therapies in patients with diseases such as malignancy associated with hypercalcemia. These include plicamycin (mithramycin), gallium nitrate, and the bisphosphonates (23). All of these agents inhibit osteoclastic activity, although their mechanism of action is unknown. In the case of the cytotoxic drugs plicamycin and gallium nitrate, it is possible that their actions are mediated through cytotoxic effects on osteoclasts or inhibition of proliferation of the osteoclast progenitors.

Bisphosphonates are very important inhibitors of osteoclastic bone resorption in vivo; they are achieving increased use in diseases associated with increased bone resorption, and particularly in osteoporosis, hypercalcemia of malignancy, Paget's disease of bone, and osteolytic bone disease. Their molecular mechanism of action is still debated. Some investigators suggest they work primarily by coating bone surfaces and rendering mineralized bone surfaces toxic to resorbing osteoclasts (64), while others postulate a cellular effect, in bone cells in the osteoclast lineage during their formation (65), or in osteoblastic cells that control osteoclastic bone resorption (66). Whatever their target, it has recently been shown that the end result is osteoclast apoptosis (18).

Sex hormone deficiency increases osteoclastic bone resorption. The mechanism is still unclear. Thus, estrogens or androgens may be used as therapy in postmenopausal women or hypogonadal men, respectively. Estrogens and androgens cause increases in all cells at all stages in the osteoclast lineage. Although relatively small numbers of estrogen receptors are present in osteoclasts (62), it is likely that the main primary cellular target is not the osteoclast, and that inhibitory effects on osteoclasts are mediated through accessory cells for bone resorption. Several cytokines have been implicated in the increased bone resorption associated with estrogen withdrawal, including interleukin-1, interleukin-6, TGF-β, and prostaglandins of the E series. As indicated earlier, evidence from in vivo studies suggest that both interleukin-1 and interleukin-6 may be involved (32,44). Because the majority of patients will not take estrogens, attempts are now being made to develop drugs that have estrogen-like effects on bone and the cardiovascular system, but not the deleterious effects of estrogens on the breast and endometrium of the uterus. One member of this group of estrogen agonists/antagonists is raloxifene (67).

REFERENCES

1. Jones SJ, Boyde A, Ali NN, Maconnachie E: A review of bone cell substratum interactions. *Scanning* 7:5–24, 1985
2. Mundy GR, Altman AJ, Gondek M, Bandelin JG: Direct resorption of bone by human monocytes. *Science* 196:1109–1111, 1977
3. Kahn AJ, Stewart CC, Teitelbaum SL: Contact-mediated bone resorption by human monocytes in vitro. *Science* 199:988–990, 1978
4. Eilon G, Mundy GR: Direct resorption of bone by human breast cancer cells in vitro. *Nature* 276:726–728, 1978
5. Boyde A, Maconnachie E, Reid SA, Delling G, Mundy GR: Scanning electron microscopy in bone pathology: Review of methods. Potential and application. *Scanning Electron Microsc* IV:1537–1554, 1986
6. Baron R, Vignery A, Horowitz M: Lymphocytes, macrophages and the regulation of bone remodeling. In: Peck WA (ed) *Bone and Mineral Research*, vol II. Elsevier, New York, 175–242, 1983
7. Roodman GD, Ibbotson KJ, MacDonald BR, Kuehl TJ, Mundy GR: 1,25(OH)₂ vitamin D3 causes formation of multinucleated cells with osteoclast characteristics in cultures of primate marrow. *Proc Natl Acad Sci* 82:8213–8217, 1985
8. Blair HC, Teitelbaum SL, Ghiselli R, Gluck S: Osteoclastic bone resorption by a polarized vacuolar proton pump. *Science* 245:855–857, 1989
9. Sly WS, Whyte MP, Sundaram V, et al.: Carbonic anhydrase II deficiency in 12 families with the autosomal recessive syndrome of osteopetrosis with renal tubular acidosis and cerebral calcification. *N Engl J Med* 313:139–145, 1985
10. Garrett IR, Boyce BF, Oreffo ROC, Bonewald L, Poser P, Mundy GR: Oxygen-derived free radicals stimulate osteoclastic bone resorption in rodent bone in vitro and in vivo. *J Clin Invest* 85:632–639, 1990
11. Davies J, Warwick J, Totty N, Philip R, Helfrich M, Horton M. The osteoclast functional antigen, implicated in the regulation of bone resorption, is biochemically related to the vitronectin receptor. *J Cell Biol* 109:1817–1826, 1989
12. Fisher JE, Caulfield MP, Sato M, Quartuccio HA, Gould RJ, Garsky VM, Rodan GA, Rosenblatt M: Inhibition of osteoclastic bone resorption in vivo by echistatin, an arginyl-glycyl-aspartyl (RGD)-containing protein. *Endocrinology* 132:1411–1413, 1993
13. Soriano P, Montgomery C, Geske R, Bradley A: Targeted disruption of the c-src proto-oncogene leads to osteopetrosis in mice. *Cell* 64:693–702, 1991
14. Boyce BF, Byars J, McWilliams S, et al.: Histological and electron microprobe studies of mineralization in aluminum-related osteomalacia. *J Clin Pathol* 45:502–508, 1992
15. Grigoriadis AE, Wang ZQ, Cecchini MG, Hofstetter W, et al.: c-fos: a key regulator of osteoclast-macrophage lineage determination and bone remodeling. *Science* 266:443–4438, 1994
16. Kahn AJ, Simmons DJ: Investigation of the cell lineage in bone using a chimera of chick and quail embryonic tissue. *Nature* 258:325–327, 1975
17. Walker DG: Control of bone resorption by hematopoietic tissue. The induction and reversal of congenital osteopetrosis in mice through the use of bone marrow mononuclear phagocytes. *J Exp Med* 156:1604–1614, 1975
18. Hughes DE, Wright KR, Uy HL, Sasaki A, Yoneda T, Roodman GD, Mundy GR, Boyce BF: Bisphosphonates promote apoptosis in murine osteoclasts in vitro and in vivo. *J Bone Miner Res* 10:1478–1487, 1995
19. Wiktor-Jedrzejczak W, Urbanowska E, Aukerman SL, et al.: Correction by CSF-1 of defects in the osteopetrotic op/op mouse suggests local, developmental, and humoral requirements for this growth factor. *Exp Hematol* 19:1049–1054, 1991
20. Zambonin Zallone A, Teti A, Primavera MV: Isolated osteoclasts in primary culture: First observations on structure and survival in cultured media. *Anat Embryol* 165:405–413, 1982
21. Rodan GA, Martin TJ: Role of osteoblasts in hormonal control of bone resorption—a hypothesis. *Calcif Tissue Int* 33:349–351, 1981
22. McSheehy PMJ, Chambers TJ. Osteoblastic cells mediate osteoclastic responsiveness to parathyroid hormone. *Endocrinology* 118:824–828, 1986
23. Mundy GR, Roodman GD: Osteoclast ontogeny and function. In: Peck W (ed) *Bone and Mineral Research*, vol V. Elsevier, New York, 209–280, 1987
24. Tsoukas CD, Provvedini DM, Manolagas SC: 1,25 dihydroxyvitamin D3: a novel immunoregulatory hormone. *Science* 224:1438–1440, 1984
25. Wener JA, Gorton SJ, Raisz LG: Escape from inhibition of resorption in cultures of fetal bone treated with calcitonin and parathyroid hormone. *Endocrinology* 90:752–759, 1972
26. Takahashi S, Goldring S, Katz M, Hilsenbeck S, Williams R, Roodman GD: Down regulation of calcitonin receptor mRNA expression by calcitonin during human osteoclast-like cell differentiation. *J Clin Invest* 95:167–171, 1995
27. Chambers TJ, Magnus CJ: Calcitonin alters the behavior of isolated osteoclasts. *J Pathol* 136:27–40, 1982

28. Pfeilschifter JP, Seyedin S, Mundy GR: Transformed growth factor inhibits bone resorption in fetal rat long bone cultures. *J Clin Invest* 82:680–685, 1988

29. Thomson BM, Saklatvala J, Chambers TJ: Osteoblasts mediate interleukin-1 stimulation of bone resorption by rat osteoclasts. *J Exp Med* 164:104–112, 1986

30. Sabatini M, Boyce B, Aufdemorte T, Bonewald L, Mundy GR: Infusions of recombinant human interleukin-1α and β cause hypercalcemia in normal mice. *Proc Natl Acad Sci* 85:5235–5239, 1988

31. Boyce BF, Aufdemorte TB, Garrett IR, Yates AJP, Mundy GR: Effects of interleukin-1 on bone turnover in normal mice. *Endocrinology* 123:1142–1150, 1989

32. Pacifici R, Rifas L, McCracken R, et al.: Ovarian steroid treatment blocks a postmenopausal increase in blood monocyte interleukin-1 release. *Proc Natl Acad Sci* 86:2398–2402, 1989

33. Bertolini DR, Nedwin GE, Bringman TS, Mundy GR: Stimulation of bone resorption and inhibition of bone formation in vitro by human tumour necrosis factors. *Nature* 319:516–518, 1986

34. Johnson RA, Boyce BF, Mundy GR, Roodman GD: Tumors producing human TNF induce hypercalcemia and osteoclastic bone resorption in nude mice. *Endocrinology* 124:1424–1427, 1989

35. Thomson BM, Mundy GR, Chambers TJ: Tumor necrosis factors alpha and beta induce osteoblastic cells to stimulate osteoclastic bone resorption. *J Immunol* 138:775–779, 1987

36. Garrett IR, Durie BGM, Nedwin GE, et al.: Production of the bone resorbing cytokine lymphotoxin by cultured human myeloma cells. *N Engl J Med* 317:526–532, 1987

37. Tashjian AH Jr, Voelkel EF, Lazzaro M, et al.: Tumor necrosis factor-alpha (cachectin) stimulates bone resorption in mouse calvaria via a prostaglandin-mediated mechanism. *Endocrinology* 120:2029–2036, 1987

38. Felix R, Cecchini MG, Fleisich H: Macrophage colony stimulating factor restores in vivo bone resorption in the op/op osteopetrotic mouse. *Endocrinology* 127:2592–2594, 1990

39. Lee MY, Eyre DR, Osborne WRA: Isolation of a murine osteoclast colony-stimulating factor. *Proc Natl Acad Sci USA* 88:8500–8504, 1991

40. Yoneda T, Kato I, Bonewald LF, Chisoku H, Burgess WH, Mundy GR: A novel osteoclastpoietic peptide: Purification and characterization. *J Bone Miner Res* 6(suppl):454, 1991

41. Feyen JHM, Elford P, Dipadova FE, Trechsel U: Interleukin-6 is produced by bone and modulated by parathyroid hormone. *J Bone Miner Res* 4:633–638, 1989

42. Black K, Garrett IR, Mundy GR: Chinese hamster ovary cells transfected with the murine interleukin-6 gene cause hypercalcemia as well as cachexia, leukocytosis and thrombocytosis in tumor-bearing nude mice. *Endocrinology* 128:2657–2659, 1991

43. Ishimi Y, Miyaura C, Jin CH, Akatsu T, Abe T, Nakamura Y, Yamaguchi A, Yoshiki S, Matsuda T, Hirano T, Kishimoto T, Suda T: IL-6 is produced by osteoblasts and induces bone resorption. *J Immunol* 145:3297–3303, 1990

44. Jilka RL, Hangoc G, Girasole G, Passeri G, Williams DC, Abrams JS, Boyce B, Broxmeyer H, Manolagas SC: Increased osteoclast development after estrogen loss—mediation by interleukin-6. *Science* 257:88–91, 1992

45. Gowen M, Mundy GR: Actions of recombinant interleukin-1, interleukin-2 and interferon gamma on bone resorption in vitro. *J Immunol* 136:2478–2482, 1986

46. Gowen M, Nedwin G, Mundy GR: Preferential inhibition of cytokine stimulated bone resorption by recombinant interferon gamma. *J Bone Miner Res* 1:469–474, 1986

47. Takahashi N, Mundy GR, Kuehl TJ, Roodman GD: Osteoclast like formation in fetal and newborn long term baboon marrow cultures is more sensitive to 1,25-dihydroxyvitamin D3 than adult long term marrow cultures. *J Bone Miner Res* 2:311–317, 1987

48. Chenu C, Pfeilschifter J, Mundy GR, Roodman GD: Transforming growth factor inhibits formation of osteoclast-like cells in long-term human marrow cultures. *Proc Natl Acad Sci* 85:5683–5687, 1988

49. Noda M, Camilliere JJ: In vivo stimulation of bone formation by transforming growth factor-beta. *Endocrinology* 124:2991–2994, 1989

50. Tashjian AH Jr, Voelkel EF, Lloyd W, et al.: Actions of growth factors on plasma calcium. Epidermal growth factor and human transforming growth factor-alpha cause elevation of plasma calcium in mice. *J Clin Invest* 78:1405–1409, 1986

51. Fell HB, Mellanby E: The effect of hypervitaminosis A on embryonic limb bones cultured in vitro. *J Physiol* 116:320–349, 1952

52. Ibbotson KJ, D'Souza SM, Smith DD, Carpenter G, Mundy GR: EGF receptor antiserum inhibits bone resorbing activity produced by a rat Leydig cell tumor associated with the humoral hypercalcemia of malignancy. *Endocrinology* 116:469–471, 1985

53. Ibbotson KJ, Harrod J, Gowen M: Human recombinant transforming growth factor alpha stimulates bone resorption and inhibits formation in vitro. *Proc Natl Acad Sci* 83:2228–2232, 1986

54. Stern PH, Krieger NS, Nissenson RA, et al.: Human transforming growth factor alpha stimulates bone resorption in vitro. *J Clin Invest* 76:2016–2020, 1985

55. Takahashi N, MacDonald BR, Hon J, Winkler ME, Derynck R, Mundy GR, Roodman GD: Recombinant human transforming growth factor alpha stimulates the formation of osteoclast-like cells in long term human marrow cultures. *J Clin Invest* 78:894–898, 1986

56. Raisz LG, Niemann I: Effect of phosphate, calcium and magnesium on bone resorption and hormonal responses in tissue culture. *Endocrinology* 85:446–452, 1969

57. Tashjian AH, Voelkel EF, Levine L, et al.: Evidence that the bone resorption-stimulating factor produced by mouse fibrosarcoma cells is prostaglandin E2: A new model for the hypercalcemia of cancer. *J Exp Med* 136:1329–1343, 1972

58. Gallwitz WE, Mundy GR, Oreffo ROC, Gaskell SJ, Bonewald LF: Purification of osteoclastotropic factors produced by stromal cells: Identification of 5-lipoxygenase metabolites. *J Bone Miner Res* 6(suppl):457, 1991

59. Mundy GR, Shapiro JL, Bandelin JG, Canalis EM, Raisz LG: Direct stimulation of bone resorption by thyroid hormones. *J Clin Invest* 58:529–534, 1976

60. Mundy GR, Rick ME, Turcotte R, Kowalski MA: Pathogenesis of hypercalcemia in lymphosarcoma cell leukemia. Role of an osteoclast activating factor-like substance and mechanism of action for glucocorticoid therapy. *Am J Med* 65:600–606, 1978

61. Lindsay R, Hart DM, Forrest C, et al.: Prevention of spinal osteoporosis in oophorectomised women. *Lancet* 2:1151–1153, 1980

62. Oursler MJ, Osdoby P, Pyfferoen J, Riggs BL, Spelsberg TC: Avian osteoclasts as estrogen target cells. *Proc Natl Acad Sci USA* 88:6613–6617, 1991

63. Girasole G, Jilka RL, Passeri G, et al.: 17 beta-estradiol inhibits interleukin-6 production by bone marrow-derived stromal cells and osteoblasts in vitro—a potential mechanism for the antiosteoporotic effect of estrogens. *J Clin Invest* 89:883–891, 1992

64. Sato M, Grasser W, Endo N, Akins R, Simmons H, Thompson DD, Golub E, Rodan GA: Bisphosphonate action—Alendronate localization in rat bone and effects on osteoclast ultrastructure. *J Clin Invest* 88:2095–2105, 1991

65. Hughes DE, MacDonald BR, Russell RGG, Gowen M: Inhibition of osteoclast-like cell formation by bisphosphonates in long-term cultures of human bone marrow. *J Clin Invest* 83:1930–1935, 1989

66. Sahni M, Guenther HL, Fleisch H, Collin P, Martin TJ: Bisphosphonates act on rat bone resorption through the mediation of osteoblasts. *J Clin Invest* 91:2004–2011, 1993

67. Black LJ, Sato M, Rowley ER, Magee DE, Bekele A, Williams DC, Cullinan GJ, Bendele R, Kauffman RF, Bensch WR, Frolik CA, Termine JD, Bryant HU: Raloxifene (LY139481 HCl) prevents bone loss and reduces serum cholesterol without causing uterine hypertrophy in ovariectomized rats. *J Clin Invest* 93:63–69, 1994

4. Bone Matrix Proteins and the Mineralization Process

John D. Termine, Ph.D., and *Pamela Gehron Robey, Ph.D.

*Lilly Research Laboratories, Eli Lilly and Company, Indianapolis, Indiana; and
Bone Research Branch, National Institutes of Health, Bethesda, Maryland

The largest proportion of the body's connective tissue mass is bone. It consists of extracellular matrix proteins and the cells that first make, then mineralize, and finally maintain them (1,2). Unlike other connective tissues, bone matrix is physiologically mineralized with small crystallites of a basic, carbonate-containing calcium phosphate called hydroxyapatite. In this regard, bone mineral most closely resembles a geological mineral crystalline form called dahlite. Further, the bone matrix is unique among connective tissues in that it is constantly regenerated throughout life as a consequence of bone turnover.

COLLAGEN

Some 85% to 90% of the total bone protein consists of collagen fibers made almost exclusively of type I collagen (unlike other tissues that contain fibers of mixed collagen types). Type I collagen is the most abundant form of collagen in the body and is widely distributed in connective tissue. Bone collagen fibers are highly insoluble as a result of many covalent intra- and intermolecular cross-links, the type and pattern of which differ from those in soft connective tissues (3). The basic building block of the bone matrix fiber network is the type I collagen molecule, which is a triple-helical, coiled coil (a supercoil), containing two identical $\alpha1(I)$ chains and a structurally similar, but genetically different, $\alpha2(I)$ chain. The collagen coil can form because every third residue in each chain's helical domain (~1000 amino acids, or 300 nm in length) is glycine. This amino acid has no bulky side chain and conveys the ability to coil. Collagen chains also contain a high proportion of proline, a cyclic amino acid, most of which immediately follow glycine. The gly-X-Y repeating triplet (where X is often proline, and Y is often a modified form of proline) makes the collagen structure unique in biology (4).

All of the information necessary to fold into native molecules (see below) and then pack into fibrous protein resides in the primary sequence of the individual collagen chain. In the matrix, individual collagen molecules pack end to end with a short space (or gap) between them, and then pack laterally in a one-quarter-stagger array, so that each molecule is offset from its neighbor by approximately one fourth of its length. This three-dimensional arrangement constitutes the fiber structure found in the bone extracellular space.

The genes for the $\alpha1(I)$ and $\alpha2(I)$ chains of collagen are found on chromosomes 17 and 7, respectively (5). As in most genes, each consists of multiple small regions (called exons) that code for protein, interspersed by larger, noncoding DNA regions (introns). The messenger RNA for each collagen chain encodes a biosynthesized precursor procollagen chain,

~160,000 Da in size. Following removal of a short (~20-amino-acid residue) signal sequence, the procollagen chains consist of propeptide extensions at the amino and carboxy termini of ~25,000 and 35,000 Da, respectively, attached to a central region (a chain of ~100,000 Da). The carboxy-terminal propeptide facilitates molecular folding of the trimeric procollagen molecule, which is secreted in an unprocessed form. Either concomitant with, or subsequent to, secretion from the cell, the procollagen peptide extensions are removed as fiber formation occurs (6). These propeptide extensions seem to assist in fibril formation and eventually become entrapped, at least in part, in the final matrix of bone (7). The propeptide extensions of type I collagen can also escape to serum, where they have proved to be useful markers of bone formation (8). The preponderance of propeptide type I collagen extensions found in serum come from bone turnover. The propeptide extensions of type III collagen are often measured (along with those of type I) to correct for nonbone collagen synthesis (8). Such propeptide extension measurements have correlated significantly with direct histomorphometric measurements of bone formation (9).

Several posttranslational modifications of collagen occur during its biosynthesis and secretion. Intracellular modifications include hydroxylation of some proline and lysine residues, addition of galactose to certain hydroxylysines, and serine phosphorylation. Extracellular modifications include cleavage of the peptide extensions from the procollagen molecule by specific peptidases, and, after fibril formation, complexation with noncollagen proteins (see below) and cross-link formation. Intra- and intermolecular covalent cross-links are formed by lysyl oxidase action on collagen lysine and/or hydroxylysine residues (10,11). In bone, multiple cross-linking sites combine extracellularly to form pyridinium ring structures (the pyridinolines), tying several collagen monomer molecules together within the fiber, thereby rendering it completely insoluble (3). These pyridinium cross-links are released only on degradation of the mineralized collagen fibrils during bone resorption. Measurement of these ringed cross-link structures in urine have proved to be good measures of bone resorption (12).

NONCOLLAGENOUS PROTEINS

Noncollagenous proteins (NCPs) account for 10% to 15% of the total bone protein content. Approximately one fourth of the bone NCP is exogenously derived, being adsorbed or entrapped in the bone matrix space (13). This fraction is largely composed of serum-derived proteins that are acidic in character and become bound to the hydroxyapatite mineral of bone. Some of these proteins may be advantageous to the tissue. For example, trapped growth factors [e.g., platelet-derived growth factor (PDGF)] could easily contribute to the regeneration of bone upon injury (13). Other proteins, such as serum albumin, may be present merely adventitiously.

On a mole-to-mole basis, however, it can be calculated that the bone cell synthesizes and secretes as many molecules of NCP as it does of collagen. Remember, triple helical collagen has a molecular weight of over 300,000, whereas most bone NCPs are approximately one-tenth that size. Thus, a considerable portion (~50%) of the osteoblast's matrix-directed biosynthetic activities are devoted to NCP molecules. These can be broken down into four general groups of protein products: (i) proteoglycans, (ii) growth-related proteins, (iii) cell attachment proteins, and (iv) γ-carboxylated (gla) proteins. These classifications are often overlapping, and most of the physiologic roles for individual bone protein constituents remain undefined at present (Table 1).

Proteoglycans are macromolecules that contain acidic polysaccharide side chains (glycosaminoglycans) attached to a central core protein. In bone, two types of glycosaminoglycan are predominately found: chondroitin sulfate, a polymer of sulfated N-acetylgalactosamine and glucuronic acid, and heparan sulfate, a polymer of sulfated N-acetylglucosamine and glucuronic acid. The bone cell heparan sulfate proteoglycan product is membrane associated and, as for all connective tissues, probably facilitates interaction of the osteoblast with extracellular macromolecules (some of which are cell attachment proteins) and heparin-binding growth factors (14,15). During development, high levels of hyaluronan, an unsulfated glycosaminoglycan that is not attached to a protein core, are also found.

Chondroitin sulfate in bone is attached to three separate core proteins (15). One of these is approximately 300,000 Da in size (resultant proteoglycan, ~600 to 800 kDa) and resembles a proteoglycan product synthesized by fibroblasts called *versican* (16). Its role is not yet understood, but it may be important in delineating areas that will become bone (17). The vast bulk of the glycosaminoglycans of bone are attached to two small (~40 kDa) core proteins that are composed of a leucine-rich repeat sequence. While they are very similar, they are separate gene products (18). *Decorin* has one attached 50,000-Da chondroitin sulfate chain and *biglycan* has two attached chains, based on their relative electrophoretic migration on sodium dodecyl sulfate gels (18). Decorin is found in all stages of bone development and biglycan is more abundant in developing (i.e., fetal or young) than in adult bone. Decorin is distributed predominantly in the extracellular matrix space of connective tissues, whereas biglycan tends to be found in pericellular locales (19). A similar developmental distribution for these two proteoglycans is found in other connective tissues (19). Decorin, so called because it binds to collagen fibrils, has been implicated in the regulation of collagen fibrillogenesis (reviewed in ref. 20). Although the exact physiologic functions of the small proteoglycans have not been definitively elucidated, they are generally assumed to be important for the integrity of most connective tissue matrices. One function might arise from their ability to bind and modulate the activity of transforming growth factor-β (TGF-β) family in the extracellular space (21,22). By this property, decorin and biglycan can influence cell proliferation and differentiation in a variety of connective tissues, including bone.

Other bone cell products (primarily glycoproteins that are differentially, posttranslationally modified) may be associated with the growth and/or differentiation of the osteoblast in an indirect or as yet undefined fashion. One of the hallmarks of the osteoblast phenotype is the synthesis of high levels of *alkaline phosphatase* (23). This enzyme is first found on the osteoblast plasmalemma, and some may be cleaved from the cell surface and adsorbed within the mineralized bone matrix space. The function of alkaline phosphatase in bone cell biology has been the subject of much speculation, but it remains undefined to the present day.

The most abundant NCP produced by bone cells is *osteonectin,* a phosphorylated glycoprotein accounting for approximately 2% of the total protein of developing bone in most animal species. The protein has high affinity for binding ionic calcium and physiologic hydroxyapatite (24). It also binds to collagen (24) and thrombospondin (25). Osteonectin protein is found in platelets (26) and in nonbone tissues that are rapidly proliferating, remodeling, or undergoing profound changes in tissue architecture (27,28). Thus, the protein is associated with growing tissue, and in nonbone systems, its transcription and synthesis are down-regulated under steady-state conditions. Osteonectin biosynthesis is up-regulated, again in nonbone systems, during wound repair, and in some conditions of cell culture. Its function(s) in bone may be multiple, with potential association with osteoblast growth and/or proliferation, as well as with matrix mineralization (see below). Using synthetic peptides specific for parts of the osteonectin molecule, a number of different activities have been identified (primarily in endothelial cells), such as binding to PDGF-AB, cell cycle regulation, and modulation of shape change (reviewed in ref. 29). However, it is not known if the effects of these synthetic peptides (taken out of the context of the entire molecule) also pertain to cells in the osteoblastic lineage.

All connective tissue cells interact with their extracellular environment in response to chemical stimuli that direct or coordinate specific cell functions, such as proliferation, migration, and differentiation. These particular interactions involve cell attachment and spreading, via transient, focal adhesions to extracellular macromolecules. This is done via the integrin family of cell surface receptors that transduce signals to the cytoskeleton (30). Bone cells synthesize at least six proteins that affect cell attachment: type I collagen; fibronectin; thrombospondin; and low levels of vitronectin (Dunlay, Grzesik, and Gehron Robey, *unpublished results*), osteopontin, bone sialoprotein (31–33), and most likely BAG-75 (34). Three of these *(thrombospondin, osteopontin, and bone sialoprotein)* are strong binders of ionic calcium and are found in the mineralized bone extracellular space (1,2). Osteopontin is a phosphoprotein that, like fibronectin and thrombospondin, is found also in nonbone tissue systems (35). Bone sialoprotein is almost exclusively found in the skeleton (36), and its appearance is tightly correlated

TABLE 1. *Stages of osteoblast maturation and their principal noncollagenous products*

Stage of maturation	Protein (M_r, kDa)	Chemical features	Potential function
Osteoprogenitors	Type I collagen (300,000)	[α1(I)$_2\alpha$2(I)], RGD	Matrix organization
	Type III collagen (300 kDa)	[α1(III)]$_3$, disulfide bonds	Matrix organization
	Versican (~1 × 10^6)	360-kDa core with EGF-like sequences, 45-kDa CS chains	"Capture space" destined to become bone
Pre-osteoblasts	Collagen I, III, versican		
	Alkaline phosphatase (200–160 kDa)	Bone/liver/kidney isoforms, tissue-specific glycosylation, disulfide-bonded dimer	Hydrolyze phosphates, ion carrier protein
	Thrombospondin (~450 kDa)	Three identical disulfide-bonded subunits of ~150 kDa, RGD	Cell attachment, growth factor binding
	Matrix gla protein (19 kDa)	Gla residues	Unknown
	Decorin (~160 kDa)	~40-kDa core with leucine repeats, 50-kDa CS chains	Collagen fibril diameter, binds to TGF-β
Osteoblasts	Alkaline phosphatase, thrombospondin, decorin		
	Fibronectin (~400 kDa)	Two non-identical disulfide-bonded subunits of ~200 KD, RGD	Major protein in serum, cell attachment
	Osteonectin (~45 kDa)	Glycosylated, phosphorylated, EF hand structure	High-and low -affinity Ca^{2+}-binding, apatite binding, matrix protein binding
	Biglycan (~280 kDa)	~40-kDa core with leucine repeats, 50-kDa CS chains	Pericellular environment, growth factor binding
	Osteopontin (~90–45 kDa)	Glycosylated, phosphorylated, RGD	Cell proliferation, cell attachment
	Bone sialoprotein (~85 kDa)	Heavily glycosylated (50%), sulfated, RGD	Cell attachment, marker of mineralization
	Type I collagen (only)	Different posttranslational modifications (gal-hyl cross-links, phosphorylation of N-propeptide), RGD	May orient nucleators of matrix mineralization
Osteocytes	Fibronectin, biglycan		
	Osteocalcin (5800)	Gla-residues, one disulfide bridge	Binds Ca^{2+}, marker of bone turnover

The proteins listed for each stage of maturation do not exist only in that stage, but they are maximally detected at that point in maturation (53). M_r, molecular weight; RGD, Arg-Gly-Asn cell attachment consensus sequence; CS, chondroitin sulfate.

with the appearance of mineral (37). Both osteopontin and bone sialoprotein bind Ca^{2+} via polyacidic amino acid sequences, and both are known to anchor osteoclasts to the bone extracellular space in cell regions called clear zones (36,38). Specific extracellular matrix receptors called integrins bind to these molecules allowing the osteoclasts to first form ruffled borders and then resorb bone (39).

Vitamin K–dependent γ-carboxylation occurs on three bone NCPs: *osteocalcin* (bone gla-protein) and *matrix gla-protein* (MGP), which are both made by bone cells (40), and protein S, which is made primarily in the liver (41). Dicarboxylic glutamyl (gla) residues also occur in blood-clotting proteins, where enhanced calcium binding to gla side chains is important to the bioactivity of these molecules. Osteocalcin (~6 kDa) is somewhat bone specific, although the related mRNA has been found in platelets and megakaryocytes (42), whereas MGP (~9 kDa) is found also in cartilage (40). In human bone, osteocalcin is concentrated in osteocytes (43) and its release may provide a signal in the bone turnover cascade (44). Osteocalcin and MGP are partially

homologous structurally (40), but it is as yet unclear how they function physiologically, either together or separately in bone tissue. Nevertheless, determination of osteocalcin in serum has proved valuable as a marker of bone turnover in metabolic disease states (45).

A number of proteins in bone appear to be associated with the life cycle and function of the osteoblast. These proteins may be *morphogens* (46), growth factors such as TGF-β1 through -β5 and insulin-like growth factors, osteoblast secretion products that can stimulate osteoblast cell growth in an autocrine or paracrine fashion (47,48). Thus, the growth potential of a bone cell may result from its own genetic activity and may involve transcription of both factors and their receptors in the same cell population.

MINERALIZATION

Two mechanisms for bone mineralization have been described, one that predominates in both calcified cartilage and primitive woven bone, the other in lamellar bone (49–52). In some instances, calcified cartilage and woven bone seem to mineralize via matrix vesicles (49), membrane-bound bodies that exocytose from the plasma membrane and migrate to the loose extracellular matrix space. The lipid-rich inner membrane of these vesicles becomes the nidus for hydroxyapatite crystal formation, and eventually crystallization proceeds to the point of obliteration of the vesicle membrane, producing a spherulite of clustered, small (50Å × 200Å × 400Å) crystals. In this context, the matrix vesicle is on a suicide mission, and its "death" leads to mineral encrustation. Recent studies indicate that osteoblasts secrete matrix components that have been preorganized within the cell, and, upon secretion, these packets of matrix proteins (including bone sialoprotein) become mineralized immediately (37). These spherulites conglomerate until a continuous mineralized mass is achieved throughout the matrix space. The driving force for this mineral cascade, once initiated, seems to be the mineral crystals themselves that are first associated with the matrix vesicle membrane. The rate of mineralization in both woven and (see below) lamellar bone seems to depend on the presence of inhibitor molecules (e.g., pyrophosphate and acidic NCPs), which in solution seem to regulate the kinetics of the mineralization process (50). Thus, in this type of calcification, the cell buds off organelles capable of mineral accumulation and then synthesizes proteins that can control the rate at which crystallization proceeds.

The extracellular matrix in nonfetal and more abundant lamellar bone is tightly packed with well-aligned collagen fibrils that are "decorated" with complexed NCPs (e.g., proteoglycan and osteonectin). Either because there is simply insufficient space for them or for developmental reasons, matrix vesicles are rarely (if ever) seen in lamellar bone. Instead, mineralization proceeds in association with the heteropolymeric (collagen–NCP complex) matrix fibrils themselves. Somewhat more mineral appears associated with aligned gap regions (or "hole" zones) of the fibers (three-dimensional channels resulting from the spaces between longitudinally associated collagen monomers), which have more room for inorganic ions that rest of the fibril structure. Other loci for the bone mineral appear to be between the collagen fibrils in a brick-and-mortar fashion (51). It is unlikely that the driving force for mineralization is bone collagen, because purified collagen appears to be a poor initiator of crystal deposition. Consequently, it is probable that the NCPs are responsible for this process. The extent of mineralization in the bone matrix space appears limited by the volume of bone occupied by its insoluble organic fibrous protein content alone. Decreased mineralization seems to occur under conditions of mineral ion deprivation, such as osteomalacia, and is fully reversible by increasing the pool of ions available for this purpose.

REFERENCES

1. Gehron Robey P, Bianco P, Termine JD: The cellular biology and molecular biochemistry of bone formation. In: Coe FL, Favus MJ (eds) *Disorders of Mineral Metabolism.* Raven Press, New York, 241–263, 1992
2. Gehron Robey P, Boskey AL: The biochemistry of bone. In: Marcus RA, Feldman D, Kelsey J (eds) *Osteoporosis.* Academic Press, New York, 95–183, 1996
3. Eyre DR, Dickson IR, Van Ness K: Collagen cross-linking in human bone and articular cartilage. Age-related changes in the content of mature hydroxypyridinium residues. *Biochem J* 252: 495–500, 1988
4. Hulmes DJ: The collagen superfamily—diverse structures and assemblies. *Essays Biochem* 27:49–67, 1992
5. Vuorio E, de Crombrugghe B: The family of collagen genes. *Annu Rev Biochem* 59:837–872, 1990
6. Fleischmajer R, Perlish JS, Olsen BR: Amino and carboxyl propeptides in bone collagen fibrils during embryogenesis. *Cell Tissue Res* 247:105–109, 1987
7. Fisher LW, Gehron Robey P, Tuross N, Otsuka A, Tepen DA, Esch FS, Shimasaki S, Termine JD: The M_r 24,000 phosphoprotein from developing bone is the NH_2-terminal propeptide of the α1 chain of type I collagen. *J Biol Chem* 262:13457–13463, 1987
8. Krane SM, Munoz AJ, Harris ED: Urinary polypeptides related to collagen synthesis. *J Clin Invest* 49:716–720, 1970
9. Parfitt AM, Simon LS, Villanueva AR, Krane SM: Procollagen type I carboxy-terminal extension peptide in serum as a marker of collagen biosynthesis in bone. Correlation with iliac bone formation rates and comparison with total alkaline phosphatase. *J Bone Miner Res* 2:427–436, 1987
10. Yamauchi M, Katz EP, Mechanic GL: Intermolecular cross-linking and stereospecific molecular packing in type I collagen fibrils of the periodontal ligament. *Biochemistry* 25:4907–4913, 1986
11. Robins SP, Duncan A: Pyridinium cross-links of bone collagen and location in peptides isolated from rat femur. *Biochim Biophys Acta* 914:233–239, 1987
12. Uebelhart D, Gineyts E, Chapuy M-C, Delmas PD: Urinary excretion of pyridinium cross-links; a new marker of bone resorption in metabolic bone disease. *Bone Miner* 8:87–96, 1990
13. Termine JD: Non-collagen proteins in bone. In: Evered D, Harnett S (eds) *Cell and Molecular Biology of Vertebrate Hard Tissues.* Ciba Foundation Synposium 136. John Wiley and Sons, Chichester, 178–190, 1988
14. Hook M, Woods A, Johansson S, Kjellen L, Couchman Jr: Functions of proteoglycans at the cell surface. In: Evered E, Whelan J (eds) *Functions of the Proteoglycans.* Ciba Foundation Symposium 124. John Wiley and Sons, Chichester, 143–156, 1986
15. Beresford JN, Fedarko NS, Fisher LW, Midura RJ, Yanagishita M, Termine JD, Gehron Robey P: Analysis of the proteoglycans synthesized by human bone cells in vitro. *J Biol Chem* 262: 17164–17172, 1987
16. Krusius T, Gehlsen KR, Ruoslahti E: A fibroblast chondroitin sulfate proteoglycan core protein contains lectin-like and growth factor-like sequences. *J Biol Chem* 262:13120–13125, 1987
17. Fisher LW: The nature of the proteoglycans of bone, In: Butler WT (ed) *The Chemistry and Biology of Mineralized Tissues.* EBSCO Media, Birmingham, AL, 188–196, 1985
18. Fisher LW, Hawkins GR, Tuross N, Termine JD: Purification and partial characterization of small proteoglycans I and II, bone sialoproteins I and II and osteonectin from the mineral compartment of developing human bone. *J Biol Chem* 262:9702–9708, 1987
19. Bianco P, Fisher LW, Young MF, Termine JD, Gehron Robey P: Expression and localization of the two small proteoglycans biglycan and decorin in developing human skeletal and nonskeletal tissues. *J Histochem Cytochem* 38:1549–1563, 1990
20. Ruoslahti E: Structure and biology of proteoglycans. *Annu Rev Cell Biol* 4:229–255, 1988
21. Yamaguchi Y, Mann DM, Rouslahti E: Negative regulation of transforming growth factor-β by the proteoglycan decorin. *Nature* 346:281–284, 1990
22. Takeuchi Y, Kodama Y, Matsumoto T: Bone matrix decorin binds transforming growth factor-β and enhances its bioactivity. *J Biol Chem* 51:32634–32638, 1994
23. Rodan GA, Heath JK, Yoon K, Noda M, Rodan SB: Diversity of the osteoblast phenotype. In: Evered D, Harnett S (eds) *Cell and Molecular Biology of Vertebrate Hard Tissues.* Ciba Foundation Symposium 136. John Wiley and Sons, Chichester, 78–85, 1988
24. Termine JD, Kleinman HK, Whitson SW, Conn KM, McGarvey ML, Martin GR: Osteonectin, a bone-specific protein linking mineral to collagen. *Cell* 26:99–105, 1981
25. Clezardin P, Malaval L, Ehrensperger AS, Delmas P, Dechavanne M, McGregor JL: Complex formation of human thrombospondin with osteonectin. *Eur J Biochem* 175:275–284, 1988

26. Stenner DD, Tracy RP, Riggs BL, Mann KG: Human platelets contain and secrete osteonectin, a major protein of mineralized bone. *Proc Natl Acad Sci USA* 83:6892–6896, 1986

27. Holland PWH, Harper SJ, McVey JH, Hogan BLM: In vivo expression of mRNA for the Ca^{+2}-binding protein SPARC (osteonectin) revealed by in situ hybridization. *J Cell Biol* 105:473–482, 1987

28. Wewer UM, Albrechtsen R, Fisher LW, Young MF, Termine JD: Osteonectin/SPARC/BM-40 in human decidua and carcinoma, tissues characterized by de novo formation of basement membrane. *Am J Pathol* 132:345–355, 1988

29. Lane TF, Sage EH: The biology of SPARC, a protein that modulates cell–matrix interactions. *FASEB J* 8:163–73, 1994

30. Ruoslahti E, Pierschbacher MD: New perspectives in cell adhesion: RGD and integrins. *Science* 238:491–497, 1987

31. Gehron Robey P, Young MF, Fisher LW, McClain TD: Thrombospondin is an osteoblast-derived component of mineralized extracellular matrix. *J Cell Biol* 108:719–727, 1988

32. Somerman MJ, Fisher LW, Foster RA, Sauk JJ: Human bone sialoprotein I and II enhance fibroblast attachment in vitro. *Calcif Tissue Int* 43:50–53, 1988

33. Grzesik WJ, Gehron Robey P: Bone matrix RGD glycoproteins: immunolocalization and interaction with human primary osteoblastic bone cells in vitro. *J Bone Miner Res* 9:487–496, 1994

34. Gorski JP: Acidic phosphoproteins from bone matrix: a structural rationalization of their role in biomineralization. *Calcif Tissue Int* 50:391–396, 1992

35. Mark MP, Prince CW, Gay S, Austin RL, Butler WT: 44kDal bone phosphoprotein (osteopontin) antigenicity at ectopic sites in newborn rats: kidney and nervous tissues. *Cell Tissue Res* 251:23–30, 1988

36. Bianco P, Fisher LW, Young MF, Termine JD, Gehron Robey P: Expression of bone sialoprotein (BSP) in developing human tissues. *Calcif Tissue Int* 49:421–426, 1991

37. Bianco P, Riminucci M, Silvestrini G, Bonucci E, Termine JD, Fisher LW, Gehron Robey P: Localization of bone sialoprotein (BSP) to golgi and post-golgi secretory structures in osteoblasts and to discrete sites in early bone matrix. *J Histochem Cytochem* 41:193–203, 1993

38. Reinholt FP, Hultenby K, Oldberg A, Heinegard D: Osteopontin—A possible anchor osteoclasts to bone. *Proc Natl Acad Sci USA* 87:4473–4475, 1990

39. Zambonin-Zallone A, Teti A, Grano M, Rubinacci A, Abbadini M, Gaboli M, Marchisio: Immunocytochemical distribution of extracellular matrix receptors in human osteoclasts; a β_3 integrin is co-localized with vinculin and talin in the podosomes of osteoclastoma giant cells. *Exp Cell Res* 182:645–652, 1989

40. Price PA: Vitamin K-dependent bone proteins. In: Cohn DV, Martin TJ, Meunier PJ (eds) *Calcium Regulation and Bone Metabolism: Basic and Clinical Aspects,* vol 9. Elsevier Science, Amsterdam, 419–425, 1987

41. Maillard C, Berruyer M, Serre CM, Dechavane M, Delmas PD: Protein S, a vitamin K-dependent protein, is a bone matrix component synthesized and secreted by osteoblasts. *Endocrinology* 130:1599–1604, 1992

42. Thiede MA, Smock SL, Petersen DN, Grasser WA, Thompson DD, Nishimoto SK: Presence of messenger ribonucleic acid encoding osteocalcin, a marker of bone turnover, in bone marrow megakaryocytes and peripheral blood platelets. *Endocrinology* 135:929–937, 1994

43. Kasai R, Bianco, P, Gehron Robey P, Kahn AJ: Production and characterization of an antibody against the human bone GLA protein (BGP/osteocalcin) propeptide and its use in immunocytochemistry of bone cells. *Bone Miner* 25:167–182, 1994

44. Glowacki J, Lian JB: Impaired recruitment of osteoclast progenitors by osteocalcin-deficient bone implants. In: Butler WT (ed) *The Chemistry and Biology of Mineralized Tissues.* EBSCO Media, Birmingham, AL, 164–169, 1985

45. Price PA, Parthemore JG, Deftos LJ: New biochemical marker for bone metabolism. *J Clin Invest* 66:878–883, 1980

46. Wozney JP: Bone morphogenetic proteins and their gene expression. In: *Cellular Molecular Biology of Bone*, Academic Press, New York, 131–168, 1993

47. Gehron Robey P, Young MF, Flanders KC, Roche NS, Kondaiah P, Reddi AH, Termine JD, Sporn MB, Roberts AB: Osteoblasts synthesize and respond to TGF-beta in vitro. *J Cell Biol* 105:457–463, 1987

48. Canalis E, McCarthy T, Centrella M: Isolation and characterization of insulin-like growth factor I (somatomedin C) from cultures of fetal rat calvariae. *Endocrinology* 122:22–27, 1988

49. Bonucci E: The locus of initial calcification in cartilage and bone. *Clin Orthop* 78:108–139, 1971

50. Glimcher MJ: The nature of the mineral component of bone and the mechanism of calcification. In: Coe FL, Favus MJ (eds) *Disorders of Bone and Mineral Metabolism.* Raven Press, New York, 265–286, 1992

51. Termine JD, Eanes ED, Conn KM: Phosphoprotein modulation of apatite crystallization. *Calcif Tissue Int* 31:247–251, 1980

52. Weiner S, Traub W: Organization of hydroxyapatite crystals within collagen fibrils. *FEBS Lett* 206:262–266, 1986

53. Aubin JE, Kahn A: The osteoblast lineage—embryologic origins and the differentiation sequence. In: Favus MJ, Christakos S, Goldring SR, et al. (ed) *Primer on the Metabolic Bone Diseases and Disorders of Mineral Metabolism,* Third edition. Lippincott-Raven Publishers, Philadelphia, 35–38, 1996

Calcium, Magnesium, and Phosphorus Homeostasis

5. Mineral Balance and Homeostasis

Arthur E. Broadus, M.D., Ph.D.

Department of Internal Medicine, Yale University, New Haven, Connecticut

Life began in a primordial sea, rich in potassium and magnesium and poor in sodium and calcium, and it is felt that the present composition of the cytosol, also rich in potassium and magnesium and poor in sodium and calcium, reflects this ancient heritage. With time, geologic changes altered the composition of the seas to one rich in sodium and calcium, and primitive organisms adapted to this altered milieu by developing ion pumps in order to maintain the asymmetry of the concentrations of monovalent and divalent cations across their plasma membranes. The evolution of these pumps and channels may be viewed as one of the most fundamental developments in cell biology.

The progression to terrestrial life carried with it a complete dependence on minerals from the environment. With this came the evolution of the mineral exchange mechanisms in intestine, kidney, and bone (which subserve systemic mineral needs) as well as the key systemic hormones, parathyroid hormone (PTH) and 1,25-dihydroxyvitamin D [1,25(OH)$_2$D] (which regulate these exchange mechanisms). This integrated regulatory system has many checks and balances and is an elegant example of biologic control.

Calcium. An adult human contains approximately 1000 g of calcium (1,2). Some 99% of this calcium is in the skeleton in the form of hydroxyapatite, and 1% is contained in the extracellular fluids and soft tissues. About 1% of the skeletal content of calcium is freely exchangeable with the extracellular fluids. Although a small percentage of skeletal content, this exchangeable pool is approximately equal to the total content of calcium in the extracellular fluids and soft tissues, and it serves as an important buffer or storehouse of calcium. The extracellular concentration of calcium ions (Ca^{2+}) is in the range of 10^{-3} M, whereas the concentration of Ca^{2+} in the cytosol is about 10^{-6} M.

Calcium plays two predominant physiologic roles in the organism. In bone, calcium salts provide the structural integrity of the skeleton. In the extracellular fluids and in the cytosol, the concentration of Ca^{2+} is critically important in the maintenance and control of a number of biochemical processes, and the concentrations of Ca^{2+} in both compartments are maintained with great constancy.

Phosphorus. An adult human contains approximately 600 g of phosphorus. Some 85% of this phosphorus is present in crystalline form in the skeleton and plays a structural role. About 15% is present in the extracellular fluids, largely in the form of inorganic phosphate ions, and in soft tissues, almost totally in the form of phosphate esters. Intracellular phosphate esters and phosphorylated intermediates are involved in a number of important biochemical processes, including the generation and transfer of cellular energy. Intracellular and extracellular concentrations of

phosphorus (as the phosphate divalent anion) are approximately 1 × 10^{-4} M and 2 × 10^{-4} M, respectively, and these concentrations are less rigidly maintained than are those of calcium and magnesium.

Magnesium. An adult human contains approximately 25 g or 2000 mEq of magnesium. About two thirds is present in the skeleton and one third in soft tissues. The magnesium in bone is not an integral part of the hydroxyapatite lattice structure but appears to be located on the crystal surface. Only a minor fraction of the magnesium in bone is freely exchangeable with extracellular magnesium. Magnesium is the most abundant intracellular divalent cation, and cellular magnesium is important as a cofactor for a number of enzymatic reactions and in the regulation of neuromuscular excitability. Approximately 1% of total body magnesium is contained in the extracellular compartment, and its concentration in plasma does not provide a reliable index of either total body or soft tissue magnesium content. The concentration of magnesium ions (Mg^{2+}) is about 5 × 10^{-4} M in the cytosol as well as in the extracellular fluids, and its concentration in both compartments is rigidly maintained.

EXTRACELLULAR MINERAL METABOLISM

Calcium. There are three definable fractions of calcium in serum: ionized calcium (about 50%), protein-bound calcium (about 40%), and calcium that is complexed, mostly to citrate and phosphate ions (about 10%) (3). Both the complexed and ionized fractions are ultrafilterable, so that about 60% of the total calcium in serum crosses semipermeable membranes. About 90% of the protein-bound calcium is bound to albumin and the remainder to globulins. Alterations in the serum albumin concentration have a major influence on the measured total serum calcium concentration. At pH 7.4, each gm/dl of albumin binds 0.8 mg/dl of calcium, and this simple relationship can be used to "correct" the total serum calcium concentration when circulating albumin is abnormal (e.g., given measured albumin and calcium concentrations of 2.0 gm/dl and 7.4 mg/dl, respectively, the corrected serum calcium concentration at an albumin concentration of 4.0 gm/dl is 9.0 mg/dl). Calcium is bound largely to the carboxyl groups in albumin, and this binding is highly pH-dependent. Acute acidosis decreases binding and increases ionized calcium, and acute alkalosis increases binding with a consequent decrease in ionized calcium. These changes are not reflected in the total serum calcium concentration and can only be appreciated by actual management of ionized serum calcium at the ambient pH. Calcium concentrations are typically recorded in mg/dl (mg%); these concentrations can be converted to molar units simply by dividing by 4 (e.g., 10 mg/dl converts to 2.5 mM).

It is the ionized fraction of calcium (Ca^{2+}) that is physiologically important and that is rigidly maintained by the combined effects of PTH and $1,25(OH)_2D$. Examples of the physiologic functions of extracellular Ca^{2+} include (i) serving as a cofactor in the coagulation cascade (e.g., for factors VII, IX, X, and prothrombin), (ii) maintenance of the normal mineral ion product required for skeletal mineralization, and (iii) contributing stability to plasma membranes by binding to phospholipids in the lipid bilayer and also regulating the permeability of plasma membranes to sodium ions. A reduction in ionized calcium increases sodium permeability and enhances the excitability of all excitable tissues; an increase in ionized calcium has the opposite effect. For example, the pH dependency of calcium binding to carboxyl groups noted above is the explanation for the reduction in ionized calcium that is responsible for the neuromuscular symptoms that characterize the hyperventilation syndrome.

Phosphorus. Serum inorganic phosphate also exists as three fractions: ionized, protein-bound, and complexed. Protein binding is relatively insignificant for phosphate, representing some 10% of the total, but about 35% is complexed to sodium, calcium, and magnesium. Thus, approximately 90% of the inorganic phosphate in serum is ultrafilterable. The major ionic species of phosphate in serum at pH 7.4 is the divalent anion (HPO_4^{2-}).

In contrast to the rigidly regulated concentration of calcium in serum, the serum phosphorus concentration varies quite widely throughout the day and is influenced by age, sex, diet, pH, and a variety of hormones. An adequate serum phosphate concentration is important in maintaining a sufficient ion product for normal mineralization.

Magnesium. About 55% of serum magnesium is ionized, with 30% being protein bound and 15% complexed. The protein-bound fraction interacts with the carboxyl groups of albumin and is influenced by pH in a fashion analogous to that of calcium. It is the ionized fraction of magnesium that is physiologically important (e.g., to plasma membrane excitability). The extracellular concentration of ionized magnesium is tightly controlled by the tubular maximum or threshold for magnesium in the nephron (4).

Only fasting measurements of serum calcium and phosphorus should be considered reliable.

CELLULAR MINERAL METABOLISM

A detailed summary of the numerous metabolic functions of calcium, magnesium, and phosphorus within cells is beyond the scope of this syllabus. This section attempts simply to highlight briefly some of the important roles of these ions in cellular physiology.

Calcium. The control of cellular calcium homeostasis is complex, and the regulation of the concentration of the calcium ion in the cytosol is as rigidly maintained as is its concentration in extracellular fluids (5). Cells are bathed in extracellular fluids containing approximately 10^{-3} M Ca^{2+}. The concentration of Ca^{2+} in the cytoplasm is approximately 10^{-6} M, or one-thousandth that in extracellular fluids. Cytosolic calcium is to some extent buffered by binding to other cytoplasmic constituents, and certain cells contain a specific calcium-binding protein that may serve as a buffer

and/or a calcium transport protein within the cytosol. The mitochondria and microsomes contain 90% to 99% of the intracellular calcium, bound largely to organic and inorganic phosphates. The calcium content of these organelles is sufficient to replenish cytosolic calcium some 500 times.

The low Ca^{2+} concentration in the cytosol is maintained by three pump-leak transport systems: an external system located in the plasma membrane and two internal systems located in the microsomal membrane and the inner mitochondrial membrane, respectively. Calcium diffuses into the cytosol across these three membranes. Each of the three pumps is oriented in a direction of calcium egress from the cytosol; each requires energy, and each shares a high affinity for calcium (K_m approximately 10^{-6} M).

The importance of these three calcium transport systems in regulating cellular calcium metabolism varies considerably from cell to cell depending on the function of a particular cell type. Several examples serve to illustrate how the details of cellular calcium homeostasis have been adapted to subserve the specific physiologic function of a given cell type.

Calcium ion is the coupling factor linking excitation and contraction in all forms of skeletal and cardiac muscle (5). In striated muscle, the microsomes are extensively developed as the sarcoplasmic reticulum, which serves as the principal storehouse of intracellular calcium in muscle and which is the most highly developed calcium transport system known. Depolarization of the plasma membrane is accompanied by the entry of a small amount of extracellular calcium into the cell, and this acts as a trigger to release large quantities of calcium stored in the sarcoplasmic reticulum. The abrupt increase in cytosolic calcium interacts with troponin, a specific calcium-binding protein, leading to a conformational change and the actin–myosin interaction that constitutes muscle contraction. The reticulum vesicles are capable of reaccumulating the large quantity of cytosolic calcium with the extreme speed required by the relaxation process.

In most mammalian cells other than muscle, the principal internal calcium pump-leak system is that of the inner mitochondrial membrane. In a number of cells, calcium serves as a second messenger, mediating the effects of membrane signals on the release of secretory products (e.g., neurotransmitters, exocrine secretions such as amylase, and endocrine secretions such as insulin and aldosterone) (5). The calcium messenger system involves a flow of information along several pathways: (i) the calmodulin pathway and (ii) the phosphoinositide C-kinase pathway. It is now recognized that in many cells the several branches of the calcium messenger system and the cyclic adenosine monophosphate (cAMP) messenger system are intimately related, and that these systems are integrated in such a way that the net cellular response to a given stimulus is determined by a complex interplay ("cross-talk") between these systems (5).

Phosphorus. The transport of phosphate ions across the plasma membrane and the membranes of intracellular organelles proceeds passively but is determined by the movement of cations, mostly calcium. The phosphate content in mitochondria is high, where it is largely in the form of calcium salts. The cytoplasmic concentration of free phosphate ions is estimated to be quite low, and the remaining portion of intracellular phosphate is either bound or in the form of organic phosphate esters. These phosphate esters play a variety of critically important roles in cellular metabolism: purine nucleotides provide the cell with stored energy; phosphorylated intermediates are concerned with energy conservation and transfer; phospholipids are major constituents of cell membranes, and the phosphorylation of proteins is an important means of regulating their function.

Magnesium. Magnesium is the most abundant intracellular divalent cation and the second most abundant intracellular cation after potassium. Approximately 60% of cellular magnesium is contained in the mitochondria, and it is estimated that only 5% to 10% of intracellular magnesium exists as free ions in the cytoplasm. The transport mechanisms responsible for maintaining the asymmetric distribution of magnesium in intracellular compartments are less well studied than the corresponding calcium transport systems, but it is clear that the cellular metabolisms of calcium and magnesium are regulated independently. Magnesium is an essential cofactor in the functioning of a wide variety of key enzymes, including essentially all enzymes concerned with the transfer of phosphate groups, all reactions that require ATP, and each of the steps concerned with the replication, transcription, and translation of genetic information.

MINERAL ION BALANCE AND MECHANISMS FOR MAINTAINING SYSTEMIC MINERAL HOMEOSTASIS

Mineral ion influx and efflux in the intestine, bone, and kidney, and the regulation of these processes by PTH and $1,25(OH)_2D$ are described in detail in other chapters in this primer. The information in the sections that follow attempts to integrate these processes at the level of the intact organism, and it describes the fine set of checks and balances that regulate mineral homeostasis *in vivo*.

The term *mineral ion balance* refers to the state of mineral homeostasis in the organism vis-à-vis the environment. In zero balance, mineral intake and accretion exactly match mineral losses. In positive balance, mineral intake and accretion exceed mineral losses. In negative balance, mineral losses exceed mineral intake and accretion. A growing child is in positive mineral balance, whereas an immobilized patient is in negative mineral balance. Formal balance studies are a relic of the past and are no longer performed, but the concept of balance is central to even a cursory understanding of systemic mineral ion homeostasis. Figure 1 is a schematic representation of calcium, phosphorus, and magnesium metabolism in a normal adult on an average diet who is in zero mineral ion balance.

Calcium. The total extracellular pool of calcium is approximately 900 mg. This pool is in dynamic equilibrium with calcium entering and exiting via the intestine, bone, and renal tubule. In zero balance, bone resorption and formation are equivalent at about 500 mg/day, and the net quantity of calcium absorbed by the intestine, approximately 175 mg per day, is quantitatively excreted into the urine. Thus, under normal circumstances, net calcium absorption provides a surplus of calcium that considerably exceeds systemic requirements.

Several points illustrated in this schema merit some emphasis. The first is the quantitative importance of the kidney in the regulation of calcium homeostasis. The filtered load of calcium is a whopping 10,000 mg/day, and 10% of this, or 1000 mg/day, is under the control of PTH-regulated reabsorption in the distal nephron. The second is the elegance of biologic control that must underlie a system in which calcium absorption and excretion are matched on essentially a milligram-per-milligram basis.

Phosphorus. The extracellular pool of orthophosphate is approximately 550 mg (Fig. 1). This pool is in dynamic equilibrium with phosphate entry and exit via the intestine, bone, kidney, and soft tissues (not depicted in the figure). In zero balance, fractional net phosphorus absorption is about two thirds of phosphorus intake; this amount represents a vast excess over systemic requirements and is quantitatively excreted into the urine.

Again, several points merit emphasis. The first is that the absorption of phosphate in the intestine is far less rigidly regulated than is the absorption of calcium. The second is the dominant role of the kidney; in this case, the threshold for phosphate reabsorption in the proximal tubule [tubular maximum for phosphate/glomerular filtration rate (TmP/GFR)] is essentially the setpoint that defines the fasting serum phosphorus concentration, and it is the setpoint that is regulated by PTH.

Magnesium. The extracellular pool of magnesium is approximately 250 mg and is in bidirectional equilibrium with magnesium fluxes across the intestine, kidney, bone, and soft tissues (Fig. 1). In zero balance, the magnesium derived from net intestinal absorption, approximately 100 mg per day, represents a systemic surplus and is quantitatively excreted. The kidney is responsible for regulating the serum magnesium concentration by a setpoint or Tm-limited process that is reminiscent of the setpoint for phosphorus, except that the TmMg is not hormonally regulated.

Two key points are made in the preceding paragraphs : (i) normally, hormonal and/or intrinsic mechanisms of mineral ion absorption in the intestine provide the organism with a mineral supply that exceeds systemic mineral needs by a considerable measure, and (ii) the renal tubule plays the dominant quantitative role in maintaining normal mineral homeostasis. Within this framework, minor fluctuations in systemic requirements are easily met by the surfeit of normal mineral absorption and do not require hormonal adjustments.

SYSTEMIC CALCIUM HOMEOSTASIS AND MAINTENANCE OF A NORMAL SERUM CALCIUM CONCENTRATION

The parathyroid chief cell is exquisitely sensitive to the ionized serum calcium concentration and is capable of responding to changes in this concentration so small that they are unmeasurable by human hands (1,6). The recently identified calcium receptor is the sensing device that is at the core of the chief cell's sensitivity to the ambient calcium concentration.

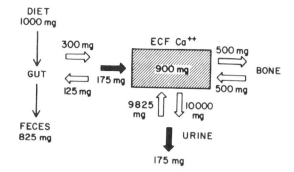

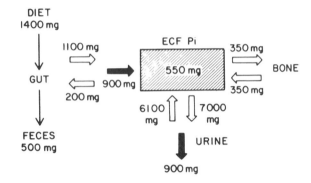

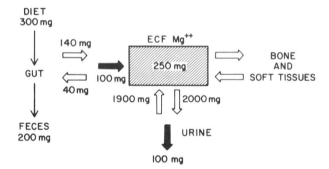

FIG. 1. Schematic representations of calcium, phosphorus, and magnesium fluxes in a normal adult in zero mineral ion balance. *Open arrows* denote unidirectional mineral fluxes, and *solid arrows* denote net fluxes; all values are given in mg/day. (From: Stewart AF, Broadus AE. Mineral metabolism. In: Felig P, Baxter JD, Broadus AE, Frohman LA (eds) *Endocrinology and Metabolism*, 2nd ed. McGraw-Hill, New York, 1317–1453, 1987.)

The integrated actions of PTH on distal tubular calcium reabsorption, bone resorption, and 1,25(OH)₂D-mediated intestinal calcium absorption are responsible for the fine regulation of the serum ionized calcium concentration. The precision of this integrated control is such that, in a normal individual, serum ionized calcium probably fluctuates by no more than 0.1 mg/dl in either direction from its normal set-point value throughout the day.

Distal tubular calcium reabsorption and osteoclastic bone resorption are the major control points in minute-to-minute serum calcium homeostasis; of these two processes, the effect of PTH on the distal tubule is quantitatively the more

important. Indeed, the 1000 mg/dl of calcium that is under PTH control as it passes through the distal nephron is clearly the centerpiece of the organism's ability to fine tune the serum calcium concentration on a minute-to-minute basis. The effects of PTH on the acute phase of bone resorption and calcium reclamation in the distal tubule together constitute a classic "short-loop" feedback system, in that the calcium so provided feeds back directly in the parathyroid chief cell.

The parathyroid–renal (PTH–1,25(OH)₂D) axis is reminiscent of the pituitary–adrenal (ACTH–cortisol) axis, and use of the axis concept and terminology is encouraged. Whereas 1,25(OH)₂D does influence PTH secretion directly as a short-loop feedback, the essence of the PTH–1,25(OH)₂D axis in practice is a long-loop feedback system in which 1,25(OH)₂D-mediated calcium absorption provides the ultimate feedback on the parathyroid chief cell. This long-loop system is the only means by which the organism can change its net capacity to obtain calcium from the environment, and it is therefore the centerpiece of the organism's response to either a prolonged or a major hypocalcemic challenge. Maximal adjustments to the rate of calcium absorption in the intestine via the PTH–1,25(OH)₂D axis require 24 to 48 hours to become fully operative, so that this system has little to do with minute-to-minute regulation.

A 12- to 15-hour fast in a normal individual represents a minor physiologic hypocalcemic challenge that requires only subtle hormonal readjustments for correction. The total quantity of calcium lost into the urine during this time is in the range of 50 to 75 mg. An unmeasurable fall in serum calcium occurs, leading to a slight increase in PTH secretion. The dip in serum calcium is corrected by an increased efficiency of calcium reclamation in the distal tubule and by the rapid resorptive response to PTH in bone; by 12 hours, only minor increases in 1,25(OH)₂D synthesis will have occurred.

An abrupt reduction in dietary calcium intake to less than 100 mg per day, or the administration of 80 mg of furosemide daily to a normal individual, represents a moderate hypocalcemic challenge; in each case, the initial deficit of calcium is in the range of 100 to 150 mg per day. A series of adjustments occurs, leading to a new steady state by 48 hours (Fig. 2). A moderate increase in the secretion rate of PTH results in: (i) increased calcium reabsorption from the distal tubule, (ii) increased mobilization of calcium and phosphorus from bone, and (iii) increased synthesis of 1,25(OH)₂D, which participates with PTH in bone resorption and increases the efficiency of calcium and phosphorus absorption in the intestine. The increased circulating concentration of PTH resets the renal tubular phosphate threshold (TmP/GFR) at a lower level so that the increased amount of phosphorus mobilized from bone and absorbed from the intestine is quantitatively excreted into the urine. In the new steady state, serum calcium has returned to normal, serum phosphorus is unchanged or slightly reduced, and a state of mild secondary hyperparathyroidism and efficient intestinal mineral absorption exists. At this point, the initial requirement for calcium mobilization from the skeleton is largely replaced by the enhanced absorption of calcium in the intestine.

The systemic mechanisms for the prevention of hypercalcemia consist largely of a reversal of the sequence just described, namely, an inhibition of PTH and 1,25(OH)$_2$D synthesis, with a reduction in calcium mobilization from bone, absorption from the intestine, and reclamation from the distal renal tubule. Whether the putative effects of calcitonin are of pathophysiologic importance in humans remains unclear. The bottleneck in the system's defense against hypercalcemia is the limited capacity of the kidneys to excrete calcium. In theory, normal kidneys can excrete a calcium load of 1000 mg or more per day. In practice, calcium excretion rates in this range are rarely seen. Limitations in the theoretical ability of the kidney to combat hypercalcemia include: (i) the fact that abnormalities in distal tubular reabsorption are actually involved in the genesis of hypercalcemia in a number of conditions (e.g., primary hyperparathyroidism), (ii) the fact that a degree of renal impairment frequently accompanies many hypercalcemic conditions, and (iii) the fact that an increased calcium concentration inhibits the ability of the renal tubule to conserve water, which may lead to a vicious cycle of dehydration, prerenal azotemia, and worsening hypercalcemia. One or more of these limitations can usually be demonstrated in any given patient with hypercalcemia.

A patient with advanced breast carcinoma metastatic to bone represents a severe hypercalcemic challenge. In such a patient, calcium is mobilized from bone by local osteolytic mechanisms, parathyroid function and 1,25(OH)$_2$D synthesis are appropriately suppressed, and the normal mechanisms of bone resorption, intestinal calcium absorption, and distal tubular calcium reabsorption are virtually eliminated. Initially, these adjustments may lead to a compensated steady state in which approximately 800 to 1000 mg per day of mobilized calcium is excreted, with a serum calcium that is high-normal or only slightly elevated. With advancing

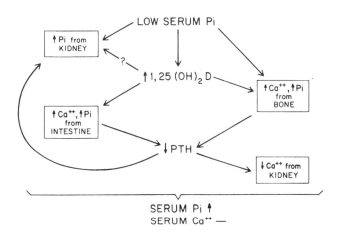

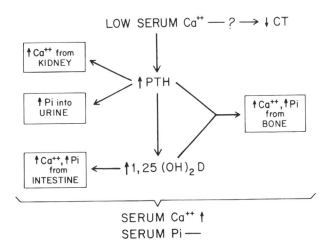

FIG. 2. The sequence of adjustments that are called into play in response to a moderate hypocalcemic challenge. (From: Stewart AF, Broadus AE. Mineral metabolism. In: Felig P, Baxter JD, Broadus AE, Frohman LA (eds) *Endocrinology and Metabolism*, 2nd ed. McGraw-Hill, New York, 1317–1453, 1987.)

FIG. 3. The sequence of adjustments initiated in response to hypophosphatemia. (From: Stewart AF, Broadus AE. Mineral metabolism. In: Felig P, Baxter JD, Broadus AE, Frohman LA (eds) *Endocrinology and Metabolism*, 2nd ed. McGraw-Hill, New York, 1317–1453, 1987.)

disease or, as often occurs, with immobilization resulting from the basic disease process or an intercurrent illness, the quantity of mobilized calcium overwhelms the renal capacity for calcium excretion, and the spiral of hypercalcemia, dehydration, azotemia, and worsening hypercalcemia begins. In this circumstance, the serum calcium may climb from 10.5 to 15 mg/dl within 48 hours.

SYSTEMIC PHOSPHORUS HOMEOSTASIS AND MAINTENANCE OF A NORMAL SERUM PHOSPHORUS CONCENTRATION

The kidney plays the dominant role in systemic phosphorus homeostasis and maintains the serum phosphorus concentration at a value very close to the tubular phosphorus threshold or TmP/GFR. Because of the normal efficiency and lack of fine regulation of phosphorus absorption in the intestine, only in unusual circumstances (e.g., prolonged use of phosphate-binding antacids) is the systemic supply of phosphorus a limiting factor in phosphorus homeostasis. Thus, most disorders associated with chronic hypophosphatemia and/or phosphorus depletion in humans result from either intrinsic (e.g., familial hypophosphatemic rickets) or extrinsic (e.g., primary hyperparathyroidism) alterations in TmP/GFR. Similarly, most conditions of chronic hyperphosphatemia result from either intrinsic (e.g., renal impairment) or extrinsic (e.g., hypoparathyroidism) abnormalities in the renal threshold for phosphorus. Acute hypophosphatemia most commonly results from the flux of extracellular phosphate ions into soft tissues.

The sequence of events initiated in the face of a hypophosphatemic challenge (Fig. 3) includes: (i) stimulation of 1,25(OH)$_2$D synthesis in the kidney, (ii) enhanced mobilization of phosphorus and calcium from bone, and (iii) a hypophosphatemia-induced increase in TmP/GFR (the exact mechanism of which is unknown). The increased circulating concentration of 1,25(OH)$_2$D leads to increases in phosphorus and calcium absorption in the intestine and provides an additional stimulus for phosphorus and calcium mobilization from bone. The increased flow of calcium from bone and the intestine results in an inhibition of PTH secretion, which diverts the systemic flow of calcium into the urine and further increases TmP/GFR. The net result of this sequence of adjustments is a return of the serum phosphorus concentration to normal without change in the serum calcium concentration.

The defense against hyperphosphatemia consists largely of a reversal of the sequence of adjustments just described. The principal humoral factor that combats hyperphosphatemia is PTH, but its action is indirect. The product of the concentrations of calcium and phosphorus in serum is referred to as the mineral ion $(Ca \times P)$ product. This product tends to be a biologic constant, in the sense that an increase in the concentration of one member leads to a reciprocal change in the concentration of the other. Thus, an acute rise in the serum phosphorus concentration produces a transient fall in the concentration of serum ionized calcium and a stimulation of PTH secretion, which reduces TmP/GFR and leads to a readjustment in serum phosphorus and calcium concentrations. A prolonged rise in the serum phosphorus concentration results in (i) an intrinsic downward adjustment in TmP/GFR that is independent of PTH and (ii) a persistent increase in PTH secretion that can ultimately lead to chief cell hyperplasia. If hyperphosphatemia is prolonged and severe (e.g., as occurs in chronic renal insufficiency), the degree of secondary hyperparathyroidism is sufficient to lead to the typical findings of parathyroid bone disease.

SYSTEMIC MAGNESIUM HOMEOSTASIS AND MAINTENANCE OF A NORMAL SERUM MAGNESIUM CONCENTRATION

The understanding of systemic magnesium homeostasis remains at a relatively primitive state. Unlike calcium and phosphorus, there appears to be no important systemic or hormonal regulation of the magnesium concentration in the extracellular fluids. Instead, maintenance of the serum magnesium concentration seems to result from the combined fluxes of magnesium at the levels of the intestine, kidney, intracellular fluids, and perhaps the skeleton. The kidney is primarily responsible for the regulation of the serum magnesium concentration.

The fractional absorption of magnesium is approximately 30%. In conditions of dietary magnesium excess, a smaller proportion may be absorbed, and in conditions of dietary magnesium deficiency, a higher proportion may be absorbed. The cellular mechanisms mediating magnesium absorption in the small intestine are poorly defined but would appear to consist of both passive and facilitated (but not active) elements. These elements do not seem to be sensitive to PTH, calcitonin, or 1,25(OH)$_2$D. Thus, the net quantity of magnesium absorbed appears to be primarily a function of magnesium intake.

Of the approximately 2000 mg of magnesium filtered per day, 96% is reabsorbed along the nephron and some 4% is excreted in the urine (fractional magnesium excretion). The mechanisms of magnesium reabsorption along the nephron at a cellular level are poorly understood, but, as is the case for calcium and phosphorus, it is possible to define a renal magnesium threshold or tubular maximum for magnesium (TmMg). The TmMg represents the net effects of magnesium reabsorption at different sites along the nephron. The TmMg is approximately 1.4 mg/dl when expressed as a function of the ultrafilterable serum magnesium concentration, or 2.0 mg/dl when expressed as a function of the total serum magnesium concentration (4). The tubular maximum functions essentially as a setpoint for reabsorption, such that magnesium filtered at a concentration above the TmMg is excreted and that filtered at a concentration beneath the TmMg is retained. As in the intestine, renal tubular magnesium handling does not appear to be regulated by systemic or hormonal mechanisms in any important way.

In summary, systemic magnesium homeostasis does not appear to be hormonally regulated and therefore reflects largely the quantitative interplay of net magnesium absorption in the intestine and the fractional excretion of magnesium by the kidney. The fractional excretion of magnesium functions as a Tm-limited process and is primarily responsible for maintaining the serum magnesium concentration within rather narrow limits. The fine regulation of the serum magnesium concentration in the absence of hormonal controls provides an excellent example of the biologic power of a Tm-limited transport process.

ACKNOWLEDGMENT

Supported in part by National Institutes of Health grant RR125.

REFERENCES

1. Bringhurst FR: Calcium and phosphate distribution, turnover and metabolic actions. In: DeGroot LJ (ed) *Endocrinology*, 3rd ed. Saunders, Philadelphia, 1015–1043, 1995
2. Krane SM: Calcium, phosphate and magnesium. In: Rasmussen H (ed) In: *International Encyclopedia of Pharmacology and Therapeutics*, vol 1. Pergamon Press, London, 19–59, 1970
3. Marshall RW: Plasma fractions. In: Nordin BEC (ed) In: *Calcium, Phosphate and Magnesium Metabolism*. Churchill Livingstone, London, 162–185, 1976
4. Rude RK, Singer FR: Magnesium deficiency and excess. *Ann Rev Med* 32:245–253, 1981
5. Rasmussen H, Rasmussen J: Calcium as intracellular messenger: From simplicity to complexity. *Curr Top Cell Regul* 31: 1–109, 1990
6. Stewart AF, Broadus AE: Mineral metabolism. In: Felig P, Baxter JD, Broadus AE, Frohman LA (eds) In: *Endocrinology and Metabolism*, 2nd ed. McGraw-Hill, New York: 1317–1453, 1987

SECTION III

Clinical Evaluation of Bone and Mineral Disorders

6. Biochemical Markers of Bone Turnover

David R. Eyre, Ph.D.

Department of Orthopedics, University of Washington, Seattle, Washington

Reliable and convenient tests for quantifying bone turnover would aid in the clinical management of osteoporosis and other metabolic bone diseases. In recent years, immunoassays for novel bone metabolites have been reported in the research literature, with data indicating improved specificity and responsiveness to bone cell activity over traditional markers (1,2). Biochemical assays for monitoring bone turnover all rely on the measurement, in serum or urine, of enzymes or matrix proteins synthesized by osteoblasts or osteoclasts that spill over into body fluids, or of osteoclast-generated degradation products of the bone matrix itself. Serum levels of skeletal alkaline phosphatase and osteocalcin are currently the most convincing formation markers. The most useful resorption markers are all products of collagen degradation that for now are best measured in urine. Table 1 lists the more commonly explored biochemical markers of bone formation and resorption.

BONE FORMATION MARKERS

Total alkaline phosphatase activity in serum is still the most used index of bone formation in clinical use (e.g., to monitor Paget's disease of bone). Immunoassays for serum osteocalcin and bone-specific alkaline phosphatase have become the preferred tools in clinical research investigations where greater specificity is required. Propeptides of type I collagen have also proven to respond as expected as serum markers of bone formation (3,4), but they presumably reflect the sum of all type I collagen synthetic activity throughout the body and so are not bone specific.

Alkaline Phosphatase

The common form of alkaline phosphatase is a cell-membrane-associated enzyme expressed by liver, bone, kidney, and placenta from a single gene. Liver and bone are the primary sources of the serum enzymes, and the molecules differ posttranslationally in their glycosylation pattern. Alkaline phosphatase is a prominent product of osteoblasts and osteoblast precursors, and it plays a key role, as yet poorly defined, in mineralization. The development of monoclonal antibodies that can select for the osteoblast enzyme, bone-specific alkaline phosphatase (BAP), by recognizing a posttranslational characteristic, has provided the basis for a more specific index of bone formation activity (5,6). An immunoassay for the protein is more attractive than approaches that separate and measure the activities of the bone-derived and liver enzymes in serum (7,8). The measure of bone formation provided by alkaline phosphatase is indirect, depending presumably on a spillover of excess or spent enzyme from active osteoblasts and probably also pre-osteoblasts, lining cells, and perhaps osteocytes. Therefore,

as with all bone-turnover assays, the quantitative relationship between serum levels of BAP and the actual rate of bone deposition may not be simple or constant within or between individuals.

Osteocalcin

Human osteocalcin (or bone Gla-protein, BGP) is a 49-residue polypeptide expressed under 1,25-dihydroxyvitamin D_3 control by osteoblasts as they actively deposit bone. Other calcified tissues, including dentin and calcified cartilage, also contain osteocalcin. Osteocalcin forms about 1% of the organic matrix of bone where it exists in close association with the surface of the mineral crystallites. Serum osteocalcin (9,10) seems to reflect primarily a spillover of osteoblast synthetic activity rather than degradation products of resorbed bone matrix. Osteocalcin in bone is probably degraded on resorption to fragments. These are probably not recognized by the latest immunoassays, which use specific monoclonal antibodies to measure only intact molecules and almost intact fragments that preserve the N-terminal sequence (e.g., in two-site assay formats) (11,12).

Although serum osteocalcin (the intact molecule) and bone-specific alkaline phosphatase immunoassays are emerging as the best indicators of bone formation activity, they do not always show parallel responses. For example, serum osteocalcin is not highly elevated and correlates poorly with either total serum alkaline phosphatase activity or levels of the bone-specific enzyme molecule in Paget's disease of bone (13). Osteocalcin levels are much lower than might be expected in this high-turnover condition. The relative lack of correlation between osteocalcin and serum alkaline phosphatase may reflect the expression of these proteins at different stages of osteoblast development and synthetic

TABLE 1. *Biochemical markers of bone remodeling*

Formation (osteoblast products)
  Propeptides of type I collagen (serum)
    C-propeptide
    N-propeptide
  Osteocalcin (serum)
  Alkaline phosphatase (serum)
    Total activity
    Bone-specific enzyme
Resorption (osteoclast products)
  Tartrate-resistant acid phosphatase (serum)
  Hydroxyproline (urine)
  Hydroxylysine glycosides (urine)
  Collagen cross-links (urine and serum)
    Total pyridinolines (Pyr and/or Dpy)
    Free pyridinolines (Pyr and/or Dpy)
    Cross-linked N- and C-telopeptides

activity (14,15). Also, since serum osteocalcin is thought to represent only a fraction of the synthetic pool, which escapes incorporation into newly formed bone matrix, the amount of this spillover fraction may change under different conditions of osteoblast physiology and pathology.

Type I Collagen Propeptides

The common types of collagen, types I, II, and III, are synthesized as procollagen molecules which have their N- and C-propeptides removed extracellularly. Propeptides of all three collagen types can be found in serum as by-products of collagen synthesis, and all have seen use as indicators in clinical studies. Immunoassays for both N- and C-propeptides of type I collagen have been developed as markers of bone formation (1–4,16). Because bone is such a major organ of turnover of collagen type I, serum levels of these propeptides may reasonably reflect total bone-forming activity in the body. Data from clinical studies on various disease states support this concept, but they indicate a relatively low specificity and lack of responsiveness in conditions where changes in bone turnover are subtle (17). Furthermore, studies that compared N- and C-propeptide assay results showed poor correlation (16).

BONE RESORPTION MARKERS

Consistently, the most promising markers of bone resorption are urinary levels of collagen degradation products (Table 1).

Hydroxyproline

Total urinary hydroxyproline (after acid hydrolysis) is the traditional index, but its usefulness is blunted by contribution from the diet, lack of specificity to bone collagen, degradative losses of the free amino acid in the liver, and relatively tedious chemical assays. More precise assays for hydroxyproline by high-performance liquid chromatography (HPLC) appear to offer greater specificity for bone metabolism than the traditional colorimetric assay (18).

Hydroxylysine Glycosides

All collagens contain glycosylated hydroxylysine residues. There are two forms, glucosylgalactosylhydroxylysine (GGHyl) and galactosylhydroxylysine (GHyl). These are also excreted in urine as the free hydroxylysine glycosides, which presumably are derived from collagen catabolism (19). The degree of glycosylation and ratio of GGHyl/GHyl varies with collagen type and tissue type. For instance, human bone collagen type and contains mostly GHyl whereas skin contains mostly GGHyl (19), suggesting that analysis of GHyl in urine may be a useful index of bone resorption. Moro et al. (20) developed an HPLC assay for GGHyl and GHyl in urine and showed appropriate changes when applied to clinical conditions of high turnover such as metastatic bone disease (21). Although bone is clearly a significant source of the pool of GGHyl

and GHyl in urine, other tissues also probably contribute. In addition, because the free amino acid glycosides, not peptides, are the primary forms in urine (19), the initial products of collagen degradation at the tissue level presumably become fully degraded in the liver and/or kidney.

Tartrate-Resistant Acid Phosphatase

Tartrate-resistant acid phosphatase (TRAP) is a prominent enzyme of osteoclasts that appears to be involved in bone matrix degradation. TRAP can dephosphorylate the protein osteopontin, for example (22). TRAP activity in serum is elevated in clinical conditions that cause increased bone turnover (23), but the degree of specificity to osteoclasts is not well defined, and it is known that other cell types produce TRAP activity (24). The development of immunoassays for the enzyme molecule (25,26) could prove more useful than enzyme activity measurements, but data are still few.

Pyridinoline Cross-links of Collagen

Urinary levels of pyridinoline have been the most studied bone resorption markers in the last decade (27,28). These complex amino acids appear not to be metabolized after tissue collagen is degraded and are excreted in urine, where they can be measured by HPLC using their natural fluorescence for detection (29). Usually, about two thirds are in the form of small peptides and the remaining are free amino acids. Two chemical forms exist: hydroxylysylpyridinoline (or simply pyridinoline, HP, or Pyr) and lysylpyridinoline (deoxypyridinoline, LP, or Dpy). These structures reflect posttranslational heterogeneity in the degree of hydroxylation of lysine residues at specific crosslinking sites in types I, II, III, and IX collagens (30).

The pyridinolines function as mature cross-links in collagen of most connective tissues other than skin. Because bone is such a major reservoir of type I collagen in the body and turns over faster than most major connective tissues, the pyridinolines in adult urine are primarily derived from bone resorption. This conclusion is supported by the observed similarity in the ratios of Pyr to Dpy in adult human bone (3.5:1) and urine (range, 2:1 to 7:1), compared with most nonbone connective tissues, in which Dpy is usually present at less than 10% of the content of Pyr (30,31). Urinary Dpy is therefore theoretically more specific than Pyr or total pyridinoline as a marker of bone degradation, and the clinical data from HPLC assay results support this (32).

However, it is important to recognize that even though the ratio of Pyr to Dpy is usually much higher in tissues other than bone, the concentration of Dpy can be as high as that in bone collagen, as it is, for example, in collagen of skeletal muscle and the vasculature (33,34). The ratio of Pyr to Dpy in vascular tissue and skeletal muscle collagen is also closer to that of bone at 6 to 8:1 (34). The absolute concentration of total pyridinolines in bone collagen is actually quite low (about 0.3 moles per mole of collagen) compared with other tissue collagens [1.5 moles/mole in cartilage; 0.5 to 1.0 moles/mole in vascular tissue, tendon, ligament, fascia, lung, intestine, liver, muscle, etc. (35)].

Therefore, because nothing is known about the turnover rates of collagen in these tissues relative to bone, it is still uncertain to what degree total pyridinolines or even Dpy can be relied on as specific markers of bone resorption. Half the total urinary pyridinolines could come from a nonbone source and still result in a ratio typically seen in urine (34).

Cross-linked N- and C-Telopeptide Assays

Figure 1 illustrates the two locations of pyridinoline cross-links in type I collagen, N-telopeptide-to-helix and C-telopeptide-to-helix. Pyridinoline-containing peptides (MW < 2 kDa) from both sites have been recovered from urine, that appear to resist further proteolysis (36). The pool of cross-linked N-telopeptides from urine had a Pyr:Dpy ratio of about 2:1, indicating an origin in bone. Similar domains prepared from human bone collagen showed that two thirds of the Dpy in collagen is located at the N-telopeptide site and one third at the C-telopeptide site (36). The α2(I) N-telopeptide was also prominently involved in crosslinking in bone collagen, which appears to be a distinguishing property over nonmineralized collagens (36). The cross-linked N-telopeptides in urine were targeted, therefore, as a particularly promising marker of bone resorption. A monoclonal antibody, mAb 1H11, was prepared which recognized small cross-linked N-telopeptides that contained the α2(I) N-telopeptide sequence QYDGKGVG, where K̇ is involved in trivalent cross-linking (36). The antibody did not recognize synthetic, individual telopeptides alone, nor the pyridinoline cross-link structure itself. The latter property may be important because of potential photolytic and other destructive losses of the 3-hydroxypyridinium ring structure of pyridinolines in urine. Moreover, the peptide antigen (NTx) becomes recognizable by the antibody only when bone collagen is degraded to small peptides, for example by bacterial collagenase or by osteoclasts. Osteoclasts were shown to gener-

ate immunoreactive NTx, but not free pyridinolines, when cultured on human bone particles in vitro (37). The antigen, therefore, appears to embody conformational features and to be a proteolytic neoepitope. A microtiter-plate enzyme-linked immunosorbent assay (ELISA) was developed that can be applied directly to urine (36,38).

Assays for collagen type I cross-linked C-telopeptides (ICTP) have also been described. The ICTP assay uses a polyclonal antibody raised against a cross-linked C-telopeptide prepared from human bone collagen (39). It recognizes antigen in serum but not in urine. Clinical evidence in support of this assay as a specific indicator of bone-resorbing activity has been disappointing (40), and the entities being recognized in serum appear not to have been characterized. Another C-telopeptide assay for urine uses a polyclonal antiserum raised against a cross-linked synthetic octapeptide (EKAHDGGR) that matches the C-telopeptide domain of the α1(I) chain of type I collagen containing the cross-linking lysine residue (41,42). This sequence was selected with the anticipation that it would be protected from degradation when embodied in pyridinoline cross-linked structures (36,41).

Free Pyridinolines

Most reports on pyridinoline levels in urine have measured the total pools of Pyr and Dpy by HPLC after acid hydrolysis to convert peptides to free amino acids (33). The free fraction of Pyr and Dpy has also been targeted. This can be done by HPLC, but an immunoassay would be more convenient and would allow direct analysis without any pretreatment steps. A polyclonal antibody-based ELISA that recognizes free Pyr was originally described (43) and further developed into both polyclonal- and monoclonal-antibody based versions (44). More recently, a monoclonal antibody-based ELISA that is specific for free Dpy has also become commercially available (51).

Clinical Results

To date, most reports on the newer bone biomarkers have presented cross-sectional data showing statistically significant increases or decreases between different subject groups (e.g., postmenopausal, premenopausal, and Paget's disease). Performance data from longitudinal studies on individual subjects are few.

Bone formation markers (intact osteocalcin and alkaline phosphatase) generally give tighter overall coefficients of variance than urinary assays. This no doubt reflects in part the added error in having to normalize urinary values to a second analyte, creatinine. Serum formation markers, on the other hand, respond more slowly to changes in bone turnover rate that occur naturally [e.g., at menopause (46)], after surgical oophorectomy (47), or on intervention with the antiresorptive agents, estrogen (48) and bisphosphonate (40). In most clinical situations, resorption and formation are coupled, but the change in formation markers lags several months behind that of resorption markers, whether turnover activity goes up or down.

Studies comparing the newer formation and resorption markers have been reported (38,40,45,49). Based on the

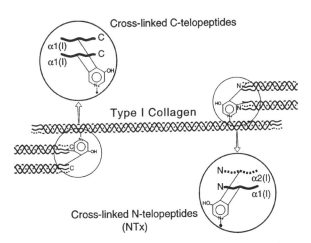

FIG. 1. Pyridinoline cross-links are located at two intermolecular sites in type I collagen fibrils, N-telopeptide-to-helix and C-telopeptide-to-helix. Both α1(I) and α2(I) N-telopeptides participate, but only α1(I) C-telopeptides. The α2(I) N-telopeptide is a favored participant in bone collagen cross-linking.

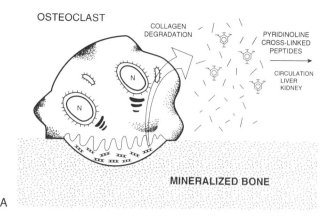

OSTEOCLAST

COLLAGEN DEGRADATION

PYRIDINOLINE CROSS-LINKED PEPTIDES

CIRCULATION LIVER KIDNEY

MINERALIZED BONE

A

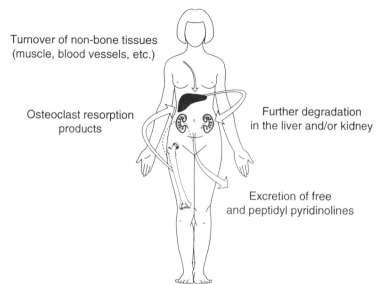

Turnover of non-bone tissues (muscle, blood vessels, etc.)

Osteoclast resorption products

Further degradation in the liver and/or kidney

Excretion of free and peptidyl pyridinolines

B

FIG. 2. Osteoclasts degrade bone collagen to peptides, including pyridinoline-containing structures **(A)**, but not to free pyridinolines, which are presumably generated from circulating peptides in the liver or kidney **(B)**.

percentage increase in postmenopausal women over premenopausal women as a measure of increased turnover, BAP was the most responsive formation marker (40). Osteocalcin was a close second, but type I collagen C-propeptide was not significantly different (40). In response to the bisphosphonate, alendronate, the formation markers, BAP, osteocalcin, and type I C-propeptide all dropped 40% to 50%, but gradually, over 6 to 12 months (40). The most responsive resorption marker was the cross-linked N-telopeptide, NTx, in urine (40). This analyte showed the greatest increase at menopause (46) and the most rapid and greatest percentage drop from baseline in bisphosphonate intervention trials (38,40,49). Total Pyr and particularly total Dpy measured by HPLC after acid hydrolysis were also responsive, but quantitatively less so than NTx (38,40). In a separate study, the cross-linked C-telopeptide (CTx) in urine was also significantly elevated postmenopausally and suppressed by both estrogen and bisphosphonate therapy (45,50). Free pyridinolines (Pyr or Dpy) measured in urine by immunoassay turn out to be unresponsive to bisphosphonate intervention compared with the cross-linked N- or C-telopeptides, total Pyr, or total Dpy by HPLC (40,45,49). The exact reason is unclear, but it is notable that osteoclasts *in vitro* do not generate free pyridinolines but do produce the immunoreactive telopeptide analyte, NTx (37). Therefore, there may be other tissue sources of the free pyridinolines and a requirement for peptide breakdown in the liver or kidney (Fig. 2). Interestingly, free pyridinoline levels in urine, as well as total pyridinolines and telopeptide markers (45), were suppressed on long-term estrogen therapy, which might be explained by the systemic effects of estrogen on other tissues in contrast with bisphosphonates which specifically target osteoclasts. Further studies are clearly needed to understand better the tissue origins and metabolic handling in the liver and kidney of these various peptide and free amino acid degradation products of collagen. Conceptually, the ideal resorption marker would be a unique product of the action of osteoclasts on bone that escapes further metabolism in the liver and is rapidly cleared by the kidney.

REFERENCES

1. Delmas PD: Clinical use of biochemical markers of bone remodeling in osteoporosis. *Bone* 13:517–521, 1992
2. Eriksen EF, Brixen K, Charles P: New markers of bone metabolism: Clinical use in metabolic bone disease. *Eur J Endocrinol* 132:251–263, 1995
3. Parfitt AM, Simon LS, Villanueva AR, Krane SM: Procollagen type I carboxy-terminal extension peptide in serum as a marker of collagen biosynthesis in bone: Correlation with iliac bone formation rates and comparison with total alkaline phosphatase. *J Bone Miner Res* 2:427–436, 1987
4. Kraenzlin ME, Mohan S, Singer F, et al.: Development of a radioimmunoassay for the N-terminal type I procollagen: Potential use to assess bone formation. *Eur J Clin Invest* 19:A86, 1989
5. Hill CS, Wolfert RL: The preparation of monoclonal antibodies which react preferentially with human bone alkaline phosphatase and not liver alkaline phosphatase. *Clin Chim Acta* 186:315–320, 1990
6. Panigrahi K, Delmas PD, Singer F, Ryan W, Reiss O, Fisher R, Miller PD, Mizrahi I, Darte C, Kress BC, et al.: Characteristics of a two-site immunoradiometric assay for human skeletal alkaline phosphatase in serum. *Clin Chem* 40:822–828, 1994
7. Behr W, Barnert J: Quantification of bone alkaline phosphatase in serum by precipitation with wheat-germ lectin: A simplified method and its clinical plausibility. *Clin Chem* 32:1960–1966, 1986
8. Bouman AA, Scheffer PG, Ooms ME, Lips P, Netelenbos C: Two bone alkaline phosphatase assays compared with osteocalcin as a marker of bone formation in healthy elderly women. *Clin Chem* 41:196–199, 1995
9. Price PA, Nishimoto SK: Radioimmunoassay for the vitamin K-dependent protein of bone and its discovery in plasma. *Proc Natl Acad Sci USA* 77:2234–2238, 1980
10. Gundberg CM, Lian JB, Gallop PM, Steinberg JJ: Urinary γ-carboxyglutamic acid and serum osteocalcin as bone markers: Studies in osteoporosis and Paget's disease. *J Clin Endocrinol Metab* 57:1221–1225, 1983
11. Garnero P, Grimaux M, Demiaux B, Preaudat C, Seguin P, Delmas PD: Measurement of serum osteocalcin with a human specific two-site immunoradiometric method. *J Bone Miner Res* 7:1389–1398, 1992
12. Deftos LJ, Wolfert RL, Hill CS, Burton DW: Two-site assays of bone GLA protein (osteocalcin) demonstrate immunochemical heterogeneity of the intact molecule. *Clin Chem* 38:2318–2321, 1992
13. Delmas PD, Demiaux B, Malaval L, Chapuy M.C, Meunier PJ: Serum bone GLA-protein is not a sensitive marker of bone turnover in Paget's disease of bone. *Calcif Tissue Int* 38:60–61, 1986

14. Deftos LJ, Wolfert RL, Hill CS: Bone alkaline phosphatase in Paget's disease. *Horm Metab Res* 23:559–561, 1991
15. Diaz-Diego EM, Diaz-Martin MA, de la Piedra C, Rapado A: Lack of correlation between levels of osteocalcin and bone alkaline phosphatase in healthy control and post-menopausal osteoporotic women. *Horm Metab Res* 27:151–154, 1995
16. Ebeling PR, Peterson JM, Riggs BL: Utility of type I procollagen propeptide assays for assessing abnormalities in metabolic bone diseases. *J Bone Miner Res* 7:1243–1250, 1992
17. Hassager C, Fabbri-Mabelli G, Christiansen C: The effect of the menopause and hormone replacement therapy on serum carboxyterminal propeptide of type I collagen. *Osteoporosis Int* 3:50–52, 1993
18. Pavori R, DeVecchi E, Fermo I, Arcelloni C, Diomede L, Magri F, Borini PA: Total urinary hydroxyproline determined with rapid and simple high-performance liquid chromatography. *Clin Chem* 38:407–411, 1992
19. Segrest JP, Cunningham LW: Variation in human urinary O-hydroxylysyl glycoside levels and their relationship to collagen metabolism. *J Clin Invest* 49:1497–1509, 1970
20. Moro L, Modricky C, Stagni N, Vittur F, de Bernard B: High-performance liquid chromatographic analysis of urinary hydroxylysyl glycosides as indicators of collagen turnover. *Analyst* 109:1621–1622, 1984
21. Moro L, Gazzarini C, Crivellari D, Galligioni E, Talamini R, de Bernard B: Biochemical markers for detecting bone metastases in patients with breast cancer. *Clin Chem* 39:131–134, 1993
22. Ek-Rylander B, Flores M, Wendel M, Heinegård D, Andersson G: Dephosphorylation of osteopontin and bone sialoprotein by osteoclastic tartrate-resistant acid phosphatase. *J Biol Chem* 269:14853–14856, 1994
23. Lau KHW, Orishi T, Wergedal JE, Singer FR, Baylink DJ: Characterization and assay of tartrate-resistant acid phosphatase activity in serum: Potential use to assess bone resorption. *Clin Chem* 33:458–462, 1987
24. Hattersley G, Chambers TJ: Generation of osteoclastic function in mouse bone marrow cultures: Multinuclearity and tartrate-resistant acid phosphatase are unreliable markers for osteoclastic differentiation. *Endocrinology* 124:1689–1696, 1989
25. Kraenzlin ME, Lau K-HW, Liang L, Freeman TK, Singer FR, Stepan J, Baylink DJ: Development of an immunoassay for human serum osteoclastic tartrate-resistant acid phosphatase. *J Clin Endocrinol Metab* 71:442–451, 1990
26. Cheung CK, Panesar NS, Haines C, Masarei J, Swaminathan R: Immunoassay of tartrate-resistant acid phosphatase in serum. *Clin Chem* 41:679–686, 1995
27. Robins SP, Stewart P, Astbury C, Bird HA: Measurement of the cross-linking compound, pyridinoline, in urine as an index of collagen degradation. *Ann Rheum Dis* 45:969–973, 1986
28. Demers LM, Kleerekoper M: Recent advances in biochemical markers of bone turnover (editorial). *Clin Chem* 40:1994–1995, 1994
29. Black D, Duncan A, Robins SP: Quantitative analysis of the pyridinium cross-links of collagen in urine using ion-paired reverse-phase high-performance liquid chromatography. *Anal Biochem* 169:197–203, 1988
30. Eyre DR: Collagen cross-linking amino acids. *Methods Enzymol* 144:115–139, 1987
31. Beardsworth LJ, Eyre DR, Dickson IR: Changes with age in the urinary excretion of lysyl- and hydroxylysyl-pyridinoline: Two new markers of bone collagen turnover. *J Bone Miner Res* 5:671–676, 1990
32. Uebelhart D, Schlemmer A, Johansen JS, Gineyts E, Christiansen C, Delmas PD: Effect of menopause and hormone replacement therapy on the urinary excretion of pyridinium cross-links. *Clin Endocrinol Metab* 72:367–373, 1991

33. Seibel MJ, Robins SP, Bilezikian JP: Urinary pyridinium cross-links of collagen: Specific markers of bone resorption in metabolic bone disease. *Trends Endocrinol Metab* 3:263–270, 1992
34. Eyre DR: The specificity of collagen cross-links as markers of bone and connective tissue degradation. *Acta Orthop Scand Suppl* 266:166–170, 1995
35. Eyre DR, Van Ness K, Koob TJ: Quantitation of hydroxypyridinium crosslinks in collagen by high performance liquid chromatography. *Analyt Biochem* 137:380–388, 1984
36. Hanson DA, Weis M-A E, Bollen A-M, Maslan SL, Singer FR, Eyre DR: A specific immunoassay for monitoring human bone resorption: Quantitation of type I collagen cross-linked N-telopeptides in urine. *J Bone Miner Res* 7:1251–1258, 1992
37. Apone S, Fevold K, Lee M, Eyre D: A rapid method for quantifying osteoclast activity *in vitro. J Bone Miner Res* 9(suppl 1): S178, 1994
38. Gertz BJ, Shao P, Hanson DA, Quan H, Harris ST, Genant HK, Chesnut CH III, Eyre DR: Monitoring bone resorption in early post-menopausal women by an immunoassay for cross-linked collagen peptides in urine. *J Bone Miner Res* 9:135–142, 1994
39. Risteli J, Elomaa I, Niemi S, Novamo A, Risteli L: Radioimmunoassay for the pyridinoline cross-linked carboxy-terminal telopeptide of type I collagen: A new marker of bone degradation. *Clin Chem* 39:635–640, 1993
40. Garnero P, Shih WJ, Gineyts E, Karpf DB, Delmas PD: Comparison of new biochemical markers of bone turnover in late post-menopausal osteoporotic women in response to alendronate treatment. *J Clin Endocrinol Metab* 79:1693–1700, 1994
41. Bonde M, Qvist P, Fledelius C, Riis BJ, Christiansen C: Immunoassay for quantifying type I collagen degradation products in urine evaluated. *Clin Chem* 40:2022–2025, 1994
42. Bonde M, Qvist P, Fledelius C, Riis BJ, Christiansen C: Applications of an enzyme immunoassay for a new marker of bone resorption (CrossLaps): Follow-up on hormone replacement therapy and osteoporosis risk assessment. *J Clin Endocrinol Metab* 80:864–868, 1995
43. Robins SP: An enzyme-linked immunoassay for the collagen cross-link pyridinoline. *Biochem J* 207:617–620, 1982
44. Seyedin SM, Kung VT, Daniloff YN, Hesley RP, Gomez B, Nielsen LA, Rosen HN, Zuk RF: Immunoassay for urinary pyridinoline: The new marker of bone resorption. *J Bone Miner Res* 8:635–641, 1993
45. Garnero P, Gineyts E, Arbault P, Christiansen C, Delmas PD: Different effects of bisphosphonate and estrogen therapy on free and peptide-bound bone cross-links excretion. *J Bone Miner Res* 10:641–649, 1995
46. Ebeling PR, Atley LM, Guthrie JR, et al: Bone turnover markers and bone density across the menopausal transition. *J Clin Endocrinol Metab* (in press) 1996
47. Prior JC, Eyre DR, Ebeling PR, Wark JD: Trabecular bone loss after premenopausal oophorectomy is not prevented by conjugated estrogen or medroxyprogesterone—a double-blind, randomized 1-year study. *J Bone Miner Res* 9(suppl 1): S394, 1994
48. Prestwood KM, Pilbeam CC, Burleson JA, Woodiel FN, Delmas PD, Deftos LJ, Raisz LG: The short-term effects of conjugated estrogen on bone turnover in older women. *J Clin Endocrinol Metab* 79(2):366–371, 1994
49. Rosen HN, Dresner-Pollak R, Moses AC, Rosenblatt M, Zeind AJ, Clemens JD, Greenspan SL: Specificity of urinary excretion of cross-linked N-telopeptides of type I collagen as a marker of bone turnover. *Calcif Tissue Int* 54:26–29, 1994
50. Garnero P, Gineyts E, Riou JP, Delmas PD: *J Clin Endocrinol Metab* 79:780–785, 1994
51. Robins SP, Woitge H, Hesley R, et al: Direct enzyme-linked immunoassay for urinary deoxypyridinoline as a specific marker for measuring bone resorption. *J Bone Miner Res* 9:1643–1649, 1994

7. Bone Density Measurement and the Management of Osteoporosis

C. Conrad Johnston, Jr., M.D., Charles W. Slemenda, Dr.P.H., and *L. Joseph Melton III, M.D.

*Department of Medicine, Indiana University School of Medicine, Indianapolis, Indiana; and *Department of Health Sciences Research, Mayo Clinic and Foundation, Rochester, Minnesota*

All agree that osteoporosis is a major public health problem (see Chapter 14). Any amelioration of the impact of osteoporosis depends on a reduction of its attendant fractures. Many interventions depend, in turn, on bone density measurement, and appropriate clinical application of technologies for this purpose should be based on the following criteria: (i) bone density can be measured accurately and safely; (ii) fractures result at least in part from low bone mass; (iii) bone density measurements can estimate the risk of future fractures; (iv) such information cannot be obtained from other clinical evaluations; (v) clinical decisions can be based on information obtained from bone density measurements; and (vi) such decisions lead either to an intervention that would result in a reduction in future fractures or to avoidance of future diagnostic efforts and therapeutic interventions, which would reduce health care costs. These principles are reviewed in the following sections, concluding with a summary of clinical indications for bone density measurements devised by the Scientific Advisory Committee of the National Osteoporosis Foundation (1).

MEASUREMENT OF BONE DENSITY

Bone mass can be measured with good accuracy and excellent precision using a number of currently available techniques (Table 1), which are described in detail elsewhere (2–7). Single-photon absorptiometry (SPA) and, more recently, single-energy x-ray absorptiometry (SXA) have been used to measure the radius and os calcis, and dual-photon absorptiometry (DPA) or dual-energy x-ray absorptiometry (DXA) can measure bone mineral density (BMD) in the spine and proximal femur, as well as other regions. Quantitative computed tomography (QCT) can give information similar to DXA (an integral measurement of the vertebral body) or can assess cancellous bone of the spine alone, which might be preferable depending upon the relative contributions of cancellous and cortical bone to strength of the vertebral body. All of these methods are far superior to standard roentgenograms, which have an accuracy error rate of 30% to 50% for assessing bone mass. Moreover, the accuracy of bone density measurements compares favorably with that of many other accepted clinical tests, including screening tests such as serum cholesterol.

To this list of technologies can be added measurement of the phalanges by radiographic densitometry, a method for measuring bone mass at a peripheral site, usually the hand. An x-ray of the hand is made with an aluminum step wedge placed on the film as a standard, against which density can be determined. This method has been demonstrated to be accurate and precise, similar to SPA and SXA (8). Measurement in the phalanges correlates with other sites as well as other methods correlate between sites (9). More important, data from National Health and Nutritional Examination Survey I suggest that its prediction of hip fracture is as good as that of other peripheral measurements, with the relative risk approximating 2 (10,11). In addition, a prospective study in which bone mass measurements were made at the end of the study indicated good prediction of vertebral deformities (12). Thus, radiographic absorptiometry should be an adequate method for rank-ordering individuals based on their risk of subsequent osteoporotic fractures, but its use for prospective follow-up to determine changes or effects of therapy has not been demonstrated (13).

Ultrasound measurements (14) also correlate with bone density measurements (15), but may provide additional information regarding bone quality (16).

Methods for measuring bone mass are very safe, with low radiation exposure. Single-photon absorptiometry produces a dose of < 15 mRem, DPA and DXA < 5 mRem, and modern QCT from 100 to 1000 mRem. These can be compared with the dose received from a chest x-ray of 20–50 mRem, full dental x-ray of 300 mRem, or abdominal computed tomography of 1–6 Rem (17,18).

RELATIONSHIP OF BONE DENSITY TO FRACTURES

There is considerable evidence that fractures result from low bone mass. Bone mineral density accounts for 75% to 85% of the variance in the ultimate strength of bone tissue (19), and such measurements also provide an accurate indication of the strength of whole bones (20–24). Because bone strength is an important determinant of fracture susceptibility, along with the likelihood of sustaining sufficient trauma, it follows that BMD is also correlated with fracture risk in patients (25). Indeed, there is a gradient of increasing fracture risk as bone mass falls that is independent of age (26), as illustrated in Fig. 1. On the left side of the figure, fracture risk is plotted against bone density for subjects of different ages, and it is clear that the risk increases with lower bone mass within each age group. However, age is also an independent predictor of subsequent fracture risk, and the contribution of age increases as subjects grow older, as can be seen on the right side of the figure. Even after adjustment for the influence of age, though, most fractures among elderly women are due at least in part to low bone density (27).

There are, of course, other risk factors for these fractures. Bone density is a good *in vivo* measure of bone strength, but is not the only determinant of skeletal fragility. Age-related changes in bone composition or an accumulation of stress

TABLE 1. *Comparison of bone densitometry techniques*

Technique	Site	Relative sensitivity	Precision (%)	Accuracy (%)	Duration of examination (min)	Absorbed dose (mRem)	Cost ($)
Standard techniques							
SPA	Proximal radius	1X	2–3	5	15	10	75
DPA	Spine, hip	2X	2–4	4–10	20–40	5	100–150
QCT	Spine	3–4X	2–5	5–20	10–20	100–1000	100–200
Newer developments							
SPA-R	Distal radius, calcaneus	2X	1–2	5	10–20	5–10	50[a]
DXA	Spine, hip	2X	1–2	3–5	5	1–3	75[a]
QCT-A	Spine, hip	3–4X	1–2	5–10	10	100–300	100[a]

[a]Projected cost.
DPA, dual-photon absorptiometry; DXA, DPA with a dual-energy x-ray source; SPA, single-photon absorptiometry; SPA-R, retilinear SPA; QCT, quantative computed tomography; QCT-A, QCT with advanced software and hardware capabilities. (From: Genant HK, Block JE, Steiger P, Glueer CC, Ettinger B, Harris ST: *Radiology* 170:817–822, 1989.)

microfractures could impair bone quality (19), and bone loss is associated with changes in the architectural arrangement of bone tissue that lead to reduced bone strength (28,29). However, these factors cannot be measured directly by non-invasive means, and it remains to be shown that their contribution is greater than can be accounted for by bone loss alone (30). More recently, it was demonstrated that each standard deviation (SD) increase in femoral neck length was associated with a 1.8-fold increase in hip fracture risk, independent of bone mass (31). Even more important is the influence of trauma, especially in falls among the elderly. Falling is particularly important in the etiology of hip and distal forearm fractures (32), but plays a role in vertebral fractures as well (33). The risk of falling increases with age (34), but not sufficiently to account for the exponential rise in hip fracture incidence, and most falls do not result in fracture (35). Although there is an age-related increase in the risk of falling directly on the hip, which is much more likely to result in hip fracture than other types of falls (36), bone density of the proximal femur is still an important determinant of the likelihood of fracture when a fall occurs (37). This situation is analogous to the etiology of coronary heart disease. As with heart disease, the causes of hip fractures are multifactorial. Measurement of any single risk factor (bone density, cholesterol) cannot completely explain the occurrence of the disease. Nonetheless, measurement of the factor identifies those who have the greatest risk of developing the disease and, thus, would benefit most from therapy.

BONE DENSITY MEASUREMENT PREDICTS FUTURE FRACTURES

There is ample evidence that bone mass measurements can stratify patients on the basis of fracture risk (25). Prospective studies show that bone density measurements in the radius, os calcis, spine, and femur can all predict the probability of fractures (38–49). More recently, ultrasound measurements were also shown to predict the incidence of vertebral fractures in a small prospective study (50). Bone density measurements at the lumbar spine or hip (two sites) with DPA and at the radius (two sites) with SPA performed comparably in predicting the risk of any moderate-trauma fracture for up to 10 years, with age-adjusted relative risks ranging from 1.4 to 1.6 per 1 SD decrease in bone mass (45). The long-term results from this small study are consistent with short-term results from much

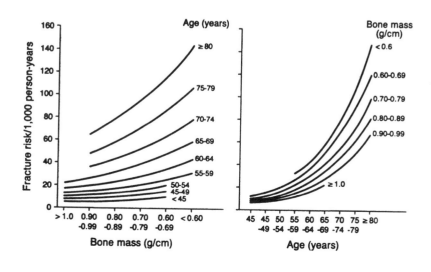

FIG. 1. Estimated incidence of fracture as a function of bone mass and age. (From: Hui SL, Slemenda CW, Johnston CC Jr: *J Clin Invest* 81:1804–1809, 1988.)

larger studies (42) and indicate that bone density measurements at any skeletal site are equally able to predict the risk of fractures in general (47). However, measurement at that particular site may be best for ascertaining the risk of a specific type of fracture, as considerable variation may be seen in bone mass assessed at one site compared with another in individual patients. Cummings et al. (44) demonstrated that bone density measured at the proximal femur was significantly better at predicting hip fractures than were measurements at other sites, as illustrated in Fig. 2.

Some confusion has resulted from the fact that bone density measurements do not clearly discriminate patients with fractures from those who have not yet experienced an osteoporotic fracture, i.e., there is overlap in the values for patients with spine, hip, and forearm fractures relative to controls (1). Because of this overlap in values, it has been argued that measuring bone mass is not helpful clinically. However, bone density measurements are not intended to be a diagnostic test for fractures—radiographs are needed instead. Rather, they measure a risk factor (reduced bone mass) for future fractures, and are properly used for risk stratification. This is again analogous to the measurement of other risk factors, such as cholesterol for coronary heart disease or blood pressure for stroke. Indeed, the relationship between bone density and the risk of fracture is as strong or stronger than the relationship between serum cholesterol and the risk of coronary heart disease (51).

FRACTURE RISK ASSESSMENT USING CLINICAL RISK FACTORS

It is commonly believed that osteoporosis-prone individuals can be identified through clinical observations, but this has never been demonstrated experimentally (52). For example, later age at menopause, estrogen or thiazide use, non-insulin-dependent diabetes, and greater height, weight, and strength were all positively associated with appendicular bone density among 9704 elderly women in the Study of Osteoporotic Fractures, whereas greater age, cigarette smoking, caffeine intake, prior gastric surgery, and a maternal history of fracture were negatively associated (53). However, models incorporating all of these independent predictors together explained only 20% to 35% of the variance in bone density at the radius or calcaneus. This low predictive power of known risk factors has been seen in other studies as well. Moreover, no one set of risk factors has been found consistently in all studies. In one evaluation of perimenopausal and early postmenopausal women (i.e., a population for whom estrogen therapy would be considered), age, height, weight, calcium and caffeine intake, alcohol and tobacco use, and a urinary marker of bone turnover were used to construct a model to predict bone density in the radius, lumbar spine, and hip (54). None of the models correctly identified more than 70% of the women with low bone mass at any site. This is not clinically acceptable, because most women with low bone mass can be correctly categorized by bone density measurements. Together, these studies demonstrate that various risk factors, although statistically significant, account for much less than half of the variability in bone mass and, therefore, do not provide adequate precision to classify individual patients (52).

An alternative approach might be to predict fractures directly and without reference to bone mass. A risk-factor score was able to discriminate those postmenopausal Dutch women who had fractures over 9 years of follow-up, but sensitivity and specificity were low (55). The lack of specificity was further revealed by the inability of various risk factors to predict vertebral fractures among a group of Japanese-American women (56). All of the women had at least two risk factors, and 91% had four or more of them. Likewise, the positive predictive value of an elevated risk-factor score was only 9% to 17% for identifying vertebral fractures among women in the United Kingdom, and most of this modest predictive power was contributed by a history of vertebral fracture per se (57). The most recent study found 16 independent risk factors for hip fracture, besides bone density, in a large population of elderly white women (58). Compared with 47% of the women who had two risk factors or fewer, the small group of women with five risk factors or more had a hip fracture incidence rate that was 17 times higher. Even in this group, however, os calcis bone density in the lowest third increased hip fracture risk by more than 40%. Thus, it appears that the assessment of some risk factors could be useful in conjunction with bone density measurements. It has been shown, for example, that the presence of fractures raises the risk of subsequent fracture

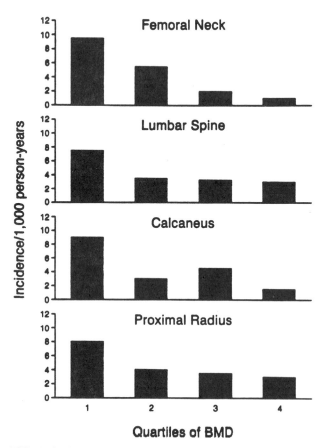

FIG. 2. Incidence of hip fracture by age-adjusted quartile of bone mineral density (BMD) measured at different skeletal sites. (From: Cummings SR, Black DM, Nevitt MC, Browner W, Cauley J, Ensrud K, Genant HK, Palermo L, Scott J, Vogt TM, for the Study of Osteoporotic Fractures Research Group: *Lancet* 341:72–75, 1993.)

above that attributable to bone mass alone (41), and combining several risk factors may have clinical utility. The individual who has slightly low bone mass, and is not at sufficient risk on that basis alone to justify an intervention, might be considered at higher risk if femoral neck length or a history of fracture were included in the assessment. However, no practical approach has yet been devised.

INDICATIONS FOR BONE DENSITY MEASUREMENTS

A task force of the National Osteoporosis Foundation has suggested the following clinical indications for bone mass measurements (1).

Estrogen-Deficient Women (Indication 1)

In estrogen-deficient women, bone density measurements can be used to diagnose significantly low bone mass to make decisions about hormone replacement or other therapy.

Rationale

Estrogen deficiency following menopause, oophorectomy, or prolonged amenorrhea from any cause is associated with accelerated bone loss. Bone loss, in turn, is associated with a greater risk of fractures. Bone loss and the associated risk of fractures can be prevented or slowed with estrogen replacement therapy (ERT). Bone density measurements are needed to determine which women have the lowest bone mass and will benefit most from treatment. Thus, measurement of bone mass will allow women to make rational decisions regarding long-term ERT for protection from osteoporosis. The same logic may apply to other treatments when estrogens are not indicated.

Background

It has been sufficiently demonstrated that there is a spectrum of bone mass in estrogen-deficient women, so that those with high or low bone density can be detected easily. As noted previously, bone mass measurements predict the risk of fractures. Therefore, decisions about ERT to prevent bone loss can be guided by measurement of bone density. A substantial proportion of postmenopausal women receive ERT for menopausal symptoms and other reasons that have little to do with osteoporosis, but treatment is typically for a limited time. It has been estimated that only 5% of postmenopausal women will get long-term ERT (10 years or more) for reasons independent of concerns about osteoporosis and, consequently, unaffected by potential bone mass measurements (1). Indeed, recent surveys indicate that only 3% to 8% of women with natural menopause are receiving ERT (59,60). Thus, the majority of postmenopausal women will have to weigh the costs and benefits of this therapy. Because ERT has side effects and potentially serious risks (61) and because patient acceptance may be a problem with the use of estrogen-progestin combinations, which often lead to cyclical bleeding, it is important to select those at

greatest risk of future fracture for long-term ERT. This determination can be made reliably only by direct measurement of bone density.

Treatment with ERT will reduce future fractures. There is compelling evidence that long-term estrogen therapy prevents bone loss and fracture. In one clinical trial of three groups of patients followed for more than 6 years after oophorectomy, estrogen (mestranol) significantly retarded bone loss for as long as estrogens were prescribed, at least 10 years (62,63). These effects of estrogen were independent of the duration of ovarian insufficiency that preceded the onset of treatment (64), and recent data show ERT to be effective in slowing bone loss up to age 70 (65). However, because the effect of treatment is to slow the rate of bone loss, greater benefits are achieved with earlier treatment because bone mass is maintained at a higher level. Similar results have been found by other investigators, as reviewed elsewhere (66). There is also evidence that ERT prevents fractures. One randomized trial showed that 38% of oophorectomized women not on treatment experienced vertebral deformity, whereas 4% of the women taking ERT had such changes (63). Randomized trials of ERT for hip fracture prevention are less feasible because of the long delay between menopause and the average age at the time of fracture. However, numerous observational studies indicate that the use of ERT is associated with at least a 25% reduction in hip fractures (61). More recently, a retrospective cohort study of 245 long-term estrogen users vs. 245 controls found a 17% reduction in fractures (67). This result was largely due to prevention of wrist and spine fractures; the difference in hip fracture risk was not significant. Data from a large prospective study, on the other hand, indicated that current users who began ERT soon after menopause had a 70% reduction in hip fracture and a 50% reduction in all limb fractures combined (68). Thus, available data show that estrogen prescribed early after menopause for a minimum of 5–10 years will reduce the risk of osteoporotic fractures by up to 50%. There are, however, suggestions that the protective effect may begin to wane after ERT is stopped (68–71).

Bone density measurements should lead to an increase in appropriate outcomes (fewer fractures). It has been estimated that, in the absence of such measurements, 15% of women over age 50 would have long-term ERT and that 10% of the entire group of perimenopausal women would experience hip fracture during their lifetimes (1). In a program emphasizing bone mass measurements in the hip to identify high-risk women, it was estimated that 22% of women would have long-term ERT and that only 8% of all perimenopausal women would experience a hip fracture during their lifetimes. Bone mass measurements would result in treating 7% more women (from 15% to 22%) with ERT and might reduce the lifetime risk of hip fracture in all women (treated plus untreated) by as much as 2% (from 10% to 8%; a relative reduction of 20%). Another analysis suggested that long-term ERT treatment of 50-year-old women with hip BMD more than 1 SD below the young normal mean might reduce the lifetime fracture risk by about 15%, from 36% to 31% (61). This use of bone density measurement to direct ERT may be more (72) or less (73) cost-effective, depending on the assumptions made about outcomes and costs.

Protocol

Women should be measured to make a diagnosis of low bone mass when ERT is being considered specifically for the prevention of bone loss or treatment of osteoporosis (74). This could include women of any age who have amenorrhea of greater than 6 months' duration. The majority of these women would be perimenopausal. In addition, younger women with prolonged amenorrhea would be eligible if prevention of bone loss was of clinical concern and ERT (including oral contraceptives) was being considered. Women who are to be prescribed long-term ERT for reasons other than prevention of bone loss or treatment of osteoporosis need not be measured. Likewise, women in whom ERT is contraindicated or who refuse to consider estrogen or some other therapy to slow bone loss do not need bone mass measurements.

Although estrogen is the only drug approved in the United States for the prevention of osteoporosis, calcitonin is approved for the treatment of patients with established osteoporosis. Calcitonin has been shown to be effective in preventing bone loss in postmenopausal women (see Chapter 12), and this may lead eventually to its approval for the prevention of osteoporosis. Likewise, a number of bisphosphonates are currently under evaluation for the treatment and prevention of osteoporosis (see Chapter 12). Published data suggest that bone mass may be increased somewhat, at least in the short term, and fracture rates reduced. This class of drugs is also likely to be effective in preventing bone loss. Because all of these drugs have beneficial therapeutic effects only on the skeleton, they should be used only on those high-risk patients who are most likely to benefit, i.e., as assessed by bone density measurement.

Bone mass can be measured in the spine by QCT, DPA, or DXA; in the hip by DPA or DXA; or in the radius or os calcis by SPA or SXA. However, the specific level of bone mass at which an intervention should be undertaken is still somewhat uncertain (see Chapter 12). An ad hoc committee of the National Osteoporosis Foundation provisionally recommended that women be considered for ERT if they are amenorrheic and their bone density is more than 1 SD below the mean for young (age 30–35) normal women. At age 50, 1 SD below the mean is close to the empirical fracture threshold of approximately $1.0 \ g/cm^2$ in the proximal femur and in the spine as assessed by DPA (1). The specific method of administration of estrogen or estrogen/progestin is discussed in Chapters 12 and 14. The length of time therapy should be continued is not certain, but a minimum of 10 years is suggested by the results of the studies reviewed earlier.

Patients whose bone mass is more than 1 SD above the mean for young normal subjects are relatively protected from osteoporosis and have a lower risk of fracture. They probably need no further measurement. If concern arises, measurement can be repeated in 5 or more years and ERT can be considered at that time. Estrogen replacement therapy is not usually indicated for patients within ± 1 SD of the mean, but they may benefit from measurements after 3–5 years to see if they have developed low bone mass (1). Further research may show that consideration of risk factors other than bone density will enhance the identification of high-risk patients within this group (48,58). For example,

some have found evidence for a subgroup of postmenopausal women who lose bone at an accelerated rate (75), and it does appear that there are more vertebral fractures (but not forearm fractures) among those losing bone most rapidly (76). Should these data be confirmed, the most efficient way to identify those at highest fracture risk could be through a combination of biochemical markers of bone turnover and bone mass measurement (77).

Roentgenographic Abnormalities (Indication 2)

In patients with vertebral abnormalities or roentgenographic osteopenia, bone density measurements would be used to diagnose spinal osteoporosis before making decisions about further diagnostic evaluation and therapy.

Rationale

Patients commonly present with roentgenographic findings consistent with spinal osteoporosis. These are either a radiologist's diagnosis of spinal osteopenia or, often, abnormalities of the thoracic or lumbar vertebrae, including anterior wedging or endplate deformities. A diagnosis of osteoporosis should prompt an evaluation to exclude treatable causes of accelerated bone loss and should stimulate aggressive therapy to prevent further bone loss or to increase spinal bone mass. The complete clinical evaluation is potentially expensive, and therapy is associated with costs and health risks. Although indiscriminate treatment of such patients would lead to the maximum reduction of fracture risk, there is evidence that many individuals with vertebral abnormalities do not have significant osteoporosis. Consequently, the costs and risks associated with the clinical workup and long-term therapy cannot be justified for them, and it becomes essential to identify among those with roentgenographic vertebral abnormalities the smaller group with reduced bone mass.

Background

There is a spectrum of bone density in patients with vertebral deformities or apparent osteopenia on roentgenograms (78). Not all patients with findings suggestive of osteopenia actually have the condition, as the roentgenographic appearance of osteopenia is notoriously inaccurate. In addition to insensitivity in detecting bone loss (79), roentgenographic osteopenia is not correlated with vertebral fractures. For example, 29% of 218 ambulatory women aged 45 or older, seen as outpatients at Henry Ford Hospital, had roentgenographic osteopenia, but only one seventh of them had vertebral wedging or compression (80). Because the appearance of osteopenia can result from technical faults on the roentgenogram, normal individuals can be misclassified. Even vertebral fractures do not provide clear evidence of osteoporosis. Some true fractures are due to episodes of severe trauma earlier in life, whereas others are not fractures at all but represent old juvenile epiphysitis, positioning problems on the roentgenogram, or normal variations in vertebral body shape (81,82).

Although changes in vertebral shape indicate a fracture, change typically cannot be assessed because of the absence of baseline roentgenograms. Thus, fractures often must be diagnosed empirically, based on deviation from expected vertebral dimensions (83). The clinical picture provides little guidance, because vertebral fracture symptoms may be nonspecific (84). Inevitably, osteoporosis will be overdiagnosed in this clinical setting. Among an age-stratified random sample of women in Rochester, Minnesota, one fourth had vertebral abnormalities of one sort or another, but 21% of these women with apparent vertebral fractures had lumbar spine BMD values above the theoretical fracture threshold of 0.97 g/cm² (Fig. 3). As noted previously, vertebral fracture is related to bone mass, and bone density measurements reflect the probability of future fractures.

Bone density measurements will lead to an increase in appropriate outcomes (reduction in inappropriate evaluation and therapy for patients without osteoporosis). Practical savings to be derived from making bone mass measurements in this setting depend on the frequency with which vertebral abnormalities are encountered. It has been estimated that 5.6 million postmenopausal women have vertebral fractures (85). If as many as one fifth of them have bone density above the fracture threshold, there is a potential for evaluating or treating a large number of middle-aged women when they in fact have normal bone mass.

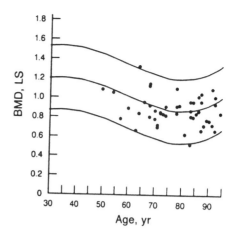

FIG. 3. Distribution of BMD of the lumbar spine (LS), by age, among Rochester, Minnesota women. The relation is best described by a cubic model: $\hat{\mu} = 0.517835 + 0.4922212 \times 10^{-1} \times age - 0.105822 \times 10^{-2} \times age^2 + 0.625726 \times 10^{-5} \times age^3$; $\sigma = 0.158749$, $r^2 = 0.33$. Values for women aged 50 years and older with one or more vertebral fractures are also indicated *(solid circles)*. (From: Melton LJ III, Kan SH, Frye MA, Wahner HW, O'Fallon WM, Riggs BL: *Am J Epidemiol* 129:1000–1011, 1989.)

Protocol

Any patient with a specific sign suggestive of spinal osteoporosis, including roentgenographic osteopenia or evidence of collapse, wedging, or ballooning of one or more thoracic or lumbar vertebral bodies, should have a bone density measurement if that patient is a candidate for therapeutic intervention or extensive diagnostic evaluation. Such measurements are not indicated for patients whose workup or treatment will not be altered by the bone density result (e.g., patients previously evaluated and for whom no specific treatment was indicated). In this setting, bone mass should be measured in the spine by DPA, DXA, or QCT. Because the BMD of compressed vertebrae may be elevated (86), any fractures in the path of the scan should be eliminated from the analysis and only intact vertebrae evaluated.

Patients with vertebral abnormalities and spinal BMD above the fracture threshold would not be considered to have fractures on the basis of osteoporosis and, consequently, would not require a workup for metabolic bone disease and would not be treated for established osteoporosis, because all such therapy is aimed at preserving bone mass or increasing it. Women with vertebral abnormalities and spinal BMD below the fracture threshold would be considered to have osteoporotic fractures and would be evaluated further.

Glucocorticoid Therapy (Indication 3)

In patients receiving long-term glucocorticoid therapy, bone density measurements would be used to diagnose low bone mass (see Chapter 17).

Rationale

Steroid therapy is required for a number of diseases, such as rheumatoid arthritis, chronic active hepatitis, inflammatory bowel disease, and asthma. This therapy has a number of serious side effects, including rapid bone loss leading to vertebral and other fractures (87). Some, but not all, steroid-treated patients experience this excessive bone loss (Fig. 4), and not all have fractures. The importance of assessment is increased because patients are frequently receiving long-term therapy. Moreover, unlike with involutional osteoporosis, patients may be children, and it must be determined whether skeletal development is lagging behind normal adolescent development patterns. Information about bone mass may permit improved patient management through more precise adjustments of dose and duration of therapy, to maximize therapeutic effects while minimizing skeletal complications.

Protocol

Patients who are to be placed on long-term (more than 1 month) glucocorticoid treatment (>7.5 mg of prednisone/day or equivalent) can have bone density measurements when it is possible to adjust the dose. Measurements of the spine using DPA, DXA, or QCT are advised because trabecular bone is primarily affected (87,88).

Primary Hyperparathyroidism (Indication 4)

In patients with asymptomatic primary hyperparathyroidism, bone density measurements would be used to diagnose low bone mass to identify those at risk of severe

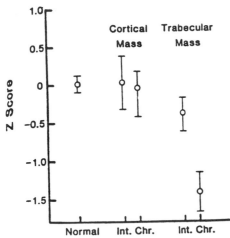

FIG. 4. Comparison of trabecular mass and cortical mass in normal controls and patients. The z-score is a function of the mean ± SD of age-adjusted and sex-adjusted values. Int., intermittent steroid use; Chr., chronic, or long-term, use. Trabecular mass in the long-term-use group was significantly smaller than in the normal ($p < 0.01$) and intermittent-use ($p < 0.03$) groups. *Bars* denote ± SEM. (From: Adinoff AD, Hollister JR: *N Engl J Med* 309:265–268, 1983.)

skeletal disease who may be candidates for surgical intervention (89).

Rationale

The clinical spectrum at presentation of primary hyperparathyroidism has changed with the advent of routine biochemical screening (90). Previously, patients presented with symptomatic bone disease, renal stones, or other complaints that alerted the physician and that led to surgical intervention. Now, many patients are asymptomatic and have no obvious complications when the diagnosis is made incidentally (90,91). The management of such asymptomatic individuals remains controversial (92). Primary hyperparathyroidism is associated with a decrease in bone mass in some patients (93), which can be detected by measurement of bone mass but not by the usual radiographic evaluation (Fig. 5). Such a reduction in bone mass may be accompanied by an increased frequency of fractures of the vertebrae, distal radius, and hip, as reviewed elsewhere (94). Thus, it can be argued that the finding of low bone mass in patients with otherwise asymptomatic hyperparathyroidism should be considered a possible indication for surgery (92). After successful surgery, bone density generally has been found to increase, although not to normal values (94). Because low bone mass is related to fracture risk, an increase in bone density should reduce the risk of subsequent fractures.

Protocol

The diagnosis of primary hyperparathyroidism should be made using accepted clinical criteria (89). Those who have no symptoms that could be attributed to primary hyperparathy-

roidism that would lead to surgery should have measurements done. Bone mass may be measured in the radius by SPA or SXA or in the spine by DPA, DXA, or QCT.

Other Potential Indications

With the improvements in technology leading to better precision and accuracy of measurements, other indications for clinical application of bone density measurements may develop.

Universal Screening for Osteoporosis Prophylaxis

Bone mass measurement for osteoporosis prophylaxis meets some of the criteria for a screening test (i.e., the disease is common; screening tests are available; effective therapy is available for patients with abnormal tests; and treatment should reduce fracture incidence). However, some patients might be receiving effective treatment for reasons unrelated to osteoporosis, whereas others might decline therapy regardless of bone density measurement. In addition, optimal screening regimens have not been determined. Consequently, most authorities have recommended against

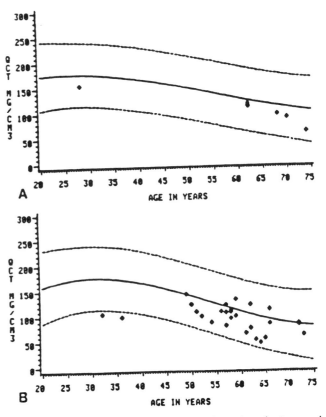

FIG. 5. Hyperparathyroid patients are plotted against normal curves as determined by QCT in males (**A**) and females (**B**). *Solid curves* indicate the cubic regression lines; *dashed lines* indicate the 95% confidence limits for the normal subjects. (From: Richardson ML, Pozzi-Mucelli RS, Kanter AS, Kolb FO, Ettinger B, Genant HK: *Skeletal Radiol* 15:85–95, 1986.)

universal (or unselective) screening (5,73,95,96). However, selective screening as outlined previously is justifiable (97).

Monitoring Bone Mass to Assess the Efficacy of Therapy

Therapeutic interventions to preserve bone mass are not always successful, and dose response may vary among patients (98). Because current methods for measuring bone density are quite precise (e.g., 1% for the spine with DXA and 1% to 2% for the radius with SPA), it may be possible to monitor responses to drugs and to alter the dose or type of drug used. Some have concluded that it is difficult to assess the true change in bone mass with two measurements taken closely enough together to provide relevant data for managing treatment (99–101). For example, two measurements of an individual 1 year apart, given a 2% SD of the difference between measurements and no actual bone loss, would yield a 95% confidence interval for the difference between the measurements extending from −5.6% to +5.6%. This results from the basic statistical fact that the variance of the difference between two measurements equals the sum of the two individual variances. Critics often note that bone loss over life is only approximately 1% per year in women and half that figure in men, and conclude that prospects are dim for monitoring changes in bone mass reliably. However, the issue is considerably more complex than this, for three reasons: (i) recent changes in technology have improved the precision of longitudinal measurement; (ii) rates of bone loss around the time of menopause may be much greater than 1%, particularly in cancellous bone; and (iii) populations for whom such monitoring might be beneficial vary greatly. Considering ERT, the example given previously implies that, even with a precision error of 1% and bone loss at 3% per year, it would require a 2-year interval between measurements to identify accurately 85% of nonresponders to a therapy expected to prevent bone loss completely. Obviously, 2 years is an unsatisfactory length of time to wait before changing or reevaluating treatments. However, if the therapies being tried cause a short-term gain in bone mass (as is common with estrogen therapy and other regimens that act by slowing bone remodeling), then differences may be accentuated and shorter intervals between measurements may be possible. At present, however, insufficient data are available for approved drugs to suggest specific protocols for follow-up.

ACKNOWLEDGMENT

This chapter was adapted from a report of the Scientific Advisory Committee of the National Osteoporosis Foundation.

REFERENCES

1. Johnston CC Jr, Melton LJ III, Lindsay R, Eddy D: Clinical indication for bone mass measurement. *J Bone Miner Res* 4(Suppl 2):1–28, 1989
2. Mazess RB: Bone densitometry for clinical diagnosis and monitoring. In: DeLuca HF, Mazess R (eds) *Osteoporosis: Physiological Basis, Assessment, and Treatment.* New York, Elsevier Science Publishing Co., Inc., 63–85, 1990
3. Sartoris DJ, Resnick D: Current and innovative methods for noninvasive bone densitometry. *Radiol Clin North Am* 28:257–278, 1990
4. Lang P, Steiger P, Faulkner K, Glüer C, Genant HK: Osteoporosis. Current techniques and recent developments in quantitative bone densitometry. *Radiol Clin North Am* 29:49–76, 1991
5. Kanis JA and the WHO Study Group: Assessment of fracture risk and its application to screening for postmenopausal osteoporosis: Synopsis of a WHO report. *Osteoporosis Int* 4:368–381, 1994
6. Wahner HW, Fogelman I: *The Evaluation of Osteoporosis: Dual Energy X-Ray Absorptiometry in Clinical Practice.* London, Martin Dunitz Ltd, 1994
7. Johnston CC, Melton LJ III: Bone densitometry. In: Riggs BL, Melton LJ III (eds) *Osteoporosis: Etiology, Diagnosis and Management.* 2nd ed. Philadelphia, Lippincott-Raven Publishers, 275–297, 1995
8. Yang S-O, Hagiwara S, Engelke K, et al: Radiographic absorptiometry for bone mineral measurement of the phalanges: Precision and accuracy study. *Radiology* 192:857–859, 1994
9. Cosman F, Herrington B, Himmelstein S, Lindsay R: Radiographic absorptiometry: A simple method for determination of bone mass. *Osteoporosis Int* 2:35–38, 1991
10. Epstein RS, Lydick E, Suppapanya N, Ross PD, Yates AJ: Baseline measurement of bone mass from hand x-rays predicts hip fractures in a national sample of white women. *Osteoporosis Int* (in press)
11. Mussolino M, Looker A, Madans J, Edelstein D, Walker R, Lydick E, Epstein R: Phalangeal bone density and hip fracture risk. *J Bone Miner Res* 10(Suppl 1):S360, 1995
12. Ross P, Huang C, Davis J, Imose K, Yates J, Vogel J, Wasnich R: Predicting vertebral deformity using bone densitometry at various skeletal sites and calcaneus ultrasound. *Bone* 16:235–332, 1995
13. Yates AJ, Ross PD, Lydick E, Epstein RS: Radiographic absorptiometry in the diagnosis of osteoporosis. *Am J Med* 98(Suppl 2A): 41S–47S, 1995
14. Kaufman JJ, Einhorn TA: Perspectives: Ultrasound assessment of bone. *J Bone Miner Res* 8:517–525, 1993
15. Ross P, Huang C, Davis J, Imose K, Yates J, Vogel J, Wasnich R: Predicting vertebral deformity using bone densitometry at various skeletal sites and calcaneus ultrasound. *Bone* 16:325–332, 1995
16. Heaney RP, Avioli LV, Chesnut CH III, Lappe J, Recker RR, Brandenburger GH: Osteoporotic bone fragility: Detection by ultrasound transmission velocity. *JAMA* 261:2986–2990, 1989
17. Kereiakes J, Rosenstein M: *Handbook of Radiation Doses in Nuclear Medicine and Diagnostic Radiology.* Boca Raton, Florida, CRC Press, 1980
18. Boshong SC: *Radiologic Science for Technologists: Physics, Biology and Protection.* 4th ed. St. Louis, CV Mosby Co., 1988
19. Melton LJ III, Chao EYS, Lane J: Biomechanical aspects of fractures. In: Riggs BL, Melton LJ III (eds) *Osteoporosis: Etiology, Diagnosis, and Management.* New York, Raven Press, 111–131, 1988
20. Eriksson SAV, Isberg BO, Lindgren JU: Prediction of vertebral strength by dual photon absorptiometry and quantitative computer tomography. *Calcif Tissue Int* 44:243–250, 1989
21. Lotz JC, Hayes WC: The use of quantitative computed tomography to estimate risk of fracture of the hip from falls. *J Bone Joint Surg* 72-A:689–700, 1990
22. Cody DD, Goldstein SA, Flynn MJ, Brown EB: Correlations between vertebral regional bone mineral density (rBMD) and whole bone fracture load. *Spine* 16:146–154, 1991
23. Myers ER, Sebeny EA, Hecker AT, Corcoran TA, Hipp JA, Greenspan SL, Hayes WC: Correlations between photon absorption properties and failure load of the distal radius in vitro. *Calcif Tissue Int* 49:292–297, 1991
24. Moro M, Hecker AT, Bouxsein ML, Myers ER: Failure load of thoracic vertebrae correlates with lumbar bone mineral density measured by DXA. *Calcif Tissue Int* 56:206–209, 1995
25. Ross PD, Davis JW, Vogel JM, Wasnich RD: A critical review of bone mass and the risk of fractures in osteoporosis. *Calcif Tissue Int* 46:149–161, 1990
26. Hui SL, Slemenda CW, Johnston CC Jr: Age and bone mass as predictors of fracture in a prospective study. *J Clin Invest* 81:1804–1809, 1988
27. Seeley DG, Browner WS, Nevitt MC, Genant HK, Scott JC, Cummings SR, and the Study of Osteoporotic Fractures Research

Group: Which fractures are associated with low appendicular bone mass in elderly women? *Ann Intern Med* 115:837–842, 1991

28. Frankel VH, Pugh JW: Biomechanics of the hip. In: Tronzo RG (ed) *Surgery of the Hip Joint.* New York, Springer-Verlag, 115–131, 1984
29. Mosekilde LI: Sex differences in age-related loss of vertebral trabecular bone mass and structure—biomechanical consequences. *Bone* 10:425–432, 1989
30. McCalden RW, McGeough JA, Barker MB, Court-Brown CM: Age-related changes in the tensile properties of cortical bone. The relative importance of changes in porosity, mineralization, and microstructure. *J Bone Joint Surg* 75-A:1193–1205, 1993
31. Faulkner KG, Cummings SR, Black D, Palermo L, Glüer C-C, Genant HK: Simple measurement of femoral geometry predicts hip fracture: The study of osteoporotic fractures. *J Bone Miner Res* 8:1211–1217, 1993
32. Nevitt MC, Cummings SR: Type of fall and risk of hip and wrist fractures: The study of osteoporotic fractures. *J Am Geriatr Soc* 41:1226–1234, 1993
33. Cooper C, Atkinson EJ, O'Fallon WM, Melton LJ III: Incidence of clinically diagnosed vertebral fractures: A population-based study in Rochester, Minnesota, 1985–1989. *J Bone Miner Res* 7:221–227, 1992
34. Winner SJ, Morgan CA, Evans JG: Perimenopausal risk of falling and incidence of distal forearm fracture. *BMJ* 298:1486–1488, 1989
35. Gibson MJ: The prevention of falls in later life. *Dan Med Bull* 34(Suppl 4):1–24, 1987
36. Hayes WC, Myers ER, Morris JN, Gerhart TN, Yett HS, Lipsitz LA: Impact near the hip dominates fracture risk in elderly nursing home residents who fall. *Calcif Tissue Int* 52:192–198, 1993
37. Greenspan SL, Myers ER, Maitland LA, Resnick NM, Hayes WC: Fall severity and bone mineral density as risk factors for hip fracture in ambulatory elderly. *JAMA* 271:128–133, 1994
38. Wasnich RD, Ross PD, Heilbrun LK, Vogel JM: Prediction of postmenopausal fracture risk with use of bone mineral measurements. *Am J Obstet Gynecol* 153:745–751, 1985
39. Hui SL, Slemenda CW, Johnston CC Jr: Baseline measurement of bone mass predicts fracture in white women. *Ann Intern Med* 111:355–361, 1989
40. Cummings SR, Black DM, Nevitt MC, Browner WS, Cauley JA, Genant HK, Mascioli SR, Scott JC, Seeley DG, Steiger P, Vogt TM, and the Study of Osteoporotic Fractures Research Group: Appendicular bone density and age predict hip fracture in women. *JAMA* 263:665–668, 1990
41. Ross PD, Davis JW, Epstein RS, Wasnich RD: Pre-existing fractures and bone mass predict vertebral fracture incidence in women. *Ann Intern Med* 114:919–923, 1991
42. Black DM, Cummings SR, Genant HK, Nevitt MC, Palermo L, Browner W: Axial and appendicular bone density predict fractures in older women. *J Bone Miner Res* 7:633–638, 1992
43. Gärdsell P, Johnell O, Nilsson BE, Gullberg B: Predicting various fragility fractures in women by forearm bone densitometry: A follow-up study. *Calcif Tissue Int* 52:348–353, 1993
44. Cummings SR, Black DM, Nevitt MC, Browner W, Cauley J, Ensrud K, Genant HK, Palermo L, Scott J, Vogt TM: The Study of Osteoporotic Fractures Research Group: Bone density at various sites for prediction of hip fractures. *Lancet* 341:72–75, 1993
45. Melton LJ III, Atkinson EJ, O Fallon WM, Wahner HW, Riggs BL: Long-term fracture prediction by bone mineral assessed at different skeletal sites. *J Bone Miner Res* 8:1227–1233, 1993
46. Ross PD, Yhee Y-K, Davis JW, Wasnich RE: Bone density predicts fracture incidence among elderly men. In: Christiansen C, Riis B (eds) *Proceedings of the Fourth International Symposium on Osteoporosis and Consensus Development Conference, Hong Kong, March 27–April 2, 1993.* Aalborg, Denmark, Handelstrykkeriet Aalborg ApS, 190–191, 1993
47. Black DM, Cummings SR: How well can bone mineral density predict different types of fractures? In: Christiansen C, Riis B (eds) *Proceedings of the Fourth International Symposium on Osteoporosis and Consensus Development Conference, Hong Kong, March 27–April 2, 1993.* Aalborg, Denmark, Handelstrykkeriet Aalborg, ApS, 300–301, 1993
48. Nguyen T, Sambrook SP, Kelly P, Jones G, Lord S, Freund J, Eis-

man J: Prediction of osteoporotic fractures by postural instability and bone density. *BMJ* 307:1111–1115, 1993
49. Kröger H, Huopio J, Honkanen R, Tuppurainen M, Puntila E, Alhava E, Saarikoski S: Prediction of fracture risk using axial bone mineral density in a perimenopausal population: A prospective study. *J Bone Miner Res* 10:302–306, 1995
50. Heaney RP, Avioli LV, Chesnut CH III, Lappe J, Recker RR, Brandenburger GH: Ultrasound velocity through bone predicts incident vertebral deformity. *J Bone Miner Res* 10:341–345, 1995
51. Johnell O: Prevention of fractures in the elderly: A review. *Acta Orthop Scand* 66:90–98, 1995
52. Ribot C, Tremollieres F, Pouilles J-M: Can we detect women with low bone mass using clinical risk factors? *Am J Med* 98(Suppl 2A):52S–55S, 1995
53. Bauer DC, Browner WS, Cauley JA, Orwoll ES, Scott JC, Black DM, Tao JL, Cummings SR, for the Study of Osteoporotic Fractures Research Group: Factors associated with appendicular bone mass in older women. *Ann Intern Med* 118:657–665, 1993
54. Slemenda CW, Hui SL, Longcope C, Wellman H, Johnston CC Jr: Predictors of bone mass in perimenopausal women: A prospective study of clinical data using photon absorptiometry. *Ann Intern Med* 112:96–101, 1990
55. van Hemert AM, Vandenbroucke JP, Birkenhäger JC, Valkenberg HA: Prediction of osteoporotic fractures in the general population by a fracture risk score: A 9-year follow-up among middle-aged women. *Am J Epidemiol* 132:123–135, 1990
56. Wasnich RD, Ross PD, MacLean CJ, Davis JW, Vogel JM: The relative strengths of osteoporotic risk factors in a prospective study of postmenopausal osteoporosis. In: Christiansen C, Johansen JS, Riis BJ (eds) *Osteoporosis 1987.* Copenhagen, Osteopress ApS, pp 394–395, 1987
57. Cooper C, Shah S, Hand DJ, Adams J, Compston J, Davie M, Woolf A (The Multicentre Vertebral Fracture Study Group): Screening for vertebral osteoporosis using individual risk factors. *Osteoporosis Int* 2:48–53, 1991
58. Cummings SR, Nevitt MC, Browner WS, Stone K, Fox KM, Ensrud KE, Cauley J, Black D, Vogt TM, for the Study of Osteoporotic Fractures Research Group: Risk factors for hip fracture in white women. *N Engl J Med* 332:767–773, 1995
59. Derby CA, Hume AL, Barbour MM, McPhillips JB, Lasater TM, Carleton RA: Correlates of postmenopausal estrogen use and trends through the 1980s in two Southeastern New England communities. *Am J Epidemiol* 137:1125–1135, 1993
60. Johannes CB, Crawford SL, Posner JG, McKinlay SM: Longitudinal patterns and correlates of hormone replacement therapy use in middle-aged women. *Am J Epidemiol* 140:439–452, 1994
61. Grady D, Rubin SM, Petitti DB, Fox CS, Black D, Ettinger B, Ernster VL, Cummings SR: Hormone therapy to prevent disease and prolong life in postmenopausal women. *Ann Intern Med* 117:1016–1037, 1992
62. Lindsay R, Hart DM, Aitken JM, MacDonald EB, Anderson JB, Clark AC: Long-term prevention of postmenopausal osteoporosis by oestrogen. Evidence for an increased bone mass after delayed onset of oestrogen treatment. *Lancet* 1:1038–1041, 1976
63. Lindsay R, Hart DM, Forrest C, Baird C: Prevention of spinal osteoporosis in oophorectomised women. *Lancet* 2:1151–1154, 1980
64. Abdalla H, Hart DM, Lindsay R: Differential bone loss and effects of long-term estrogen therapy according to time of introduction of therapy after oophorectomy. In: Christiansen C, Arnaud CD, Nordin BEC, Parfitt AM, Peck WA, Riggs BL (eds) *Osteoporosis 2.* Copenhagen, Aalborg Stifsbogtrykkeri, 621–624, 1984
65. Kohrt WM, Birge SJ Jr: Differential effects of estrogen treatment on bone mineral density of the spine, hip, wrist and total body in late postmenopausal women. *Osteoporosis Int* 5:150–155, 1995
66. Riggs BL, Melton LJ III: The prevention and treatment of osteoporosis. *N Engl J Med* 327:620–627, 1992
67. Maxim P, Ettinger B, Spitalny GM: Fracture protection provided by long-term estrogen treatment. *Osteoporosis Int* 5:23–29, 1995
68. Cauley JA, Seeley DG, Ensrud K, Ettinger B, Black D, Cummings SR, for the Study of Osteoporotic Fractures Research Group: Estrogen replacement therapy and fractures in older women. *Ann Intern Med* 122:9–16, 1995
69. Weiss NS, Ure CL, Ballard JH, Williams AR, Daling JR:

Decreased risk of fractures of the hip and lower forearm with postmenopausal use of estrogens. *N Engl J Med* 303:1195–1198, 1980

70. Kiel DP, Felson DT, Anderson JJ, Wilson PWF, Moskowitz MA: Hip fracture and the use of estrogens in postmenopausal women: The Framingham Study. *N Engl J Med* 317:1169–1174, 1987

71. Paganini-Hill A, Chao A, Ross RK, Henderson BE: Exercise and other factors in the prevention of hip fractures: The leisure world study. *Epidemiology* 2:16–25, 1991

72. Tosteson AN, Rosenthal DI, Melton LJ III, Weinstein MC: Cost effectiveness of screening perimenopausal white women for osteoporosis: Bone densitometry and hormone replacement therapy. *Ann Intern Med* 113:594–603, 1990

73. U.S. Congress, Office of Technology Assessment: *Effectiveness and Costs of Osteoporosis Screening and Hormone Replacement Therapy, Volume I: Cost-Effectiveness Analysis.* OTA-BP-H-160. Washington, DC, U.S. Government Printing Office, August 1995

74. Rubin SM, Cummings SR: Results of bone densitometry affect women's decisions about taking measures to prevent fractures. *Ann Intern Med* 116:990–995, 1992

75. Christiansen C, Riis BJ, Rødbro P: Prediction of rapid bone loss in postmenopausal women. *Lancet* 1:1105–1108, 1987

76. Hansen MA, Overgaard K, Riis BJ, Christiansen C: Role of peak bone mass and bone loss in postmenopausal osteoporosis: 12-year study. *BMJ* 303:961–964, 1991

77. Riis BJ: Cost effective techniques for assessment of present and future bone mineral status: The practical integration of bone mass and biochemical markers. In: Christiansen C, Riis B (eds) *Proceedings of the Fourth International Symposium on Osteoporosis and Consensus Development Conference, Hong Kong, March 27-April 2, 1993.* Aalborg, Denmark, Handelstrykkeriet Aalborg ApS, 297–299, 1993

78. Melton LJ III, Kan SH, Frye MA, Wahner HW, O'Fallon WM, Riggs BL: Epidemiology of vertebral fractures in women. *Am J Epidemiol* 129:1000–1011, 1989

79. Epstein DM, Dalinka MK, Kaplan FS, Aronchick JM, Marinelli DL, Kundel HL: Observer variation in the detection of osteopenia. *Skeletal Radiol* 15:347–349, 1986

80. Smith RW Jr, Rizek J: Epidemiologic studies of osteoporosis in women of Puerto Rico and southeastern Michigan with special reference to age, race, national origin and to other related or associated findings. *Clin Orthop* 45:31–48, 1966

81. Doyle FH, Gutteridge DH, Joplin GF, Fraser R: An assessment of radiological criteria used in the study of spinal osteoporosis. *Br J Radiol* 40:241–250, 1967

82. Gallagher JC, Hedlund LR, Stoner S, Meeger C: Vertebral morphometry: Normative data. *Bone Miner* 4:189–196, 1988

83. Black DM, Palermo L, Nevitt MC, Genant HK, Epstein R, San Valentin R, Cummings SR, for the Study of Osteoporotic Fractures Research Group: Comparison of methods for defining prevalent vertebral deformities: The study of osteoporotic fractures. *J Bone Miner Res* 10:890–902, 1995

84. Ettinger B, Black DM, Nevitt MC, Rundle AC, Cauley JA, Cummings SR, Genant HK, and The Study for Osteoporotic Fractures Research Group: Contribution of vertebral deformities to chronic back pain and disability. *J Bone Miner Res* 7:449–456, 1992

85. Melton LJ III, Lane AW, Cooper C, Eastell R, O'Fallon WM, Riggs BL: Prevalence and incidence of vertebral deformities. *Osteoporosis Int* 3:113–119, 1993

86. Ryan PJ, Evans P, Blake GM, Fogelman I: The effect of vertebral collapse on spinal bone mineral density measurements in osteoporosis. *Bone Miner* 18:267–272, 1992

87. Lukert BP, Raisz LG: Glucocorticoid-induced osteoporosis: Pathogenesis and management. *Ann Intern Med* 112:352–364, 1990

88. Laan RF, Buijs WC, van Erning LJ, Lemmens JA, Corstens FH, Ruijs SH, van de Putte LB, van Riel PL: Differential effects of glucocorticoids on cortical appendicular and cortical vertebral bone mineral content. *Calcif Tissue Int* 52:5–9, 1993

89. Bilezikan JP: Primary hyperparathyroidism. In: Favus MJ, Christakos S, Goldring SR, et al. (eds) *Primer on the Metabolic Bone Diseases and Disorders of Mineral Metabolism, Third edition.* Lippincott-Raven Publishers, Philadelphia, 181–186, 1996

90. Heath H III: Clinical spectrum of primary hyperparathyroidism: Evolution with changes in medical practice and technology. *J Bone Miner Res* 6(Suppl 2):S63–S70, 1991

91. Bilezikian JP: Primary hyperparathyroidism: Another important metabolic bone disease of women. *J Women's Health* 3:21–32, 1994

92. Anonymous: Consensus Development Conference Statement. *J Bone Miner Res* 6(Suppl 2):S9–S13, 1991

93. Richardson ML, Pozzi-Mucelli RS, Kanter AS, Kolb FO, Ettinger B, Genant HK: Bone mineral changes in primary hyperparathyroidism. *Skeletal Radiol* 15:85–95, 1986

94. Khosla S, Melton LJ III: Secondary osteoporosis. In: Riggs BL, Melton LJ III (eds) *Osteoporosis: Etiology, Diagnosis, and Management.* 2nd ed. Philadelphia, Lippincott-Raven Publishers, 183–204, 1995

95. Canadian Task Force on the Periodic Health Examination: The periodic health examination: 2. 1987 update. *Can Med Assoc J* 138:618–626, 1988

96. U.S. Preventive Services Task Force: Screening for postmenopausal osteoporosis. In: *Guide to Clinical Preventive Services: Report of the U.S. Preventive Services Task Force.* Baltimore, Williams & Wilkins, 239–243, 1989

97. Compston JE, Cooper C, Kanis JA: Bone densitometry in clinical practice. *BMJ* 310:1507–1510, 1995

98. Stevenson JC, Hillard TC, Lees B, Whitcroft SIJ, Ellerington MC, Whitehead MI: Postmenopausal bone loss: Does HRT always work? In: Christiansen C, Riis B (eds) *Proceedings of the Fourth International Symposium on Osteoporosis and Consensus Development Conference, Hong Kong, March 27-April 2, 1993.* Aalborg, Denmark, Handelstrykkeriet Aalborg ApS, 497–498, 1993

99. Heaney RP: En recherche de la différence (P < 0.05). *Bone Miner* 1:99–114, 1986

100. Cummings SR, Black D: Should perimenopausal women be screened for osteoporosis? *Ann Intern Med* 104:817–823, 1986

101. Davis JW, Ross PD, Wasnich RD, MacLean CJ, Vogel JM: Long-term precision of bone loss rate measurements among postmenopausal women. *Calcif Tissue Int* 48:311–318, 1991

8. Radiology of Osteoporosis and Other Metabolic Bone Diseases

Harry K. Genant, M.D.

Skeletal Section, Department of Radiology, University of California, San Francisco, San Francisco, California

Osteoporosis represents the most common form of metabolic bone disease, and its radiologic features are presented herein. The list of processes that are associated with or result in a generalized deficient quantity of bone (osteoporosis) is extensive (see Table 1). Histologically, the end result in each of these disorders is a deficient amount of osseous tissue, although different pathogenic mechanisms may be involved. In essence, the generalized osteoporoses represent a heterogeneous group of conditions encompassing many pathogenetic mechanisms, variably associated with low, normal, or increased bone-remodeling states.

Many terms have been used to describe the radiographic features of diminished bone density, such as "osteoporosis," "demineralization," "undermineralization," "deossification," and "osteopenia." The latter, osteopenia (meaning "poverty of the bone"), has become acceptable as a nonspecific, gross descriptive term for generalized or regional rarefaction of the skeleton.

The anatomic distribution of osteopenia or osteoporosis depends on the underlying cause. Osteopenia can be generalized, affecting the whole skeleton, or regional, affecting only a part of the skeleton, usually the appendicular skeleton. Typical examples of generalized osteopenias are involutional and postmenopausal osteoporosis, and osteoporosis caused by endocrine disorders such as hyperparathyroidism, hyperthyroidism, osteomalacia, and hypogonadism. Regional forms of osteoporosis result from factors affecting any part of the appendicular skeleton, such as disuse, reflex sympathetic syndrome, and transient osteoporosis of large joints. The distribution of osteopenia may vary considerably among different diseases and may be suggestive of a specific diagnosis. Focal osteopenia primarily reflects the underlying cause, such as inflammation, fracture, or tumor, and is not the subject of this chapter.

A number of characteristic radiographic features make the diagnosis of osteopenia or osteoporosis possible. However, the quantification of osteopenia by conventional radiography is inaccurate because it is influenced by many technical factors, such as radiographic exposure, film development, soft-tissue thickness of the patient, and others (1). It has been estimated that as much as 20% to 40% of bone mass must be lost before a decrease in bone density can be seen in lateral radiographs of the thoracic and lumbar spine (2,3). Finally, the diagnosis of osteopenia from conventional radiographs also depends on the experience of the reader and subjective interpretation (4). Therefore, the sensitivity of conventional radiography to detect early bone loss based on increased radiolucency is generally considered to be low (4–6).

In summary, a radiograph may reflect the amount of bone mass, histology, and gross morphology of the skeletal part examined. The principal findings of osteopenia are increased

TABLE 1. *Disorders associated with radiographic osteoporosis (osteopenia)*

I. Primary osteoporosis
    1. Involutional osteoporosis (postmenopausal and senile)
    2. Juvenile osteoporosis
II. Secondary osteoporosis
  A. Endocrine
    1. Adrenal cortex
      a. Cushing's disease
    2. Gonadal disorders
      a. Hypogonadism
    3. Pituitary
      a. Hypopituitarism
    4. Pancreas
      a. Diabetes mellitus
    5. Thyroid
      a. Hyperthyroidism
    6. Parathyroid
      a. Hyperparathyroidism
  B. Marrow replacement and expansion
    1. Myeloma
    2. Leukemia
    3. Metastatic disease
    4. Gaucher's disease
    5. Anemias (sickle cell, thalassemia)
  C. Drugs and substances
    1. Corticosteroids
    2. Heparin
    3. Anticonvulsants
    4. Immunosuppressants
    5. Alcohol
  D. Chronic disease
    1. Chronic renal disease
    2. Hepatic insufficiency
    3. Gastrointestinal malabsorption
    4. Chronic inflammatory polyarthropathies
    5. Chronic debility/immobilization
  E. Deficiency states
    1. Vitamin D
    2. Vitamin C (scurvy)
    3. Calcium
    4. Malnutrition
  F. Inborn errors of metabolism
    1. Osteogenesis imperfecta
    2. Homocystinuria

radiolucency and changes in bone microstructure (e.g., rarefaction of trabeculae, thinning of the cortices), eventually resulting in changes of the gross bone morphology, i.e., the recurrence of fractures. Further characteristics of osteopenic and osteoporotic disease conditions and specific techniques for their radiologic assessment are described in greater detail later.

PRIMARY OSTEOPOROSIS

Involutional, Postmenopausal, or Senile Osteoporosis

The term *involutional osteoporosis* has been used to describe the condition of gradual, progressive bone loss, often accompanied by fractures, seen in postmenopausal women and, with increasing age, in both men and women. It has been suggested that this broad category of involutional osteoporosis may represent two distinct syndromes—postmenopausal osteoporosis (type I) and senile osteoporosis (type II) (7–9). Gallagher (10) added a third type, meaning secondary osteoporosis. Even though the importance of estrogen deficiency for postmenopausal osteoporosis has been established, the distinction between the first two types of osteoporosis is not entirely accepted. Distinctions between postmenopausal and senile osteoporosis may sometimes be arbitrary, and the assignment of fracture sites to the different types of osteoporosis is uncertain.

Postmenopausal osteoporosis is believed to represent that process occurring in a subset of postmenopausal women, typically between the ages of 50 and 65 years. This group is characterized by accelerated trabecular bone resorption related to estrogen deficiency and is identified by a fracture pattern that involves predominantly the spine and wrist. Accelerated and disproportionate loss of trabecular bone in these areas structurally weakens the bone and predisposes these individuals to fractures. In senile osteoporosis, there is a proportionate loss of cortical and trabecular bone, in contrast to the disproportionate loss of trabecular bone in postmenopausal osteoporosis. Senile osteoporosis is characterized by fractures of the hip, proximal end of the humerus, tibia, and pelvis in elderly women and men, usually 75 years of age or older. The etiology of senile osteoporosis is speculative. However, factors that play a role include an age-related decrease in bone formation, diminished adrenal function, reduced intestinal calcium absorption, and secondary hyperparathyroidism.

Radiologic-Pathologic Findings

In the normal physiologic state in the adult, the rates of bone formation and bone resorption are roughly equal (i.e., coupled), allowing the total amount of osseous tissue to remain constant. In osteoporosis (11,12), this equilibrium is lost such that bone resorption predominates. This is reflected radiographically as various patterns of trabecular and cortical bone resorption, ultimately leading to osteopenia.

Trabecular bone resorption in the axial skeleton, particularly in postmenopausal osteoporosis, results in marked thinning and dissolution of transverse trabeculae, with relative preservation of the primary trabeculae or those aligned with the axis of stress. In areas in which trabecular bone predominates, such as the spine and pelvis, the combination of osteopenia and reinforcement of primary trabeculae may produce a striated bony appearance (Fig. 1). The reinforced primary trabeculae have a sharp appearance in osteoporotic bones, which occasionally aids in distinguishing osteoporosis from osteomalacia. In the latter, the trabeculae may appear indistinct or "fuzzy" as a result of irregular resorption from accompanying secondary hyperparathyroidism and from trabeculae that become coated by a layer of partially unmineralized osteoid. The loss of trabecular bone mass also accentuates the cortical outline, producing the so-called "picture framing" or "empty box" seen in osteoporosis of the vertebral bodies (Fig. 2). The vertebral bodies become weakened and the intervertebral disc may protrude into the adjacent vertebral body. The degree of protrusion varies, ranging from bending and buckling of the endplates (biconcave appearance) to herniation of disc material into the vertebral body (Schmorl's node formation) (Fig. 3). In more advanced cases, complete compression fractures of the vertebral bodies occur (Fig. 4).

Bone loss in the appendicular skeleton is initially most apparent radiographically at the ends of long and tubular bones, because of the predominance of cancellous bone in these regions. Endosteal resorption of bone has a prominent role, particularly in senile osteoporosis. The net result of this chronic process is widening of the medullary canal and thinning of the cortices, which is most pronounced in the appendicular skeleton (Fig. 5). In late stages of senile osteoporosis, the cortices are "paper thin" and the endosteal surfaces are smooth (Fig. 6). In rapidly evolving postmenopausal osteoporosis, on the other hand, accelerated endosteal and intracortical bone resorption may be seen and can be directly assessed by high-resolution radiographic techniques (Fig. 7).

When there is an overall loss of bone mass and progressive osteopenia, the skeletal system becomes weakened and fractures occur. These fractures are commonly seen in the vertebral bodies, femoral neck (Fig. 8), femoral intertrochanteric region (Fig. 9), distal radius, ribs, and pelvis. These may be the result of minor trauma or even normal stress on the abnormal bone (insufficiency fracture). Vertebral body and wrist fractures are generally seen at an earlier age than fractures of the femur (type II osteoporosis). Occasionally, these osteoporotic fractures are not identified on initial radiographs but are found by radionuclide bone scan, computed tomography (Fig. 10), magnetic resonance imaging, or by follow-up radiographic studies, as healing occurs. The radiologic appearance in the setting of partial healing may suggest a metastatic neoplastic process, particularly with fractures of the vertebrae, sacrum, hip, and pelvis (Fig. 11).

Idiopathic Juvenile Osteoporosis

The etiology of this rare disorder (13,14) is not known. Patients typically present before puberty with osteoporosis that is progressive initially and later stabilizes.

Radiologic-Pathologic Considerations

Bone formation is thought to proceed normally while, presumably, there is an increase in osteoclastic activity, yielding increased bone resorption (14). This causes a decrease in the quantity of bone (osteoporosis) while the quality of remaining bone is normal. This osteoporosis becomes most evident in the thoracic and lumbar spine with anterior wedging and biconcave deformities (Fig. 12) of the

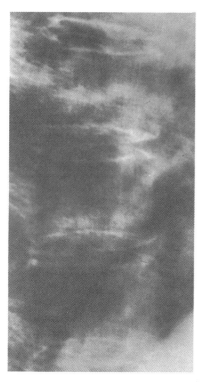

FIG. 1. Moderate postmenopausal osteoporosis of the thoracic spine with overall loss of bone density. The cortices are thinned and the vertebral bodies have a "striated" appearance due to loss of secondary trabeculae and reinforcement of sharply defined primary trabeculae.

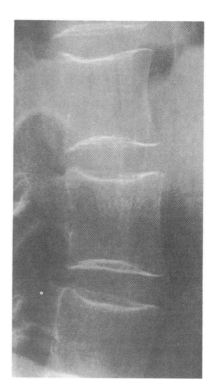

FIG. 2. Because of the loss of trabecular bone, there is accentuation of the cortices, resulting in the appearance of "picture framing" in this patient with postmenopausal osteoporosis.

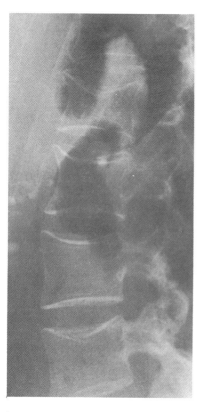

FIG. 3. Moderate osteoporotic fractures with endplate deformities of the lumbar spine due to involutional osteoporosis.

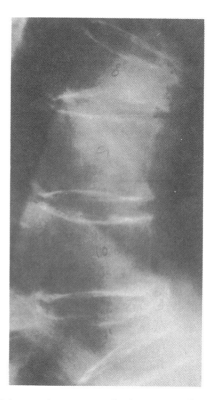

FIG. 4. Advanced osteoporotic fractures of the thoracic spine. Wedging and compression fractures have occurred as a result of involutional osteoporosis.

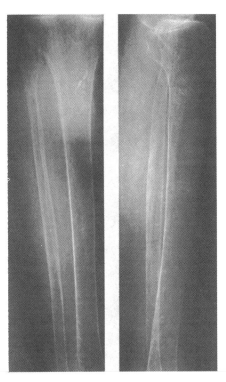

FIG. 5. Advanced involutional osteoporosis of the tibia and fibula producing marked thinning of the cortices due to chronic endosteal resorption and widening of the medullary space.

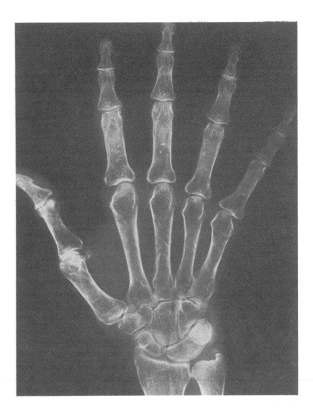

FIG. 6. High-resolution radiographs of a proximal phalanx showing endosteal scalloping and intracortical striation, indicating aggressive bone resorption in a recently (2 years previously) oophorectomized woman.

vertebral bodies are also found, and the condition should be distinguished from juvenile epiphysitis, or Scheuermann's disease (Fig. 13). Although fractures may be seen in the diaphysis of long bones, they occur more characteristically at the metaphysis. Presumably this is because the bony abnormality is more evident at sites of active bone turnover. Slipped capital femoral epiphyses may be seen.

The disorder is usually self-limited; however, if a large amount of osseous tissue is lost, the radiographic appearance may not return to normal. Laboratory values are typically normal, and diagnosis is made by exclusion.

SECONDARY OSTEOPOROSIS

Cushing's Disease (Endogenous and Exogenous)

Cushing's disease (7,13,15–20) is the result of an excess of adrenocortical steroids. This excess may be endogenous or exogenous. Endogenous Cushing's disease is caused by adrenal hyperplasia in the vast majority of cases, with other less frequent causes being tumors of the adrenal and pituitary glands. Exogenous Cushing's disease results from excessive corticosteroid medication and is far more common than the endogenous form.

Radiologic-Pathologic Considerations

As in osteoporosis, the equilibrium between bone formation and bone resorption is disrupted such that resorption

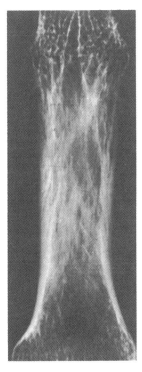

FIG. 7. Advanced involutional osteoporosis with generalized cortical thinning and uniform trabecular resorption.

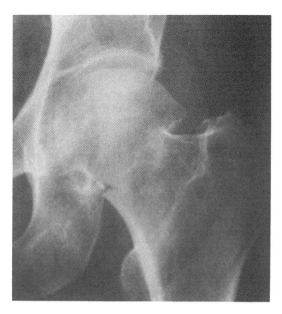

FIG. 8. Femoral neck fracture with mild valgus impaction in a patient with involutional osteoporosis.

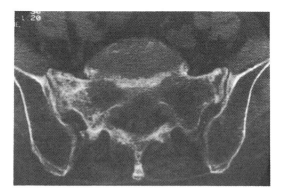

FIG. 10. Insufficiency fractures of the sacral ala due to advanced involutional osteoporosis.

predominates. Thus, the typical findings of osteoporosis are seen. Wedge, biconcave, and compression fractures are also seen. Histologically, exuberant endosteal callus formation is seen in compressed vertebrae and is manifested radiographically by increased density in the bony tissue adjacent to the vertebral endplate, referred to as "marginal condensation" (Fig. 14). This excessive callus formation is also evident in fractures involving other bones, including the ribs (which are commonly fractured in Cushing's disease).

Additional findings sometimes seen in Cushing's disease include a mottled appearance of the skull secondary to osteoporotic involvement. Osteonecrosis, particularly of the femoral heads (Fig. 15), is not uncommon in cases of exogenous steroid administration but occurs infrequently in the endogenous cases, for unknown reasons (7,21,22). Other less common findings seen only in exogenous Cushing's disease are joint infections, neuropathic-like joints, tendon rupture, delayed skeletal maturation, and decreased osteophyte formation (13,18).

Osteomalacia

Osteomalacia (13,23,24) is characterized by defective mineralization of osteoid in mature cortical and cancellous bone. It is a general term describing similar histopathologic and radiologic changes as are seen in a large group of diverse disorders. The etiology of osteomalacia in these disorders is also diverse, and may or may not be the result of a defect in vitamin D metabolism.

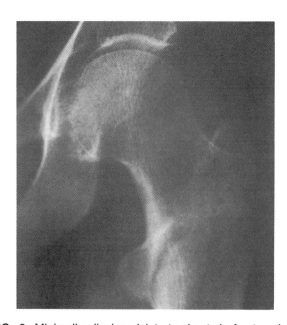

FIG. 9. Minimally displaced intertrochanteric fracture in a patient with late involutional osteoporosis.

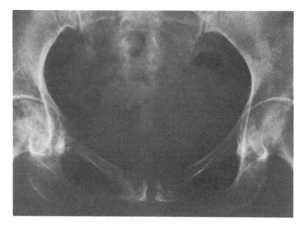

FIG. 11. Pelvic ring insufficiency fractures of the right pubic and ischial bones in a patient with involutional osteoporosis. Irregular resorption and reactive callus simulate a neoplastic process.

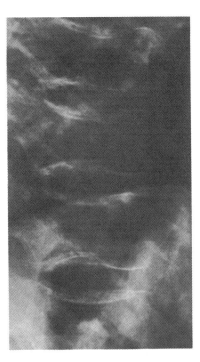

FIG. 12. Advanced idiopathic juvenile osteoporosis with biconcave vertebral deformities.

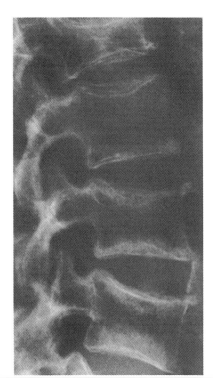

FIG. 14. Exogenous Cushing's disease. A lateral view of the lumbar spine demonstrates osteoporosis and biconcave vertebral bodies. The increased density adjacent to the vertebral endplates, called "marginal condensation," is the result of exuberant endosteal callus formation.

Radiologic-Pathologic Considerations

The primary abnormality in osteomalacia is the presence of excessive amounts of inadequately mineralized osteoid. This material is seen coating the trabeculae and thus accounts for the "fuzzy" appearance of these structures.

Focal accumulations of osteoid are seen to occur in compact bone at right angles to the long axis. Radiographically,

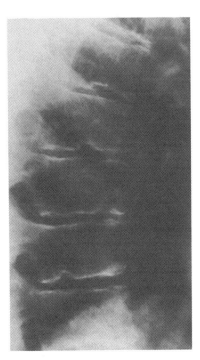

FIG. 13. Scheuermann's disease or juvenile epiphysitis with multiple discrete Schmorl's nodes and mild wedge deformities in the thoracic spine.

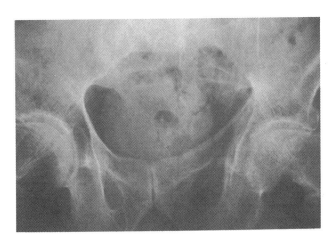

FIG. 15. Advanced osteomalacia showing generalized osteopenia, with bending deformities of the proximal femurs accompanied by medial pseudofractures of the femoral necks.

these are known as *Looser zones* or pseudofractures and are a distinguishing sign of osteomalacia, although they may occur in Paget's disease and, rarely, in simple osteoporosis (25). The exact etiology of Looser zones is unclear, although they probably represent partial insufficiency fractures. They are often symmetrical in distribution and are principally seen in the pubic rami, femoral necks (Fig. 15), scapulae, ribs, long bones, and metatarsals. Although they may remain unchanged for months or even years, true fractures may develop in these areas because they represent an area of weakened bone.

Intracortical bone resorption or cortical tunneling is observed in the tubular and long bones. High-resolution magnification techniques demonstrate these findings in the phalanges and metacarpals as a manifestation of the frequently associated secondary hyperparathyroidism (Fig. 16A). Intracortical resorption or tunneling is the most sensitive, although nonspecific, radiographic abnormality in osteomalacia, far more common than radiographic pseudofractures.

Radiologic thinning and loss of secondary trabeculae occur, resulting in decreased bone density and a coarsened appearance of the trabecular pattern, especially in the spine (Fig. 16B). Overall, the bones lose intrinsic strength, and bowing of long bones may occur. Scoliosis occasionally develops, and the vertebral bodies may assume a biconcave appearance (Fig. 17). Bone "softening" in other areas of the body may result in basilar invagination, protrusio acetabuli, and a triradiate appearance of the pelvis (13,24) (Fig. 15).

In some disorders causing osteomalacia, such as those associated with renal osteodystrophy, the massive amounts of osteoid present in the bones can become partially mineralized, typically in the presence of severe secondary hyperparathyroidism with a high serum calcium-phosphorus product. This results in increased bone density, particularly in the spine, giving the "rugger jersey" appearance (26,27) (Fig. 18). The exact mechanism of osteosclerosis in renal osteodystrophy, however, remains unclear.

Rickets

Like the term osteomalacia, rickets (13,24,28) is a general term used to describe the histopathologic and radiologic changes resulting from a group of diverse disorders. The final common pathway of these disorders is a loss of orderly maturation and mineralization of cartilage cells at the growth plate, resulting in similar pathologic and radiologic changes. Rickets represents osteomalacia in the growing skeleton.

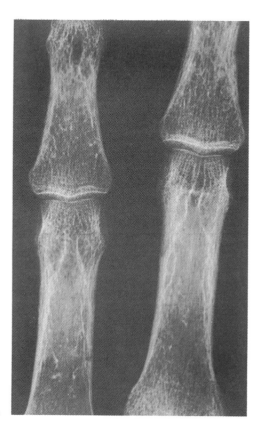
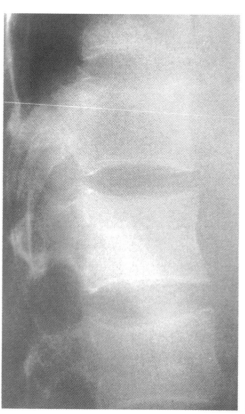

A

B

FIG. 16. Osteomalacia secondary to intestinal malabsorption. **A:** High-resolution radiograph of the hand demonstrates osteopenia accompanied by increased intracortical tunneling due to associated secondary hyperparathyroidism. **B:** Lateral view of the spine in this patient demonstrates osteopenia with indistinct cortical and trabecular outlines. Biconcave deformities of the vertebral bodies are also evident.

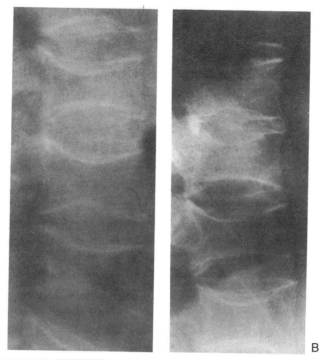

A

B

FIG. 17. Lateral views of the lumbar **(A)** and thoracic **(B)** spine in a patient with osteomalacia demonstrate moderate osteopenia involving the vertebral bodies. The trabeculae in the vertebral bodies appear indistinct, and there is evidence of bone softening with bowing of the endplates.

Radiologic-Pathologic Considerations

The radiologic findings at the physeal plate reflect the altered pathophysiology (29). The normal, ordered maturation and mineralization of cartilage cells become disrupted. This occurs predominantly in the hypertrophic zone, where the number of chondrocytes is seen to increase and the normal columnar formation of the cells is lost. There is a continued buildup of cells, resulting in the earliest radiographic finding of widening and lengthening of the growth plate (Fig. 19). Defective mineralization of the chondrocytes in the zone of provisional calcification yields the irregular metaphyseal margins seen on radiographs. Similar defective mineralization occurring in the zones of primary and secondary spongiosa produces a "frayed" appearance of the metaphyseal trabecular bone. As the cell mass in the hypertrophic zone continues to increase, it protrudes into the weakened metaphyseal region, causing cupping and widening of the metaphyses (Fig. 20). While this process is occurring on the metaphyseal side of the growth plate, similar processes are occurring on the epiphyseal side. The defective maturation and mineralization seen here result in an epiphysis that is osteopenic and has irregular, indistinct borders.

In the metaphysis and diaphysis, there is also defective mineralization of osteoid. In these areas, where mature bone is present, the radiographic findings of osteomalacia are produced.

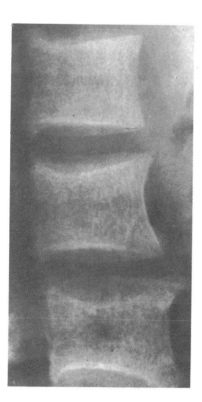

FIG. 18. Lumbar spine in renal osteodystrophy demonstrates mottled subchondral bands of sclerosis, the "rugger jersey" spine.

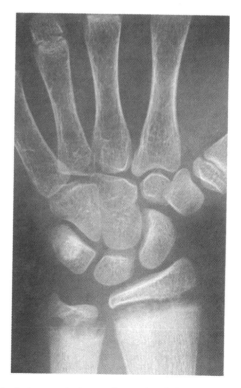

FIG. 19. Anteroposterior radiograph of the wrist in a child with rickets and osteopenia. Widening of the growth plates of the distal radius and ulna is evident. In addition, the zone of provisional calcification in both the radius and ulna is indistinct and the metaphyseal margins appear irregular. The cortices of the metacarpals are abnormally thin.

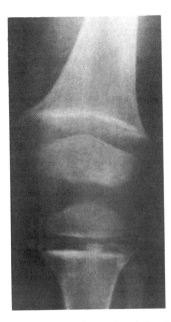

FIG. 20. Anteroposterior radiograph of the knee in rickets demonstrates diffuse osteopenia. The growth plates have widened and protrude into the weakened metaphyseal region, causing cupping and widening of the metaphyses. Note also the irregular, indistinct borders of the femoral epiphysis.

Additional radiographic findings include prominence of the growth plates at the costochondral junctions, producing the "rachitic rosary." The squared configuration of the skull seen occasionally results from excessive osteoid buildup in addition to abnormal remodeling. Because of the weakened nature of the bones, there is often bowing resulting from normal weight bearing and muscular stresses. Scoliosis, slipped capital femoral epiphyses, a triradiate configuration of the pelvis, and basilar invagination also may be seen.

Primary Hyperparathyroidism

This disorder stems from a primary defect in the parathyroid glands resulting in increased secretion of parathyroid hormone (PTH), causing an elevation of serum calcium and a reduction in serum phosphorus. The serum calcium becomes elevated, in part, by the action of PTH on bone by activation of the osteoclastic system and remodeling of osseous tissue. The resultant bony changes give the radiographic picture of primary hyperparathyroidism (13,26,30–32).

Radiologic-Pathologic Considerations

One of the effects of the elevated levels of PTH and a hallmark of this disorder is resorption of bone, or osteitis fibrosa. The resorption is believed to be the result primarily of stimulation of the osteoclast and occurs at many different sites (intracortical, endosteal, subchondral, subligamentous, and trabecular). Subperiosteal bone resorption,

which is most characteristic of hyperparathyroidism (13,31), is seen in approximately 10% of patients, most commonly on the radial aspect of the middle phalanges of the second and third digits (Fig. 21). Other sites commonly affected include the phalangeal tufts and the metaphyseal remodeling zones of the medial aspects of the proximal humerus, femur, and tibia.

Cortical striations and intracortical tunneling due to osteoclastic bone resorption (31) may be seen in more than half of the patients and are best detected in the tubular bones of the hands using magnification techniques (Fig. 22).

Erosions involving the sacroiliac joints, symphysis pubis, and ligamentous insertions; resorption of the distal or medial ends of the clavicle; and the development of "aggressive" Schmorl's nodes may all be attributed in part to subchondral resorption in these sites of high bone turnover.

In patients with primary hyperparathyroidism, the skull occasionally has a characteristic "pepper-pot" pattern, which results from trabecular resorption and remodeling of the space (13,31). Erosions of the calcaneus and inferior aspect of the distal clavicles are evidence of subligamentous resorption of these sites.

The combined effect of all these patterns of bone resorption is osteopenia in the majority of patients. Detection of this osteopenia by noninvasive bone mineral measurement becomes important for early diagnosis, as very few patients show diagnostic radiographic appearances of hyperparathyroidism on clinical presentation. Rarely, patients may demonstrate diffuse osteosclerosis (26).

Brown tumors (osteoclastomas) represent focal, bone-replacing lesions that occur most often in the metaphyses and diaphyses, though epiphyseal involvement may be seen (Fig. 23). They contain collections of giant cells that

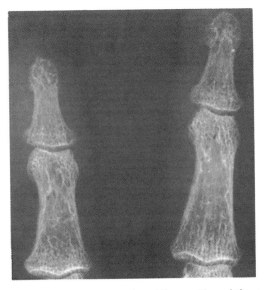

FIG. 21. Primary hyperparathyroidism with subtle subperiosteal bone resorption of the radial aspects of the middle phalanges, and irregular resorption of the tufts.

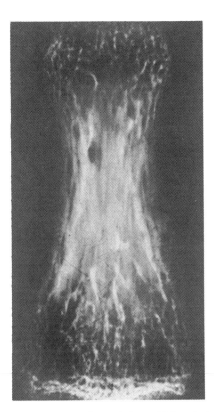

FIG. 22. High-resolution view of the middle phalanx shows marked subperiosteal and intracortical bone resorption in primary hyperparathyroidism.

are usually responsive to PTH, as the majority of lesions demonstrate healing with removal of the adenoma. They may occur as solitary lesions or involve multiple bones.

Osteogenesis Imperfecta

Osteogenesis imperfecta (13,33–35) is an inherited disorder of connective tissue that is usually transmitted in an autosomal dominant pattern. The defect in this disorder usually involves a mutation in the type I collagen gene. The classic clinical triad in this disease is (i) fragility of the bones, (ii) blue sclerae, and (iii) deafness. Two forms are recognized: the *congenita* form, in which life expectancy is usually short, and the *tarda* form, in which life expectancy is normal.

Radiologic-Pathologic Considerations

The abnormal collagen production seen in this disorder results in a primary defect in bone matrix. This and defective mineralization result in an overall loss of bone density involving both the axial and appendicular skeleton. The long bones may be either thin and gracile, as is usually the case in the tarda form, or they may be short and thick, as seen almost exclusively in the congenita form (Fig. 24). Multiple fractures (usually transverse) occur predominantly in the lower extremities, typically producing bowing deformities.

This bowing may indicate the severity of the disease, as it tends to correlate with the number of fractures. Avulsion fractures are also common.

Fracture healing is usually normal, but may demonstrate exuberant callus and pseudarthrosis. Inevitably, the extremities become shortened, which accounts in part for the short stature seen in most cases (33). Premature degenerative changes are often seen in the joints, primarily from intraarticular fractures and ligamentous laxity.

The skull and axial skeleton also show typical changes. Wormian bones (Fig. 25), enlargement of the paranasal sinuses, platybasia, and basilar impression are frequent findings. Severe kyphoscoliosis, biconcave vertebral bodies, wedge-shaped vertebral bodies, triradiate pelvis, and protrusio acetabuli may be present (Fig. 26).

Scurvy

Scurvy is the consequence of prolonged vitamin C deficiency. This deficiency causes a reduced formation of collagen and osteoid, and thus a reduced formation of bone (36,37). In contrast to rickets, calcification of the osteoid is not disturbed. Today in North America and Europe, scurvy is a rare disease that affects mainly young children and the elderly.

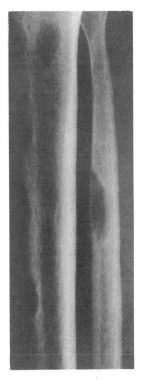

FIG. 23. Multiple brown tumors in primary hyperparathyroidism. Lateral radiograph of the leg in this patient with primary hyperparathyroidism demonstrates multiple brown tumors involving the tibia and fibula. The well-defined lytic appearance of these lesions is characteristic of brown tumors.

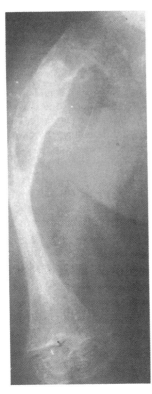

FIG. 24. Osteogenesis imperfecta (congenita form). An anteroposterior radiograph of the femur in this infant demonstrates bowing and thickening due to multiple fractures and exuberant callus formation.

Radiologic-Pathologic Considerations

In children, the decreased bone formation at the growth plates may produce characteristic radiographic findings. The zone of provisional calcification of the growth plate may be wide and dense, and therefore may be seen as a

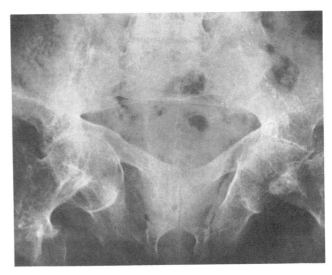

FIG. 26. A 50-year-old woman with osteogenesis imperfecta (tarda form). An anteroposterior pelvic radiograph demonstrates diffuse osteopenia. The pelvis has a triradiate configuration, and there is bilateral protrusio acetabuli.

transverse sclerotic line (white line of Frankl). Similar to the white line of Frankl, a zone of increased density may surround the ossification center in the epiphysis (Wimberger's sign). In addition to the characteristic findings at the growth plates, diffuse osteopenia and cortical thinning may be present (37,38). Elevation of the periosteum may be seen in long tubular bones of the lower extremities and generally indicates severe subperiosteal hemorrhage (Fig. 27). In adults, the radiographic signs of scurvy are less specific. These findings include diffuse osteopenia, thinned cortices, and insufficiency fractures of the spine and the appendicular skeleton.

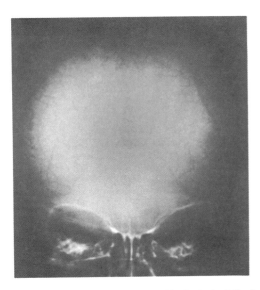

FIG. 25. Osteogenesis imperfecta. Typical skull findings in patients with osteogenesis imperfecta include numerous unfused ossification centers (wormian bones).

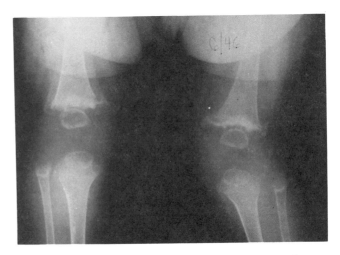

FIG. 27. Lower extremities of a child with scurvy demonstrate diffuse osteopenia, cortical thinning, transverse bands of dense calcifications adjacent to the growth plates, and periosteal new bone surrounding the diaphyses of the femur and tibia, indicating extensive subperiosteal hemorrhage.

ACKNOWLEDGMENT

Portions of this chapter have appeared in the following: Vogler JB, Genant HK: Metabolic and endocrine disease. In: Grainger RG, Allison DJ (eds) *Diagnostic Radiology—An Anglo-American Textbook of Imaging.* 2nd ed. London, Churchill Livingstone, 1992. Genant HK, Block JE: Postmenopausal and senile osteoporosis: Clinical epidemiology and detection. In: Viamonte M (ed) *Geriatric Radiology.* Baltimore, Williams & Wilkins, 1992. Genant HK, Vogler JB, Block JE: Radiology of osteoporosis. In: Riggs BL, Melton LJ (eds) *Osteoporosis: Pathogenesis, Diagnosis and Etiology.* New York, Raven Press, 1992.

REFERENCES

1. Heuck F, Schmidt E: Die quantitative Bestimmung des Mineralgehaltes des Knochens aus dem Röntgenbild. *Fortschr Röntgenstr* 93:523–554, 1960
2. Lachmann E, Whelan M: The roentgen diagnosis of osteoporosis and its limitations. *Radiology* 26:165–177, 1936
3. Virtama P: Uneven distribution of bone mineral and covering effect of non-mineralized tissue as reasons for impaired detectability of bone density from roentgenograms. *Ann Med Int Fenn* 49:57–65, 1960
4. Finsen V, Anda S: Accuracy of visually estimated bone mineralization in routine radiographs of the lower extremity. *Skeletal Radiol* 17:270–275, 1988
5. Epstein DM, Dalinka MK, Kaplan FS, Aronchick JM, Marinelli DL, Kundel HL: Observer variation in the detection of osteopenia. *Skeletal Radiol* 15:347–349, 1986
6. Williamson MR, Boyd CM, Williamson SL: Osteoporosis: Diagnosis by plain chest film versus dual photon bone densitometry. *Skeletal Radiol* 19:27–30, 1990
7. Steiner E, Jergas M, Genant HK: Radiology of osteoporosis. In: Marcus R (ed) *Osteoporosis.* San Diego, Academic Press, 1019–1054, 1995
8. Albright F: Osteoporosis. *Ann Intern Med* 27:861–882, 1947
9. Riggs BL, Melton LJ: Evidence for two distinct syndromes of involutional osteoporosis. *Am J Med* 75:899–901, 1983
10. Gallagher JC: The pathogenesis of osteoporosis. *Bone Miner* 9:215–227, 1990
11. Riggs BL, Melton LJ: Involutional osteoporosis. *N Engl J Med* 314:1676–1685, 1986
12. Parfitt MA: Morphologic basis of bone mineral measurements: Transient and steady state of effects of treatment in osteoporosis. *Miner Electrolyte Metab* 4:273–287, 1980
13. Resnick D, Niwayama G (eds): *Diagnosis of Bone and Joint Disorders.* 2nd ed. Philadelphia, WB Saunders, 1988
14. Jowsey J, Johnson KA: Juvenile osteoporosis: Bone findings in seven patients. *J Pediatr* 81:511–517, 1972
15. Bondy PK: The adrenal cortex. In: Bondy PK, Rosenberg LE (eds) *Metabolic Control and Disease.* 8th ed. Philadelphia, WB Saunders, 1427, 1980
16. Jaffe HL: *Metabolic, Degenerative and Inflammatory Diseases of Bones and Joints.* Philadelphia, Lea & Febiger, 1972
17. Sissons HA: The osteoporosis of Cushing's syndrome. *J Bone Joint Surg* 38B:418–433, 1956
18. Bockman RS, Weinerman SA: Steroid-induced osteoporosis. *Orthop Clin North Am* 21:97–107, 1990
19. Rosenberg EF: Rheumatoid arthritis, osteoporosis, and fractures related to steroid therapy. *Acta Med Scand* 162(Suppl 34):211–224, 1958
20. Curtiss PH, Clark WS, Herndon CH: Vertebral fractures resulting from cortisone and corticotropin therapy. *JAMA* 156:467–469, 1954
21. Madell SH, Freeman LM: Avascular necrosis of bone in Cushing's syndrome. *Radiology* 83:1068–1070, 1964
22. Heimann WG, Freiberger RH: Avascular necrosis of the femoral and humeral heads after high-dosage corticosteroid therapy. *N Engl J Med* 263:672–675, 1969
23. Pitt MJ: Rachitic and osteomalacic syndromes. *Radiol Clin North Am* 19:581–599, 1981
24. Steinbach HL, Noetzli M: Roentgen appearance of the skeleton in osteomalacia and rickets. *AJR* 91:955, 1964
25. Perry GM, Weinstein RS, Teitelbaum SL, Avioli LV, Fallon MD: Pseudofractures in the absence of osteomalacia. *Skeletal Radiol* 8:17–19, 1982
26. Genant HK, Baron JM, Straus FH II, Paloyan E, Jowsey J: Osteosclerosis in primary hyperparathyroidism. *Am J Med* 59:104–113, 1975
27. Sundaram M: Renal osteodystrophy. *Skeletal Radiol* 18:415–426, 1989
28. Pitt MJ: Rickets and osteomalacia are still around. *Radiol Clin North Am* 29:97–118, 1991
29. Park EA: Observations on the pathology of rickets with particular reference to the changes at the cartilage-shaft junctions of growing bones. *Bull NY Acad Med* 15:495, 1939
30. Genant HK, Heck LL, Lanzl LH, Rossmann K, Horst JV, Paloyan JE: Primary hyperparathyroidism. A comprehensive study of clinical, biochemical and radiographic manifestations. *Radiology* 109:513–524, 1973
31. Steinbach HL, Gordan GS, Eisenberg E, et al: Primary hyperparathyroidism: A correlation of roentgen, clinical and pathologic features. *AJR* 86:329–343, 1961
32. Pugh DG: Subperiosteal resorption of bone; roentgenologic manifestation of primary hyperparathyroidism and renal osteodystrophy. *AJR* 66:577–586, 1951
33. King JD, Bobechko WP: Osteogenesis imperfecta. An orthopaedic description and surgical review. *J Bone Joint Surg* 53B:72–89, 1971
34. Kivirikko KI: Collagens and their abnormalities in a wide spectrum of diseases. *Ann Med* 25:113–126, 1993
35. Sillence DO, Senn A, Danks DM: Genetic heterogeneity in osteogenesis imperfecta. *J Med Genet* 16:101–116, 1979
36. Rosenberg AE: The pathology of metabolic bone disease. *Radiol Clin North Am* 29:19–35, 1991
37. Shamash R, Laufer D, Tulchinsky V: Scurvy—a disease not only of historical interest. *Br J Oral Maxillofac Surg* 26:258–260, 1988
38. Genant HK, Vogler JB, Block JE: Radiology of osteoporosis. In: Riggs BL, Melton LJ (eds) *Osteoporosis Etiology, Diagnosis and Management.* New York, Raven Press, 181–220, 1988

SECTION IV

Clinical Aspects of Osteoporosis

IV. Introduction

Sundeep Khosla, M.D. and *Michael Kleerekoper, M.D., F.A.C.E.

*Department of Endocrinology, Mayo Clinic and Mayo Medical School, Rochester, Minnesota; and *Department of Internal Medicine,
Wayne State University School of Medicine, and Harper Hospital, Detroit Michigan*

Metabolic bone diseases can be divided into two broad categories: osteoporosis, in which there is a decrease in bone mass and microarchitectural deterioration of the skeleton, and osteomalacia, where the primary defect is in the mineralization of bone. As the names imply, in osteoporosis the bones are porous and brittle, while in osteomalacia the bones are malacic or soft, but not particularly brittle. This section follows this classification, and Chapters 9 through 22 deal with the problem of osteoporosis.

The term *osteoporosis* actually refers to a syndrome, with many causes and a number of clinical forms. Osteoporosis is generally categorized as primary or secondary, based on the absence or presence of associated medical diseases, surgical procedures, or medications known to be associated with accelerated bone loss. Describing the osteoporoses with a number of short, focused chapters has many practical advantages from the educational standpoint of this primer. However, the reader is reminded that most often patient care cannot be so neatly pigeon-holed. Thus, the chapters in the first part of this section deal separately with the different forms of primary and secondary osteoporosis, but information from several chapters may be relevant to any individual patient. Postmenopausal osteoporosis, the most common form of primary osteoporosis, is discussed in Chapters 9 through 15. These chapters review the epidemiology, pathogenesis, and prevention of this disease, including current concepts of the proper role of exercise and nutrition in preventing this disorder. Chapter 14 discusses the evaluation and management of osteoporosis. There, the reader is also referred to Chapters 7 and 8 of Section III, dealing more specifically with bone densitometry and radiology, as well as to Chapter 6 on biochemical markers of bone turnover. These earlier chapters deal more with the technical aspects of these diagnostic modalities, whereas Chapter 14 is intended to focus on the clinical evaluation of patients with osteoporosis. Because hip fracture represents a special problem and the most serious manifestation of this disease, it is dealt with separately (Chapter 15). It is also becoming clear that although osteoporosis may be more common in women, men also develop this disorder, as discussed in Chapter 18. Children and adolescents also develop an uncommon and relatively poorly understood form of primary osteoporosis, juvenile osteoporosis (Chapter 16). The remaining chapters in this part of the section deal with the secondary causes of osteoporosis, including steroid and drug-induced osteoporosis (Chapter 17) and bone loss related to excessive thyroid hormone (Chapter 19).

...demiology of Osteoporosis

...hard D. Wasnich, M.D.

...Osteoporosis Center, Honolulu, Hawaii

A ... ...oporosis as a
... ...low bone mass
... ...one tissue, leading
... ...sequent increase in
... ...hing characteristic of
... ...ollagen ratio, which dis-
... a disease characterized by
... in relation to collagen.
... prevalent metabolic bone dis-
... and other developed countries.
... ...rs to the number of people in the
... ...ven time have already had fractures
... ...osis. Vertebral fracture prevalence
... ...ed 65 has been estimated to be 27% in
N... ...nd 21% among Danish women at age 70
(3).

Incide... refers to the number of *new* fracture cases in a population within a specified time. For example, among Japanese–American women in Hawaii, 5% of 80-year-old women will experience a new vertebral fracture each year. In general, data concerning the prevalence and incidence of hip, wrist, and other nonvertebral fractures are more reliable than vertebral fracture data. That is because many vertebral fractures are not clinically evident; therefore only populations that have been surveyed by periodic spine x-rays yield accurate prevalence data.

Vertebral fracture data are further hampered by the absence of a clear radiographic definition of vertebral fracture (4).

Osteoporotic fractures increase with age; wrist fractures show a rising incidence in the 50s, vertebral fractures in the 60s, and hip fractures in the 70s (Fig. 1). There is at least a two fold higher incidence among women compared with men for all age-related fracture sites. Because life expectancy is longer for women, there are proportionately more older women than men, resulting in a greater fracture prevalence among women than would be predicted from the age-adjusted incidence ratio.

Interesting geographic and ethnic differences exist. For example, hip fracture rates are higher in white populations regardless of geographic location (5). In contrast, hip fracture rates are lower among blacks in the United States and South Africa, and also among Japanese both in Japan and in the United States (6,7).

Frequently, but not always, ethnic and geographic differences in fracture prevalence can be explained by differences in bone density. The strong relationship between diminishing bone density and the risk of fragility fractures is well established. The risk of new vertebral fractures increases by a factor of 2.0–2.4 for each standard deviation (SD) decrease of bone density, irrespective of the site of bone density measurement (8). Similar findings have been found for hip and other nonvertebral fractures. It has therefore been proposed by a World Health Organization (WHO) expert panel that women with bone density values more than 2.5 SD below the young adult mean value be considered as osteoporotic (9). If they also have one or more fragility fractures, they would be classified as severe, or established, osteoporosis. Those women with bone density values between 1 and 2.5 SD below the young adult mean values would be classified as osteopenic.

Because surveys of bone density are easier to obtain than are accurate fracture incidence data, they may provide better estimates of osteoporosis prevalence. Based on the WHO diagnostic categories, Melton has estimated that 54% of postmenopausal white women in the United States have osteopenia, and another 30% have osteoporosis (10). Thus white women alone account for 26 million people who are at risk for fracture. The addition of men and nonwhite women would increase the total considerably. This number compares to 30 million to 54 million Americans who have hypertension.

The aging of the world population, when combined with the exponential, age-related increases in fracture incidence, portend drastic increases in the costs of osteoporosis. Cummings et al. have estimated that the cost of hip fractures alone in the United States could reach $240 billion within 50 years (11). Although there is an increased mortality rate following both hip and vertebral fractures, the worst consequence of osteoporosis might not be the increased mortality but rather the fact that most patients must *live* with the disease for many years, with its associated loss of independence and impaired quality of life (12). This is particularly true for vertebral fractures, which begin at an earlier age than hip fractures and affect many more women and men.

RISK FACTORS

Major risk factors for osteoporosis, such as age and bone density, have been established by virtue of their direct and strong relationship to fracture incidence. These more potent risk factors might be categorized as clinical risk indicators (8). However, a majority of the suspected or established risk factors for osteoporosis are based on their relationship to bone density as a surrogate indicator of disease presence and are therefore only as valid as the surrogate indicator. This category of risk factors might be categorized as etiologic; the utility of these risk factors is more likely to be in the realm of public health than in the management of individual clinical patients.

Most risk factors fall into five major categories: age, or age-related; genetic; environmental; endogenous hormones and chronic diseases; and physical characteristics of bone (Table 1).

The relative contribution of individual risk factors is much influenced by the age at which they are expressed. For example, estrogen deficiency during the adolescent years can be catastrophic to the growing skeleton. It also has a significant impact at age 50, but for some women the impact is negligible. After age 70 or 80, estrogen deficiency

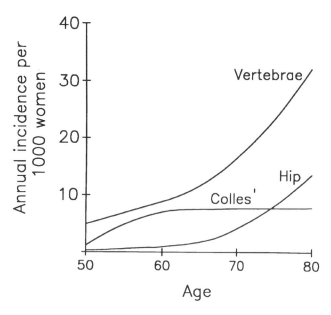

FIG. 1. Representation of the incidence rates for vertebral, Colles', and hip fractures in women.

TABLE 1. *Risk factors for osteoporosis*

Age, or Age-Related
    Each decade associated with 1.4–1.8-fold increased risk
Genetic
    Ethnicity: Caucasians and Oriental > blacks and
        Polynesians
    Gender: Female > male
    Family history
Environmental
    Nutrition; calcium deficiency
    Physical activity and mechanical loading
    Medications, e.g., corticosteroids
    Smoking
    Alcohol
    Falls (trauma)
Endogenous Hormones and Chronic Diseases
    Estrogen deficiency
    Androgen deficiency
    Chronic diseases, e.g., gastrectomy, cirrhosis,
        hyperthyroidism, hypercortisolism
Physical Characteristics of Bone
    Density (mass)
    Size and geometry
    Microarchitecture
    Composition

may be overshadowed by other risk factors. This concept is illustrated in Fig. 2. The clinical utility of bone density is derived from the fact that it is a composite, cumulative index of multiple other risk factors, both past and present, and including both genetic and lifestyle influences.

HETEROGENEITY

Because of its multifactorial etiology, it is not surprising that osteoporosis is a heterogeneous disorder. The relative contributions of age and estrogen deficiency have been emphasized in the past, but it is difficult to differentiate these two factors in most patients. It is also increasingly apparent that there are multiple, other contributing etiologies, including those that are unknown or poorly understood. Furthermore, the *predominant* etiology may vary substantially from patient to patient. Lastly, the major contribution of peak bone mass to ultimate fracture risk indicates that risk factors that are expressed during childhood

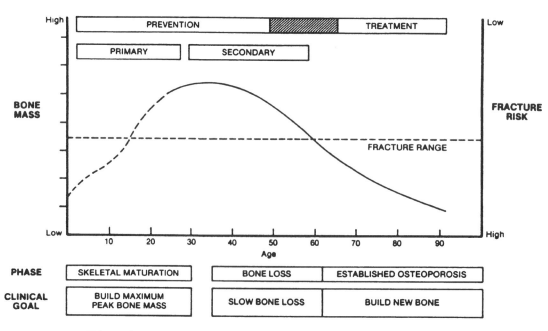

FIG. 2. Schematic lifetime representation of bone mass and fracture risk.

and adolescence may contribute as much to lifetime fracture risk as do aging and menopause. In any case, *treatable* (and preventable) etiologies are of greater clinical and public health importance, particularly if they are also common, such as low bone density.

CLINICAL IMPLICATIONS

Ultimately, knowledge gained from epidemiologic studies should influence public health practice and clinical management of individual patients. These two applications are different, and are sometimes confused, perhaps because the correct interpretation and application of epidemiologic findings to clinical practice is not always intuitively apparent. For example, estrogen deficiency following menopause is a consistently demonstrated risk factor in population studies. However, there are many women who do not show significant bone loss in the years soon after menopause, and there are a minority, perhaps 25% to 30% of women, who never experience a fracture in their lifetime. These women generally have high bone density prior to the age of menopause and/or show less bone loss after menopause. For these women, estrogen deficiency is not a major risk factor and providing estrogen replacement to these women provides no demonstrable skeletal benefit. Thus, risk factors that apply to population groups may not necessarily apply to every (or any) individual. For example, black males have an increased risk of hypertension; however, it would not be considered prudent to treat all black men for hypertension in the absence of an objective indicator of disease.

THE MEANING OF A FRACTURE

Aside from the clinical and socioeconomic consequences of a fracture, there is another, crucial implication of a fragility fracture in an individual patient. The very presence of a fracture is a potent risk factor for future fractures, independent of bone density (13,14). Although the explanation for this finding is uncertain, in the spine it may be partially explained by altered load distribution on neighboring vertebral bodies. This would also help explain why vertebral fractures tend to cluster in the midthoracic and lower thoracic/upper lumbar spine.

However, one important implication is that the clinical goal of fracture risk management should be prevention of the first fracture. Because chronologically hip fractures are usually the last fracture to occur, more emphasis should be placed on early identification of women at high fracture risk and preventive measures initiated well prior to *any* fracture.

CUMULATIVE FRACTURE RISK

The concept of lifetime fracture risk has typically been applied to populations. Thus an average 50-year-old white woman has an approximate 17% lifetime risk of hip fracture (15). However, depending on levels of bone density and other risk factors, this figure will vary substantially between individuals.

The term "remaining lifetime fracture probability" (RLFP) has been used to describe an individual's fracture risk. RLFP is calculated from age, bone density, life expectancy, and anticipated future bone loss (16). The concept of cumulative fracture risk is important when deciding whether to employ pharmacologic agents to prevent future fractures. For such clinical decisions, measures of bone density alone are insufficient; current age must also be considered. The reason is that a woman whose bone density value is −1 SD (*T* score −1.0 and therefore osteopenic) at age 80 may not benefit from drug treatment because of her limited life expectancy and future bone loss. However, a 50-year-old with a similar, but normal, bone density, say −0.9 SD (*T* score −0.9), may gain a substantial benefit from drug intervention.

For this reason, the concept of RLFP may be a useful means of incorporating multiple risk factors into a single index of risk severity, which can better guide clinical decision making.

REFERENCES

1. Consensus development conference V, 1993. Diagnosis, prophylaxis, and treatment of osteoporosis. *Am J Med* 646–650, 1994
2. Melton, LJ III. Epidemiology of vertebral fractures in women. *Am J Epidemiol* 129:1000–1011, 1989
3. Jensen GF, Christiansen C, Boesen J, Hegedus V, Transbol I. Epidemiology of postmenopausal spinal and long bone fractures. *Clin Orthop* 166:75–81, 1982
4. Cooper C, O' Neill T, Silman A, on behalf of the European Vertebral Osteoporosis Study Group. *Bone* 14:589–597, 1993
5. Melton LJ, Riggs BL: Epidemiology of age-related fractures. In: Avioli LV (eds) *The Osteoporotic Syndrome: Detection, Prevention, and Treatment.* Grune and Stratton, New York, 45–72, 1983
6. Solomon L. Osteoporosis and fracture of the femoral neck in the South African Bantu. *J Bone Joint Surg* 50:B2–13, 1968
7. Ross PD, Norimatsu H, Davis JW, et al: A comparison of hip fracture incidence among native Japanese, Japanese-Americans, and American-Caucasians. *Am J Epidemiol* 133:801–809, 1991
8. Wasnich R. Bone mass measurement: prediction of risk. *Am J Med* 95:65–105, 1993
9. Kanis JA, Melton LJ III, Christiansen C, Johnston CC, Khaltaev N. The diagnosis of Osteoporosis. *J Bone Min Res* 9:1137–1141, 1994
10. Melton LJ III. How many women have osteoporosis now? *J Bone Miner Res* 10:175–177, 1995
11. Cummings SR, Rubin SM, Black D. The future of hip fractures in the United States. *Clin Orthop* 252:163–166, 1990
12. Barrett-Connor E. The economics and human costs of osteoporotic fracture. *Am J Med* 98:3–8, 1995
13. Ross PD, Davis JW, Epstein R, Wasnich RD. Pre-existing fractures and bone mass predict vertebral fracture incidence in women. *Ann Intern Med* 114:919–923, 1991
14. Wasnich RD, Davis JW, Ross PD. Spine fracture risk is predicted by non-spine fractures. *Ost Int* 4:1–5, 1995
15. Black D, Cummings S, Melton LJ. Appendicular bone mineral and a woman's lifetime risk of hip fracture. *J Bone Min Res* 7:639–646, 1992
16. Wasnich RD, Ross PD, Vogel JM, Davis JW. *Osteoporosis. Critique and Practicum.* Banyan Press, Honolulu, 1989

10. Pathogenesis of Postmenopausal Osteoporosis

Robert P. Heaney, M.D., F.A.C.P., F.A.I.N.

Creighton University, Omaha, Nebraska

Osteoporosis is defined elsewhere in this volume as a condition of skeletal fragility characterized by reduced bone mass and microarchitectural deterioration of bone tissue, with a consequent increase in risk of fracture. Decreased bone mass is thus visualized as a risk factor for fracture. The term osteoporosis is also used to designate a bone mass value more than 2.5 standard deviations below the young adult mean. Osteoporosis thus designates both one of the risk factors for fragility and the fragility condition itself. It is in this way analogous to hypertension, in which the term designates both the blood pressure level and the condition of increased risk of untoward vascular events.

It is useful to see both sides of this ambivalent definition because ultimately pathogenesis of osteoporosis involves the development not just of low bone mass but of the other causes of bony fragility as well. The interplay of the multiplicity of causal factors is illustrated well in Fig. 1, which sets forth age-specific fracture risk gradients for various values of forearm bone mass density (BMD). Three features stand out: (i) risk rises with declining bone mass; (ii) risk also rises with age, even when bone mass is held constant; and (iii) the gradients are steeper with advancing age, i.e., a given deficiency of bone makes a bigger difference in an older person than in a younger one. As Fig. 1 suggests, the age effect is, if anything, larger than the bone mass effect.

What does it mean to say that age increases fracture risk? This effect is a composite of other changes that accumulate with age: falling more often, falling in such a way as to strike vulnerable bony parts, loss of soft tissue protection over bony prominences, accumulation of unremodeled fatigue damage in the bony tissue, loss of critical trabecular connectivity, and possibly other factors. The pathogenesis

of falls is neurologic and pharmacotherapeutic, and is beyond the scope of this chapter. Similarly, the loss of soft tissue mass with advancing age is a nutritional problem and is covered in the chapter devoted to that topic. That leaves three contributors to osseous fragility: decreased bone mass, accumulated fatigue damage, and loss of trabecular connectivity. We will examine first how each makes bone fragile and then in turn will touch on what is known of the pathogenesis of each of these fragility components.

Before doing so it is necessary to mention yet another pathogenetic factor, i.e., bone geometry, which also has a major effect on fracture risk. One example is hip axis length, the distance from the lateral surface of the trochanter to the inner surface of the pelvis, along the axis of the femoral neck. Short hip axis length results in an architecturally stronger structure for any given bone density (2). This is probably the reason why Japanese and other Orientals have about half the hip fracture rate of Caucasians, despite similar bone density values. Likewise, large vertebral body endplate areas result in lower spine pressure values for individuals of the same body size. Those with small vertebral bodies are thus more likely to fracture. Finally, the force sustained by a bone when struck in falling is a function of body height. Other things being equal, a tall person striking the lateral surface of the hip in falling is more likely to sustain a fracture than a short person. Such geometric factors both contribute to individual fracture risk and explain a substantial portion of the population-level variance in fracture rate. In each situation, however, the ultimate pathogenesis of the fracture is the fall and the force sustained by the bone on impact.

DECREASED BONE MASS

For a given material density and bony architecture, bone strength rises as approximately the square of structural density. Thus, any factor decreasing bone mass will of necessity weaken bone: a 30% reduction, such as is common in osteoporosis, will decrease strength by about 50%. Bone mass and density are the most obvious of the bone strength factors, and certainly the best studied. It is often said that mass is the most important factor as well, but this is probably not correct. Simulations suggest that mass explains less than half of the observed fracture risk (3), and clinical studies have demonstrated that expressed fragility (e.g., in the form of a prior vertebral fracture) is a stronger predictor of future fracture than low bone mass by itself (4). The reasons for this non-mass-related fragility will be discussed later.

Low bone mass (or density) is plainly a multifactorial condition involving (i) genetic predisposition, (ii) failure to achieve genetic potential during growth, (iii) excessive leanness, (iv) disuse, (v) gonadal hormone deficiency, (vi) inadequate calcium and vitamin D intake, (vii) lifestyle and

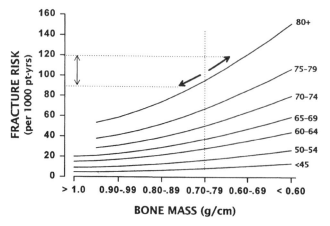

FIG. 1. Age-specific fracture risk gradients for forearm bone mineral density, redrawn from Hui et al. (1). Note that bone density declines to the right. (Copyright Robert P. Heaney, 1995. Reproduced with permission.)

medical factors (e.g., smoking, alcohol abuse, corticosteroids), (viii) remodeling errors, and (ix) miscellaneous factors. Several of these contributing causes are themselves related. For example, excessive leanness is frequently associated with both ovarian dysfunction and low calcium intake. Nevertheless, each appears to make a contribution in its own right. Most are covered in greater detail in other chapters.

Here it is necessary principally to recall that bone tissue is continually renewing itself, which means not just replacing tissue but seeking always to restore optimal mass density. This process is controlled by a classical negative feedback loop in which some cellular apparatus, most likely resident in the osteocytes, senses the degree of bending under routine loading of a part (typically on the order of 0.1% to 0.15% in any given dimension) and adjusts the local balance between bone formation and bone resorption so as to increase or decrease local bone stiffness and achieve that reference level of bending.

Failure to reach the genetic potential for bone density is most often a result of inadequate exercise and insufficient calcium intake (alone or in combination). In other words, suboptimal loading results in suboptimal stimulation of bone deposition. The result is that bone mass falls short of the genetic limit. Low calcium intake operates in a similar way: it limits how much bone density can be achieved within the envelope produced by growth and exercise (Chapter 13).

Weight is the single largest determinant of density in mature adults, explaining roughly half the population-level variance. It is not known how it operates. Almost certainly the effect involves more than just increased mechanical loading from carrying around the extra poundage, because lean mass is better correlated with bone density than is either fat mass or total body weight. The bone of heavy individuals behaves as if it had a lower setpoint for the reference level of bending under load. As a partial consequence of the increased bone density, fracture risk in obese women is about one third that of normal weight women.

By contrast, gonadal hormone loss, such as occurs in women at menopause, with anorexia nervosa or athletic amenorrhea, and gradually in aging men, appears to raise the setpoint of the bone mass regulatory system. After hormone loss, bone mass is sensed as being excessive. The relatively sharp drop across menopause is sufficient to result in remodeling carrying away about 15% of the bone over a period of 5+ years. (The quantity varies from region to region; 15% is what is typically found for the spine.) This loss is not specifically related to exercise or diet and would stop at the 15% quantum if diet and exercise were adequate. However, calcium requirement rises with age, food intake falls, and exercise usually decreases as well. As a result, bone loss typically continues and even accelerates with advancing age.

Smoking and alcohol abuse affect bone in uncertain ways. Alcohol is directly toxic to osteoblasts and is often associated with decreased calcium and vitamin D intakes and with excessive urinary loss of calcium. Calcium and vitamin D are covered in Chapter 13.

Remodeling errors are of two main types. First is excavation of overlarge haversian spaces in cortical bone. Radial

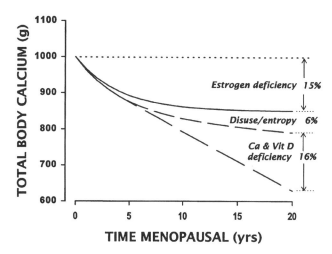

FIG. 2. Diagrammatic partition of age-related bone loss in a typical postmenopausal woman. The estrogen deficiency loss assumes no postmenopausal hormone replacement. The magnitude of the calcium deficiency loss is typical; it may be nonexistent in some individuals or substantially greater than shown in others. (Copyright Robert P. Heaney, 1991. Reproduced with permission.)

infilling is regulated by signals from the outermost osteocytes and is generally no more than 90 μM. Hence, large external diameters, which may simply occur randomly, lead to large central haversian canals, which then accumulate with age, leading to increased cortical porosity. In a similar way, osteoclast penetration of trabecular plates, or severing of trabecular beams, removes the scaffolding needed for osteoblastic replacement of resorbed bone. In both ways random remodeling errors (in addition to the other factors cited) tend to reduce both cancellous and cortical bone density and structural integrity. These remodeling errors represent a kind of entropy.

An illustrative partition of postmenopausal loss is set forth in Fig. 2, which superimposes entropic and nutritional losses on estrogen deficiency loss. The estrogen- and calcium-related losses are preventable. The entropic loss is not. Note that in the early menopausal years estrogen deficiency dominates. Note also that later, if calcium and vitamin D intakes are not adequate, nutritional loss can account, in the last analysis, for more bone loss than did menopausal estrogen loss.

BONE QUALITY AND ARCHITECTURE

We noted above that the strength of a bony structure rises roughly as the square of density, assuming constant intrinsic strength of the bony material. Here is where fatigue damage, trabecular connectedness, and other architectural factors enter into consideration. Fatigue damage weakens the material, changing its intrinsic strength, and trabecular disconnection weakens the structure. Both cause local volumes of bone to deform more under loading, thereby producing a signal greater than the reference level of bending.

Fatigue damage consists of ultramicroscopic rents in the basic bony material, resulting from the inevitable bending that occurs when a structural member is loaded. Fatigue damage is the principal cause of failure in mechanical engineering structures, and designers usually compensate by increasing the massiveness of a structure so that it bends little and thus has a larger margin of safety. Bones, by contrast, are designed to bend more and therefore have a relatively narrow margin of safety (about 2 times over peak physiologic loads). They solve the fatigue damage problem by the remodeling apparatus, which detects and removes fatigue-damaged bone. Fractures related to fatigue damage occur whenever the damage occurs faster than remodeling can repair it or whenever the remodeling apparatus is defective. March fractures and the fractures of radiation necrosis are well-recognized examples of fractures due to these two mechanisms. Fatigue damage definitely occurs in normal bone, under ordinary usage, though it is less certain as to precisely what role it may play in predisposing to osteoporotic fracture. It would, on the other hand, be surprising if bone were the only structural material known in which fatigue damage was not an important factor in failure. Furthermore, there is suggestive evidence for certain fractures (notably hip) that remodeling repair may be defective specifically at the site that ultimately fractures (5). Why remodeling surveillance or effectiveness might fail locally is not known. Nevertheless, it is clear that such failure would lead to accumulation of fatigue damage and, therefore, to local weakening of bone.

Bone structures loaded vertically, such as the vertebral bodies and femoral and tibial metaphyses, derive a substantial portion of their structural strength from a system of horizontal, cross-bracing trabeculae, which support the vertical elements and limit lateral bowing and consequent snapping under vertical loading. Severance of such trabecular connections is known to occur preferentially in postmenopausal women (6) and is considered to be a major reason for the large female/male preponderance of vertebral osteoporosis. That long, unsupported vertical trabeculae are susceptible to

fracture is reflected in the extraordinarily high prevalence of trabecular fracture callus sites in vertebral bodies examined at autopsy—typically 200–450 healing or healed fractures per vertebral body. While many of these will be well-enough healed at any given time to be structurally competent, others will be fresh and structurally weak. Such fractures are asymptomatic and their accumulation both reflects the impact of lost trabecular connections and greatly weakens the cancellous structure of the vertebral body. The incident fracture prediction ability of prior vertebral fractures (4) is probably due in part to the presence of such otherwise undetected trabecular defects. That is why prior fracture seems to predict future fracture even when bone density is relatively high. The reason for preferential osteoclastic severance of horizontal trabeculae is not known. It is sometimes attributed to overaggressive osteoclastic resorption, but that seems more descriptive than explanatory.

REFERENCES

1. Hui SL, Slemenda CW, Johnston CC Jr. Age and bone mass as predictors of fracture in a prospective study. *J Clin Invest* 81: 1804–1809, 1988
2. Faulkner KG, Cummings SR, Black D, Palermo L, Glüer C-C, Genant HK. Simple measurement of femoral geometry predicts hip fracture: the study of osteoporotic fractures. *J Bone Min Res* 8:1211–1217, 1993
3. Heaney RP. Is there a role for bone quality in fragility fractures? *Calcif Tissue Int* 53:S3–S5, 1993
4. Ross PD, Davis JW, Epstein RS, Wasnich RD. Pre-existing fractures and bone mass predict vertebral fracture incidence in women. *Ann Intern Med* 114:919–923, 1991
5. Eventov I, Frisch B, Cohen Z, Hammel I. Osteopenia, hematopoiesis and osseous remodeling in iliac crest and femoral neck biopsies: a prospective study of 102 cases of femoral neck fractures. *Bone* 12:1–6, 1991
6. Kleerekoper M, Villanueva AR, Stanciu J, Sudhaker R, Parfitt AM. The role of three-dimensional trabecular microstructure in the pathogenesis of vertebral compression fractures. *Calcif Tissue Int* 37:594–597, 1985

11. Physical Activity and Regulation of Bone Mass

Robert Marcus, M.D.

Department of Medicine, Stanford University, and Veterans Affairs Medical Center, Palo Alto, California

The primary function of bone is to provide a strong and resilient structure that permits resistance against gravitational and other forces while providing structural rigidity for locomotion. To accommodate both requirements, bone adapts to the mechanical demands that are placed on it. This principle, known as Wolff's law, may be paraphrased to state that bone accommodates the loads imposed on it by altering its mass and distribution of mass. When habitual loading increases, bone is gained; when loading decreases, bone is lost. What appears to be optimized by this adaptive response is the distribution of load-related strain, or deformation, within bones. As an example of how effective and broadly applicable this process is, it is remarkable that when animals with diverse loading patterns engage in typical activities (running, jumping, and so forth), peak long bone strains consistently fall within a fairly narrow range of 2000–3500 microstrain (1 strain = 1% deformation; 3000 microstrain = 0.12% deformation) (1).

Habitual loading can be described as the sum of all individual daily loading events, with each event further characterized by its intensity and number of repetitions. Load magnitude seems to outweigh load repetitions as an influence on bone mass (2). The relationship between mechanical loading and bone mass is curvilinear, with a much steeper slope at very low levels of loading. Thus, the most easily demonstrable interaction between physical activity and bone mass is the substantial *loss* of bone that occurs with immobilizaton. Completely immobilized patients may lose 40% of their original bone mass in 1 year, whereas standing upright with postural shifting for 30 minutes each day may completely prevent the deleterious skeletal effects of bed rest. By contrast, the amount of bone that can be gained by active people who increase their level of exercise is very limited, accounting for only a few percent increase over a year's time.

BONE MASS IN ATHLETES

Trained athletes have higher bone mass than nonathletes (3), with the largest effect seen when the regimen includes strength training (4). Much of this literature may be confounded by the possibility that the musculoskeletal characteristics of athletes may differ from those of the general population even prior to training. This may explain why the results of exercise intervention studies have been relatively meager compared to differences reported in comparative studies. That there is certainly some skeletal effect of training emerges from the exaggerated increases in bone mineral density (BMD) that are observed in the racquet vs. the non-racquet forearms of elite tennis players (5).

PHYSICAL ACTIVITY AND BONE MASS IN NONATHLETES

A critical issue is whether the skeletal benefits enjoyed by elite athletes also extend to ordinary mortals. Bone *acquisition* by children (6), adolescents (7), and young women (8) seems clearly to reflect habitual physical activity. In contrast, a few (9,10), but certainly not all (11,12), cross-sectional studies in adults have shown a positive relationship of BMD to current or previous self-reported levels of physical activity. The validity of such studies is severely constrained by major difficulties in assessing a person's true physical activity level but is hampered even more when attempting to extrapolate rough indices of overall physical exertion to estimate skeletal loading. It may be that some of the most important daily loading events for the skeleton are not even recognized by a person who maintains an exercise record. This would be particularly true for such activities as pushing against a heavy door, lifting a box of canned goods, or some other occupational activity.

RESPONSE OF BONE TO EXERCISE

With one notable exception (13), well-controlled randomized exercise trials using strength (14–17) and endurance (15,16) activities have reported significant but modest positive effects of exercise on lumbar spine BMD of young women. Increases averaged 1% to 3% and were achieved during the first year, with few if any gains thereafter (16,17). Improvement in hip BMD was found in only one study, which continued for 2 years (17). Another study showed that strength training maintains lumbar spine BMD of recently menopausal women, but no such protection was found at other skeletal sites (18).

In older individuals, walking exercise has been correlated to BMD, but intervention studies have not found brisk walking either to increase BMD or to protect against loss (19). Some, but not all, intervention trials using resistance or mixed endurance/resistance exercise have shown significant gains in bone mass in older men and women (20–23). One intriguing report described an 8% gain in spine BMD for older women who participated in resistance exercise for 1 year and who were also taking estrogen replacement therapy (23). Other studies of older people, while not reporting significant *gains* in bone mass, do indicate that exercise may constrain the rate of bone *loss* (24).

SPECIAL ASPECTS OF EXERCISE AND BONE: AMENORRHEA, GYMNASTS, AND SWIMMERS

Optimal skeletal maintenance requires an adequate hormonal, mechanical, and nutritional milieu. Deficits in one sphere are not adequately compensated by overzealous attention to the others. Amenorrheic women athletes lose bone and have increased risk for fracture despite herculean training schedules (25,26). Despite initial views that cortical bone is spared in these women, recent data show significant deficits at all appendicular sites except the radius (27).

Competitive women gymnasts have a high prevalence of oligo- and amenorrhea. It would be expected that they would also suffer deficits in BMD. However, these athletes actually show higher than predicted BMD at all sites (28). One aspect of gymnastics training may explain this finding: whereas runners load their lumbar vertebrae with 3–5 body weights with each step, dismounting from parallel bars or other high-impact gymnastics activities gives vertebral loading of 15–20 body weights. Thus, the experience in gymnasts may provide insight to the type of mechanical loads that are most osteotrophic. By contrast, even though collegiate swimmers also participate in muscle strength training, they have lower bone mass than do other athletes or even sedentary individuals of similar age (29). This may be explained by the fact that elite swimmers spend ~25 buoyant hours per week, time taken from their possible weight bearing activity.

CONTRIBUTION OF EXERCISE TO BONE HEALTH OF OLDER PEOPLE

The modest BMD results with strength training should not trivialize the importance of exercise for protecting older people against falls. More than 90% of hip fractures follow as the immediate consequence of a fall onto the hip. Among the important risk factors for falls, muscle strength is perhaps most susceptible to improvement with strength training (30). Many older patients and their physicians ask about which exercise is best for the skeleton. One must realize that only one of five adult Americans exercises as little as once each week and that the 6-month attrition rate for people who start exercising is >50%. Thus, it serves no purpose to recommend a rigorous program to most people. Most important is to stimulate them to participate safely in any activity in a frequent, regular, and sustained manner. Therefore, for sedentary and/or frail elderly, a program of walking, low-impact or water aerobics, or other pleasant, nonthreatening, and safe activity is recommended. If after several months the patient wishes to do more rigorous activity, a referral to a physical therapy department for initiation of muscle strength exercise is warranted.

REFERENCES

1. Rubin CT, Lanyon LE: Dynamic strain similarity in vertebrates: an alternative to allometric limb bone scaling. *J Theoret Biol* 107: 321–327, 1984
2. Whalen RT, Carter DR, Steele CR: The relationship between physical activity and bone density. *Trans Orthop Res Soc 33rd Mtg* 12:464–470, 1987
3. Snow-Harter C, Marcus R: Exercise, bone mineral density, and osteoporosis. *Exercise Sport Sci Rev* 19:351–388, 1991
4. Block JE, Genant HK, Black D: Greater vertebral bone mineral mass in exercising young men. *West J Med* 145:39–42, 1992
5. Huddleston AL, Rockwell D, Kulund DN, et al: Bone mass in lifetime tennis players. *JAMA* 244:1107–1109, 1980
6. Slemenda CW, Miller JZ, Hui SL, Reister TK, Johnston CC Jr: Role of physical activity in the development of skeletal mass in children. *J Bone Min Res* 6:1227–1233, 1991
7. Ruiz JC, Mandel C, Garabedian M: Influence of spontaneous calcium intake and physical exercise on the vertebral and femoral bone mineral density of children and adolescents. *J Bone Min Res* 10:675–682, 1995
8. Recker RR, Davies KM, Hinders SM, Heaney RP, Stegman MR, Kimmel DB: Bone gain in young adult women. *JAMA* 268: 2403–2408, 1992
9. Aloia JF, Vaswani AN, Yeh JK, Cohn SH: Premenopausal bone mass is related to physical activity. *Arch Intern Med* 148:121–123, 1988
10. Snow-Harter C, Whalen R, Myburgh K, Arnaud S, Marcus R: Bone mineral density, muscle strength, and recreational exercise in men. *J Bone Min Res* 7:1291–1296, 1992
11. Sowers MR, Wallace RB, Lemke JH: Correlates of mid-radius bone density among postmenopausal women: a community study. *Am J Clin Nutr* 41:1045–1053, 1985
12. Mazess RB, Bardin HS: Bone density in premenopausal women: effects of age, dietary intake, physical activity, smoking, and birth-control pills. *Am J Clin Nutr* 53:132–142, 1991
13. Rockwell J, Sorensen A, Baker S, Leahey D, Stock J, Michaels J, Baran D: Weight training decreases vertebral bone density in premenopausal women: a prospective study. *J Clin Endocrinol Metab* 71:988–993, 1990
14. Gleeson PB, Protas EJ, LeBlanc AD, Schneider VS, Evans HJ: Effects of weight lifting on bone mineral density in premenopausal women. *J Bone Min Res* 5:153–158, 1990
15. Snow-Harter C, Bouxsein ML, Lewis BT, Carter DR, Marcus R: Effects of resistance and endurance exercise on bone mineral status of young women: a randomized exercise intervention trial. *J Bone Min Res* 7:761–769, 1992
16. Friedlander AL, Genant HK, Sadowsky S, Byl NN, Glüer C-C: A two year program of aerobics and weight training enhances bone mineral density of young women. *J Bone Min Res* 10:574–585, 1995
17. Lohman T, Going S, Pamenter R, et al: Effects of resistance training on regional and total bone mineral density in premenopausal women: a randomized prospective study. *J Bone Min Res* 10: 1015–1024, 1995
18. Pruitt LA, Jackson RD, Bartels RL, Lehnhard HJ: Weight-training effects on bone mineral density in early postmenopausal women. *J Bone Min Res* 7:179–185, 1992
19. Cavanaugh DJ, Cann CE: Brisk walking does not stop bone loss in postmenopausal women. *Bone* 9:201–204, 1988
20. Simkin A, Ayalon J, Leichter I: Increased trabecular bone density due to bone-loading exercises on postmenopausal osteoporotic women. *Calcif Tiss Int* 40:59–63, 1987
21. Dalsky G, Stocke KS, Eshani AA, et al: Weight-bearing exercise training and lumbar bone mineral content in postmenopausal women. *Ann Intern Med* 108:824–828, 1988
22. Menkes A, Mazel S, Redmond RA et al: Strength training increases regional bone mineral density and bone remodeling in middle-aged and older men. *J Appl Physiol* 74:2478–2484, 1993
23. Notelovitz M, Martin D, Tesar R, et al: Estrogen therapy and variable-resistance weight training increase bone mineral in surgically menopausal women. *J Bone Min Res* 6:583–590, 1991
24. Prince RL, Devine A, Dick I, et al: The effects of calcium supplementation (milk powder or tablets) and exercise on bone density in postmenopausal women. *J Bone Min Res* 10:1068–1075, 1995
25. Drinkwater BL, Nilson K, Chesnut CH III, Bremner WJ, Shainholtz, Southworth MB: Bone mineral content of amenorrheic and eumenorrheic athletes. *N Engl J Med* 311:277–281, 1984
26. Marcus R, Cann C, Madvig P, et al: Menstrual function and bone mass in elite women distance runners. Endocrine and metabolic features. *Ann Intern Med* 102:158–163, 1985
27. Myburgh KH, Bachrach LK, Lewis B, Kent K, Marcus R: Low

bone mineral density at axial and appendicular sites in amenor-rheic athletes. *Med Sci Sports Exerc* 25:1197–1202, 1993

28. Robinson TL, Snow-Harter C, Taaffe DR, Gillis D, Shaw J, Mar-cus R: Gymnasts exhibit higher bone mass than runners despite similar prevalence of amenorrhea. *J Bone Min Res* 10:26–35, 1995

29. Taaffe DR, Snow-Harter C, Connolly DA, Robinson TL, Brown MD, Marcus R: Differential effects of swimming versus weight-bearing activity on bone mineral status of eumenorrheic athletes. *J Bone Miner Res* 10:586–593, 1995

30. Cummings SR, Nevitt MC, Browner WS, et al: Risk factors for hip fracture in white women. *N Engl J Med* 332:767–773, 1995

12. Prevention of Osteoporosis

Robert Lindsay, Ph.D., M.B., Ch.B., F.R.C.P.

Department of Clinical Medicine, Columbia University, New York, New York; and Department of Medicine, Helen Hayes Hospital, West Haverstraw, New York

An ounce of prevention is worth more than any amount of treatment.

The definition of osteoporosis developed for the World Health Organization (WHO) is an operational one based on bone mass measurement. This definition is clearly stated to provide a diagnostic label and not necessarily provide an indication of the need for intervention. For the purposes of this chapter, "prevention" means intervention to prevent declining bone mass, irrespective of whether the patient can be classified as having osteoporosis by the WHO definition (below 2.5 standard deviation (SD) from the mean for young normal individuals). The assumption is that prevention of bone loss will reduce fracture risk the only benefit of intervention that is important to the patient. Strategies to prevent fracture in someone who already has osteoporotic fractures or to rebuild the skeleton are beyond the scope and dealt with as treatment.

The phenomenon of bone loss that precedes fractures in osteoporosis is associated in cancellous bone with disruption of the microarchitecture that includes complete loss of trabecular elements, a process that is considered mostly irreversible. It is clear, therefore, that the most efficient method of tackling these skeletal changes is by prevention. Both public health strategies and those that must be undertaken on an individual basis are important, with safety, at least as much as efficacy and low cost, determining those that might be instituted as public health priorities. Since, almost by definition, those individuals to be targeted for prevention are asymptomatic, the first priority is the identification of those at risk. Thus, the approach to osteoporosis is similar to that for hypertension or hypercholesterolemia.

IDENTIFICATION OF "AT-RISK" INDIVIDUALS

As in many other disorders of aging a large number of factors (Table 1) have been incriminated in the pathogenesis of fractures among the elderly (1). Some clearly change the onset, duration, or rate of bone loss in individuals, whereas others increase fracture risk by modifying the risk of injury. Yet others may be linked by association that is statistically significant without any demonstrable cause-and-effect relationship. A rough clinical evaluation of risk can be obtained by assessment of comparatively few such factors. The general factors include being female, Caucasian or Asian, and becoming postmenopausal (with surgical or early natural menopause probably conferring greater risk). For those fulfilling these criteria, a personal history of fracture after age 50 or a history of hip, wrist, or vertebral fracture in a first-degree relative, low-body-weight, and cigarette consumption adds to the risk (with each confer-

ring additional risk). These features can easily be obtained by history and simple physical.

Superimposed on these are of course a wide variety of factors, including chronic illness, disuse, and drugs (steroids, diuretics, thyroid hormone, gonadotropin-releasing hormone agonists, Dilantin, tetracyclines, aluminum, and methotrexate).

In general, for each patient, the more risk factors present (1) and the longer the duration of their presence, the greater the risk of future problems (1,2). For example, a 55-year-old woman (postmenopausal) who has a family history, a prior fracture, is thin, and smokes has a relative risk of further fracture that is about 16 times the average for 55-year-old postmenopausal women. Physicians can use the presence of these factors in two ways. First, they can be used to sensitize the patient and the physician to the likelihood of osteoporosis and to target these individuals for further investigation and/or treatment. Second, those risk factors that are amenable to elimination or alteration should be discussed with the patient. Many risk factors (e.g., smoking, alcohol excess, physical inactivity) also contribute to development of diseases in organ systems other than bone and should be discussed in those terms.

Practically, menopause is the most common time when evaluation of the patient for osteoporosis begins, although nutritional and lifestyle habits should be changed as early in life as possible. No combination of these risk factors can indicate skeletal status for the individual patient, although they can be used to determine fracture risk. The analogy is hypertension for which there is also a list of risk factors, but no assemblage of these predicts an individual patient's blood pressure (although they may be predictive of risk of stroke). Nevertheless, risk factor review is a useful "initial" approach to the patient.

Skeletal Status

The best-documented risk factor to date is skeletal status. While on a population basis both the starting bone mass and the subsequent rate of loss of bone tissue must contribute to risk of fracture, for any individual we usually use bone mass at the time of consultation as the principal determinant of fracture risk. Fracture prevalence and incidence have been shown to be greater in those with low bone mass at any age and several studies indicate that low bone mass is predictive of an increased fracture risk (3,4). This suggests that a single measurement of bone mass will provide information that can be used clinically to determine risk of osteoporosis. Because hip measurements provide the best estimate of the most important osteoporotic fractures (hip and spine), this site is preferred if available. When required clinically, however, most would agree that any measurement is better than none. For a complete review of the techniques available for bone mass measurement, the reader is referred to Chapter 7. The clinician should learn the use of the techniques available in his or her area. The analogies in clinical practice are the measurement of blood pressure as a risk assessment for cerebrovascular accident, cholesterol, or lipoprotein fractionation as risk factors for coronary heart disease.

There is no absolute value of bone mass that indicates a need for treatment. Rather such information should be added to the entire clinical profile of any individual to establish the requirement to intervene. The presence of one or more risk factors would, for example, influence the decision to treat, as would the benefits, risks, and cost of intervention.

CLINICAL PROTOCOL

Prevention of bone loss in asymptomatic women is generally achieved using two complementary approaches: behavior modification (public health approach) and pharmacologic intervention. Again, this is similar to the management of hypertension and hypercholesterolemia.

The initial approach to the patient is based on modification of the risk factor profile. Elimination of secondary causes of osteoporosis is a mandatory part of this initial evaluation (Chapters 17, 19, 20, and 22). For prevention of primary (postmenopausal) osteoporosis, alterations in nutrition and lifestyle form the preliminary approach, on the assumption that a reduction in risk factor profile will be beneficial. Reductions in alcohol consumption and elimination of cigarette use are amenable to intervention and these measures are particularly beneficial to the patient's general health.

Calcium Supplementation

Although calcium is a nutrient and adequate intake should be obtained from nutritional sources (5), in practice it is difficult for many people to achieve a dietary intake >800 mg/day (the current recommended daily allowance). Self-

TABLE 1. *Proposed risk factors for osteoporosis*

Genetic
    Race
    Sex
    Familial prevalence
Nutritional
    Low calcium intake
    High alcohol
    High caffeine
    High sodium
    High animal protein
Lifestyle
    Cigarette use
    Low physical activity
Endocrine
    Menopausal age (oophorectomy)
    Obesity

imposed calorie restrictions and the avoidance of cholesterol results in limitation of dairy produce, the major source of dietary calcium in the Western world. Other sources of calcium include green vegetables, nuts, and certain fish. Bioavailability of calcium from foods is ~30%, with only calcium in spinach being unavailable for absorption.

In providing advice about calcium intake the intent is to ensure that the majority of the population obtain sufficient calcium to maintain calcium balance. Recommendations include an intake of 800 mg until age 10; 1200 mg during adolescence; and 1000 mg thereafter, increasing to 1200 mg during pregnancy and lactation, and 1500 mg if at increased risk of osteoporosis or if over age 65 (6). To achieve such intakes, it is commonly necessary to resort to calcium supplementation. Most individuals require only 500–1000 mg/day as a supplement to dietary sources to realize these intakes.

There are many forms of calcium available as supplement, and the advice to the patient should be as simple as possible. First, it is important that the calcium be bioavailable. Some studies suggest that name brands are in general more soluble than generic varieties, although most of the latter are clearly adequate. Because calcium absorption is better in an acid environment for the carbonate, we recommend that the supplement be taken with food (for carbonate), although there is a school of thought that argues for the supplement to be taken at night to reduce the proposed nocturnal surge in bone resorption. The addition of a modest calcium supplement to each meal is a regimen to which the patient can easily adhere. Both calcium carbonate and citrate offer the highest calcium content per unit tablet weight (40% and 30%, respectively). Absorption of calcium as the citrate is slightly more efficient and not dependent on gastric acidity. However, this may not be biologically important for most patients, and citrate is generally more expensive.

At the recommended dietary intakes, calcium supplementation is virtually free of side effects. If eructation, intestinal colic, and constipation occur with the carbonate, then citrate is a useful alternative. Care should be taken in prescribing calcium supplements to patients with a history of renal stones. If urine calcium excretion is not increased, the citrate salt may be used.

Several clinical trials have demonstrated the effect of calcium supplementation on bone mass. In general, the results confirm a weak "antiresorptive" effect with some prevention of loss. The effects are most obvious in the elderly but can be seen in some premenopausal populations. The effect is more modest in the years immediately following menopause, when estrogen loss is driving bone loss. The consequences of an adequate calcium intake are reductions in the risk of fracture that are modest but consistent. The modest effectiveness, inexpensiveness, freedom from side effects, and prevalence of inadequate intake all argue for increased calcium intake as a public health measure.

Vitamin D

Some studies indicate a modest effect of supplemental vitamin D on bone mass in at-risk populations, such as the elderly, the institutionalized, and those with disorders likely to impair vitamin D supply or metabolism. Intakes of 400–800 U/day of vitamin D_3 are easy to obtain (many multivitamin preparations have 400 U of D) and are safe. High doses (>1000 U/day) are not recommended. The effect of vitamin D supplementation by itself on fracture frequency is not known, as it is usually supplied with calcium and combinations have been shown to reduce the risk of hip fracture. Vitamin D metabolites and analogs are currently not recommended for prevention of osteoporosis.

Physical Activity

It has long been assumed that adequate physical activity is associated with the prevention of osteoporotic fractures, but the evidence is sparse, largely because of the difficulty in conducting good-quality controlled trials in this area. There is no doubt that at the extremes of activity effects on bone and fracture are evident, but it is within the range of normal activity that the doubts persist. However, because physical activity is associated with a number of health benefits and well-being, it remains an important feature of osteoporosis prevention.

Changing the pattern of physical activity may be difficult, especially for patients who are less positively motivated. This is especially true when discussing prevention with patients, who are, by definition, asymptomatic. Most of the patients seen in our clinic are at a relatively low level of fitness and may require formal cardiovascular evaluation before beginning an exercise program. We suggest that the exercise activity chosen be fun to improve compliance. In the absence of proven benefit for any specific exercise for prevention of osteoporosis, any weight-bearing activity suffices (6). Recreational therapy, which has a social component, may serve to improve patient compliance. However, even simple activities such as walking are useful and can be added to the daily routine with minimal difficulty. Back-strengthening exercise is probably also of value, and patients may be referred to a trainer for specific instructions because there may be limitations of exercises that force spinal flexion. In addition to any potential beneficial effects on the skeleton, continued activity in patients' daily lives reduces the risk of falls, trauma from falls, and fracture.

Pharmacologic Therapy to Prevent Bone Loss

A considerable body of data supports the concept that estrogen administration to postmenopausal women reduces skeletal turnover and reduces the rate of bone loss (7). Epidemiologic data indicate that estrogen use is associated with a reduction in the risk of fracture, especially fractures of the hip and wrist (Colles' fracture). Risk reduction averaged over several studies appears to be on the order of 50%. For vertebral fractures the interpretation of the few prospective data available suggest that estrogens also reduce the risk of vertebral fracture by as much as 75%.

Several general guidelines can be given for the use of estrogen for this indication. Because estrogens primarily reduce the rate of bone loss, the earlier therapy is begun, the more likely the bone mass and structure will be preserved.

However, recent data suggest that estrogen therapy reduces the rate of bone loss in estrogen-deficient women independent of age, with reduction in bone loss among older individuals, at least up to the eighth decade (8). The minimum effective dose of estrogen for most individuals is 0.625 mg conjugated equine estrogen or its equivalent (9). Efficacy has been demonstrated for several other estrogens, including estradiol and estrone sulfate. It is also apparent that the route of administration is not important, and several studies have demonstrated that transdermal estrogen is effective (10).

The effects of estrogen continue for as long as treatment is provided, whereas bone loss ensues when treatment is discontinued at a rate comparable to the rate of bone loss that occurs immediately after ovariectomy. Prospective controlled clinical trials have confirmed the long-term efficacy of estrogen for bone loss prevention for at least 10 years. It appears, however, that long-term administration—possibly lifelong—is required to reduce fracture risk, perhaps because of the bone loss that occurs when treatment is stopped (11).

Practical Aspects of Estrogen Administration

Although menopausal symptoms remain the most frequent indication for estrogen therapy, prevention of osteoporosis is becoming a more widely recognized indication for therapy for postmenopausal women. Treatment of menopause is accompanied by an excellent symptomatic response to therapy. For control of bone loss, however, the majority of patients are in the asymptomatic phase of bone loss. The physician always faces problems of acceptance and compliance in providing therapy for an asymptomatic phase of a disease whether it be hypertension, hypercholesterolemia, or osteoporosis. The epidemiologic data that indicate that estrogens may reduce the risk of ischemic heart disease add another benefit for estrogen use. The more recent suggestion that estrogens improve cognitive function and reduce the risk of Alzheimer's disease among aging women is preliminary and requires more detailed study. The potential complications of endometrial and breast malignancies must also be discussed with each patient.

When the patient presents for an assessment of the risk of osteoporosis we begin with evaluation of the risk factors. The presence of enough risk factors may be sufficient to precipitate both patient and physician into treatment, especially above 60 years of age where there is more imminent risk of fracture. For most individuals, when therapy is being considered specifically for osteoporosis prevention a bone mass measurement should be performed. This allows determination of the future risk of fracture for the individual patient. The lower the bone mineral density, the greater the likelihood that therapy is required. The level of bone mass that requires intervention varies with age and the presence or absence of risk factors. Nomograms that allow treatment decisions based on age, Z or T scores, and risk factors are being developed at present. However, when bone mass falls into the diagnostic range for osteoporosis, after evaluation for secondary causes of bone loss, treatment with hormone replacement therapy should be considered. When bone mass is above this level, a wait-and-see approach can be proposed, especially for younger individuals with no risk factors. With increasing age and presence of risk factors a more aggressive approach can be recommended.

In our clinic we include a discussion about the other effects of estrogen. Estrogens, given unopposed by progestins, increase the risk of endometrial hyperplasia and carcinoma. There is more doubt about the effect of estrogen on breast cancer, but long-term therapy (>15 years) may increase the risk slightly (10% to 30%) (12). On the other hand, estrogens alleviate menopausal symptoms, improve urogenital atrophy, and appear to reduce the risk of ischemic heart disease by as much as 50% (13). In addition, they may reduce the risk of thrombotic stroke modestly, and more recently have been suggested to reduce the risk of Alzheimer's disease. Estrogens have been associated with improved overall mortality. Thus, the implications of estrogen use are considerably more complex than simply effects on the skeleton.

The specific protocol for estrogen use remains a subject of considerable discussion and controversy. Some general recommendations can be made. All patients should have a mammography and be taught breast self-examination before therapy is initiated. The schedule for mammography in this age range should be based on the National Cancer Institute's guidelines and be independent of the decision to treat, but treatment certainly mandates it. If the patient has gone through a natural menopause and still has her uterus, combination or sequential therapy with a progestin is used to protect the endometrium (14). There is no rationale at present for progestin in patients who have undergone hysterectomy. There is no evidence that addition of a progestin will negatively impact on the estrogen effect on the skeleton. One study using norethindrone acetate, a 19-nortestosterone derivative, suggested that there may be an additive effect when given along with estrogens (15). For younger women just after menopause, we favor a sequential regimen. Estrogen is given every day, with rest periods at the end of each month only for those who have significant mastalgia with therapy, whereas the progestin is given from the first of each calendar month for at least 12 days (2 weeks is often simpler). Most patients will have some endometrial shedding, which may be fairly light, between the 11th and 21st of each month (16). Recurrent bleeding not on that schedule requires investigation. The progestin dose should be the minimum required for endometrial protection. For medroxyprogesterone acetate, the most commonly used progestin in the United States, 5 mg/day is the minimum, but it must be increased to 10 mg if bleeding is out of schedule. Norethindrone is available in 5 mg tablets in the United States, but this is an excessive dose. If there are symptoms with medroxyprogesterone acetate, norethindrone [one-half tablet a day (2.5 mg)] may be tried, or two tablets a day of a progestin only oral contraceptive containing 0.35 mg norethindrone per tablet. The latter is an expensive regimen even when used for only 2 weeks each month. The estrogen dose required to reduce bone loss in most individuals is 0.625 mg conjugated equine estrogen or its equivalent (9). The 0.05-mg estradiol patch also appears sufficient (10). Because some patients will continue to lose bone on these doses (perhaps as much as 5% to 15%), measurement of bone mass after 1 year with the highly precise dual-energy x-ray

absorptionmetry (DXA) technique may be advantageous. It is not clear if those individuals who lose bone on estrogen therapy are nonresponders or partial responders who will subsequently respond to an increase in the daily dose.

Older women and those who wish to avoid monthly vaginal bleeding may consider a combined continuous regimen. In this regimen the estrogen and progestin are both given each day of the month. The estrogen dose is similar to that recommended above, but the progestin dose may be reduced by half. This regimen is associated with some irregular, unheralded bleeding in the first 2–6 months of treatment in ~50% of patients, but close to 80% will become amenorrheic thereafter. Because the early bleeding is often light and may just be spotting, many patients will suffer this temporary inconvenience in return for the promise of no further bleeding. Long-term endometrial safety data using the combined regimen are sparse.

Side effects of therapy include occasional weight gain and, rarely, an idiosyncratic increase in blood pressure. Therefore, blood pressure should be measured in all patients after 3 months of therapy. Progestin side effects include irritability and mood swings, often described as being premenstrual, which may become sufficiently troublesome to require the progestin dose to be reduced to the minimum. Increased risks of deep vein thrombosis and gallstones are recorded as side effects but rarely seen. The relationship between estrogen use and breast cancer has been outlined above.

For prevention of osteoporosis, treatment should be continued for as long as feasible, at least 5–10 years, and possibly lifelong. As a practical issue we review each patient on at least an annual basis and evaluate with her the benefits and her concerns regarding treatment. Modifications can be made at this time. We now use repeat measurements of bone mass by DXA to monitor patients to ensure that bone loss is not progressing. This can also be used as an aid to compliance, which is notably poor with estrogens, primarily because of bleeding and the perceived risk of cancer. An alternative to bone mass measurement is to measure the biochemical indices of bone remodeling before and at some time, often 3 months, after the institution of treatment. Estrogens are associated with a reduction in alkaline phosphatase (especially the bone-specific isoenzyme), osteocalcin, and urinary hydroxyproline, deoxypyridinoline, and pyridinoline crosslinks (17). A biochemical response usually indicates a skeletal response but may not be absolutely predictive.

The high rate of poor compliance noted by some authors appears most often associated with failure to educate the patient adequately about the expected results of therapy and the potential problems. In practice, once patients are established on therapy for 6 months to 1 year, they usually are comfortable remaining on treatment for many years thereafter.

The main contraindication to estrogen therapy is the presence or history of an estrogen-dependent tumor, especially breast malignancy. Other relative contraindications include undiagnosed vaginal bleeding, a prior history of endometrial malignancy (3 years posthysterectomy), active thromboembolic disease, and grossly abnormal liver or renal function. Hypertension and diabetes are not contraindications but must be controlled before therapy is begun.

Alternatives to Estrogen

Calcitonin

Salmon calcitonin is a Food and Drug Administration (FDA)–approved alternative to estrogen for the treatment but not prevention of osteoporosis (17). Salmon calcitonin can be delivered by an intranasal spray, which obviates the problems of parenteral administration. The indication for its use is osteoporosis as a second-line therapy for those who cannot or should not take estrogens. The recommended dose is 200 U/day as a single nasal administration (18). However, larger doses may be required for prevention, especially in the immediate postmenopausal period (probably 400 U/day). Controlled data documenting the effect of calcitonin on fractures are somewhat sparse. Side effects of nasal administration are usually mild with local nasal irritation being the most frequent. Flushing and nausea are more usually associated with parenteral administration but may occur especially with higher doses by intranasal route. With long-term use antibody formation occurs in a significant proportion of patients and has been suggested to be responsible for reduced long-term efficacy, although with no definitive proof that this is so. The major advantages to calcitonin are its safety, its specificity to bone, and the fact that it can be used in male patients.

Bisphosphonates

These agents are derivatives of pyrophosphate but are not metabolized by the body (19). The bisphosphonates are potent inhibitors of bone remodeling; however, the mode of action of these drugs is still not entirely clear, and each of the bisphosphonates may affect remodeling with subtle but important differences. The agents appear to be well tolerated and to date are without significant side effects, apart from upper gastrointestinal distress that is related to their irritant effect on the mucosa, and some generalized aches that occur in some individuals in the early weeks of treatment. The major advantages of bisphosphonates include the oral route of administration and their specificity for the skeleton. One bisphosphonate, alendronate, is approved by the FDA for treatment of osteoporosis (designated in the package insert as a *T* score below –2.0), but not prevention. Clinical trials suggest a reduction in the risk of vertebral fracture of 48% and a 30% (20) reduction in the risk of peripheral fractures, although the latter was not statistically significant. Because of their ease of use and their low level of side effects, bisphosphonates may become important therapies in the prevention of osteoporosis of all types. The concerns with these agents is their poor intestinal absorption (generally less than 1% of ingested dose) and their long residence time in bone. Long-term data will be required to determine if the latter is problematic. The former requires dosing on an empty stomach. The recommendations for alendronate dosing are that it should be given first thing in the morning with 6–8 ounces of water (not coffee or juice) and that a minimum of one-half hour be allowed before any additional food or drink is taken. The recommended dose is 10 mg/day.

Since both calcitonin and bisphosphonates are agents that affect the skeleton specifically and are more expensive than estrogens (cost of drug), guidelines for their use differ, and both at present should probably be reserved for the highest risk groups.

Certain progestins by themselves appear to have bone-sparing effects but are unlikely to be used in prevention. The addition of a progestin to estrogen, as previously noted, does not negatively impact on the skeletal effect of the estrogen, and certain progestins may enhance the bone-sparing effects of estrogens (15). For postmenopausal patients with a history of breast cancer, there is some evidence that the so-called antiestrogen tamoxifen in doses usually used to prevent cancer recurrence (20–30 mg/day) (20,21) may reduce the rate of bone loss and prevent osteoporosis, a potentially serious problem for this group of patients. Tamoxifen is not FDA-approved for osteoporosis prevention, and patients who are on tamoxifen should have bone mass carefully monitored so that a bone-specific agent can be added early should bone loss occur.

CONCLUSIONS

The initial approach to osteoporosis prevention consists of identification of those subjects likely to be at risk; behavior modification to eliminate risk factors and improved nutrition and lifestyle; and estrogen intervention, which remains the cornerstone of prevention for the postmenopausal patient. Calcitonin (nasal spray) and oral bisphosphonates are alternatives available for those at greatest risk or those who cannot or will not take hormone replacement therapy.

REFERENCES

1. Riggs BL, Melton LJ III: Involutional osteoporosis. *N Engl J Med* 314:1676–1686, 1986
2. Consensus Development Conference: Prophylaxis and treatment of osteoporosis. *Osteo Int* 1:114–126, 1991
3. Hui SL, Slemenda CW, Johnston CC Jr: Baseline measurement of bone mass predicts fracture in white women. *Ann Intern Med* 111:355–361, 1989
4. Johnston CC Jr, Melton LJ III, Lindsay R, et al: Clinical indications for bone mass measurement. *J Bone Min Res* 4:1–28, 1989
5. Heaney RP: Effect of calcium on skeletal development, bone loss, and risk of fractures. *Am J Med* 91:23S–28S, 1991
6. Dalsky GP, Stocke KS, Ehsani AA, et al: Weight-bearing exercise training and lumbar bone mineral content in postmenopausal women. *Ann Intern Med* 108:824–828, 1988
7. Lindsay R: Sex steroids in the pathogenesis and prevention of osteoporosis. In: Riggs BL (ed) *Osteoporosis: Etiology, Diagnosis and Management.* Raven Press, New York, 333–358, 1988
8. Lindsay R, Tohme J: Estrogen treatment of patients with established postmenopausal osteoporosis. *Obstet Gynecol* 76:290–295, 1990
9. Lindsay R, Hart DM, Clark DM: The minimum effective dose of estrogen for prevention of postmenopausal bone loss. *Obstet Gynecol* 63:759–763, 1984
10. Stevenson JC, Cust MP, Gangar KF, Hillard TC, Lees B, Whitehead MI: Effects of transdermal versus oral hormone replacement therapy on bone density in spine and proximal femur in postmenopausal women. *Lancet* 336:265–269, 1990

11. Cauley JA, Seeley DG, Ensrud K, Ettinger B, Black D, Cummings SR: Estrogen replacement therapy and fractures in older women. *Ann Intern Med* 122:9–16, 1995
12. Hulka BS: Hormone-replacement therapy and the risk of breast cancer. *Cancer* 40:289–296, 1990
13. Barrett-Connor E, Bush TL: Estrogen and coronary heart disease in women. *JAMA* 265:1861–1967, 1991
14. Voight LF, Weiss NS, Chu J, et al: Progestogen supplementation of exogenous estrogens and the risk of endometrial cancer. *Lancet* 338:274–277, 1991
15. Christiansen C, Riis BJ: 17β-Estradiol and continuous norethisterone: a unique treatment for established osteoporosis in elderly women. *J Clin Endocrinol Metab* 71:836–841, 1990
16. Padwick ML, Pryse-Davies J, Whitehead MI: A simple method for determining the optimal dosage of progestin in postmenopausal women receiving estrogen. *N Engl J Med* 315:930–934, 1986
17. Uebelhart D, Schlemmer A, Johansen JS, Gineyts E, Christiansen C, Delmas PD: Effect of menopause and hormone replacement therapy on the urinary excretion of pyridinoline cross-links. *J Clin Endocrinol Metab* 72:367–373, 1991
18. Overgaard K, Hansen MA, Jensen SB, Christiansen C. Effect of salcatonin given intranassaly on bone mass and frature rates in established osteoporosis: a dose–response study. *Br Med J* 305:556–561, 1992
19. Fleisch H: The possible use of bisphosphonates in osteoporosis. In: DeLuca HF, Mazess R (eds) *Osteoporosis: Physiological Basis, Assessment and Treatment.* Elsevier, New York, 323–330, 1990
20. Turken S, Siris E, Seldin D, Lindsay R: Effects of tamoxifen on spinal bone density. *JNCI* 81:1086–1088, 1989
21. Love RR, Mazess RB, Barden HS, et al: Effects of tamoxifen on bone mineral density in postmenopausal women with breast cancer. *N Engl J Med* 326:852–856, 1992

13. Nutrition and Osteoporosis

Robert P. Heaney, M.D., F.A.C.P., F.A.I.N.

Creighton University, Omaha, Nebraska

Nutrition plays a role in pathogenesis, prevention, and treatment of osteoporosis (1). The nutrients known with certainty to be important are calcium, vitamin D, protein, and calories. Phosphorus, certain trace minerals (manganese, copper, and zinc), and vitamins C and K, while involved in bone health generally, are less certainly involved in osteoporosis. Bone cells, of course, are as dependent on total nutrition—including all the vitamins and trace minerals—as any other cell or tissue types. However, current bone mass and bone strength are dependent on cell activity over a many year period, and hence acute nutrient deficiencies, while undoubtedly impairing current cellular competence, tend to have less effect on overall bone strength, which is our concern here in a primer on osteoporosis. The major exceptions to this generalization are the nutrients calcium and vitamin D.

CALCIUM

Calcium is the principal cation of bone mineral. Bone constitutes a very large nutrient reserve for calcium which, over the course of evolution, acquired a secondary, structural function that dominates our concern with respect to osteoporosis. As noted elsewhere (see "Pathogenesis" Chapter 10), bone strength varies as the approximate second power of bone density. While reserves are designed to be used in times of need, it nevertheless must be recognized that any decrease in bone mass produces a corresponding decrease in bone strength.

Bone mass is limited both by the genetic program and by experienced mechanical loading. However, neither limit can be reached if calcium intake is insufficient. Bone resorption, as noted elsewhere in this volume, is controlled by parathyroid hormone, which in turn is concerned with maintenance of extracellular fluid calcium ion levels. Whenever absorbed calcium intake is insufficient to meet either the demands of growth or the drain of dermal and excretory losses, resorption will increase and bone mass will be reduced.

The intake of calcium that is optimal for growth and adult maintenance has been estimated at a National Institutes of Health (NIH) Consensus Conference in 1994 (2) to be 800–1000 mg/day during childhood, 1200–1500 mg/day from age 12 to 24, 1000 mg/day from age 25 to time of estrogen deprivation or age 65 (whichever comes first), and 1500 mg/day thereafter. These intakes are mostly above 1989 Recommended Dietary Allowances (RDAs) and are specific for the United States (and probably Canada as well). The difference is larger than the numbers alone indicate. An RDA is a value for a population and is intended to be an intake at or above the actual requirement of 90% to 95% of the individuals making up the population. (Thus many individuals could have intakes below the RDA which would still be fully adequate for their own needs. Conventionally, nutritionists have considered as cause for concern only individual values less than two thirds of the RDA.) An optimal intake value, by contrast, applies to individuals.

The specific applicability of the National Institutes of Health (NIH) values to North America is a function of the effect of other nutrients on the calcium requirement. High intakes of both protein and sodium, such as are typical of the United States, increase urinary calcium loss and thereby increase the calcium intake requirement. On low intakes of both nutrients, such as might be found in certain Third World environments, the adult requirement can be less than 500 mg/day. This is part of the reason why requirements seem to vary across different countries and cultures.

Low calcium intakes in childhood are associated with increased risk of osteoporosis later in life as well as increased fracture risk even in adolescents (1,3). Calcium intakes are positively correlated with bone mass at all ages, but most especially in old age when the requirement rises and the calcium intake tends to drop (thereby widening the gap between need and supply). Calcium supplementation reduces both bone loss and fracture rate in the elderly (4–8). Only in the few years immediately following estrogen withdrawal at menopause is calcium without much effect (9). (This is largely because bone loss then is due mainly to estrogen deficiency, not to nutrient deficiency.) The abnormal parathyroid secretory physiology, high circulating parathyroid hormone (PTH) levels, and elevated biomarkers for bone resorption typical of the elderly are all reversible with a high calcium intake (10). These hallmarks of the aging calcium economy, once considered due to aging itself, are now recognized as manifestations of calcium privation. Thus, at one and the same time, low calcium intakes are pathogenetic for osteoporosis and high intakes are prophylactic.

Prophylaxis is provided by meeting the NIH recommendations, either by natural foods (principally low-fat dairy products, tofu, a few greens, and a few crustaceans) or by calcium-fortified foods (such as fortified fruit juices, bread, yogurt, breakfast cereals, potato chips, rice, and so forth). Calcium-rich foods, especially milk, tend to be less expensive per calorie than the calcium-poor foods they would displace in the diet. Hence calcium administered in this way has a negative cost and such dietary change has a very favorable cost–benefit relationship.

Supplements may also be indicated. Calcium carbonate is the salt most widely used in the United States. Like all calcium sources (including food), supplements should be taken with meals to ensure optimal absorption. Even for relatively less soluble salts such as the carbonate, gastric acid is not necessary if the supplement is taken with food. Brand name or chewable products have proved over the years to be the most reliable.

Calcium is also of critical importance as cotherapy in the treatment of established osteoporosis. Agents capable of increasing bone mass (such as fluoride and the newer bisphosphonates) cannot achieve their full effect if calcium intake is limiting. Certain agents, such as fluoride (and possibly PTH) with a preferential trophic effect for axial cancellous bone, will actually take bone from other regions of the skeleton to meet the needs of new bone formation in the central skeleton when ingested calcium is not adequate. Because of poor absorption efficiency in the elderly in general and in many osteoporotics in particular, therapeutic intakes must be well above the NIH maintenance figure of 1500 mg/day, probably 2000–2500 mg/day. Unless the number and variety of calcium-fortified foods increases substantially, supplements will be the obvious choice here.

Vitamin D

Vitamin D is important for bone, certainly for its role in facilitating calcium absorption, but probably for other reasons as well. (One of the best attested effects of 1,25(OH)$_2$D is the prompt rise in serum osteocalcin that follows administration of the hormone.) Vitamin D also facilitates PTH-mediated bone resorption.

Serum 25(OH)D levels decline with age. This is partly due to decreased solar exposure. Intestinal calcium absorption also decreases with age due to decreased 1α-hydroxylation of 25(OH)D, and decreased responsiveness of the intestinal mucosa to circulating 1,25(OH)$_2$D. Vitamin D supplementation in the elderly reduces fractures of all types (11). It takes about 600 IU/day to maintain 25(OH)D levels in healthy young males (which is more than the Recommended Daily Allowance, or RDA, of 200 IU), and the vitamin D requirement is probably higher still in the elderly. Hence it seems prudent to recommend intakes of 800 IU in all elderly individuals with or without osteoporosis. If individuals succeed in raising their calcium intakes through increased milk consumption, they will at the same time improve their vitamin D status because fluid milks in the United States are fortified with vitamin D at a level of 100 IU per serving.

Protein and Calories

Total nutrition, and specifically adequacy of protein and energy intake, is important in several ways. First, malnutrition predisposes to falls. Second, soft tissue mass over bony prominences (e.g., lateral hip) distributes the energy sustained in falls and thereby reduces point loads on bone. Finally, adequacy of protein intake is a major factor in determining outcome after hip fracture. Patients with hip fracture are commonly malnourished, enter the hospital with low serum albumin levels, and typically become more severely hypoproteinemic during hospitalization. Serum albumin levels are the single best predictor of survival or death following hip fracture (12). Protein supplementation of hip fracture patients has been shown to improve outcome dramatically (fewer deaths, less permanent institutionalization, more return to independent living) (13,14). Unfortunately, most hospital standards of care for hip fracture patients lack a nutritional component.

Phosphorus

Phosphorus intake is generally above the RDA in North Americans; hence phosphorus depletion is not common. (There has even been some concern expressed that there is too much phosphorus in the American diet. That is probably not the case.) However, low phosphorus intakes are relatively common among the elderly (i.e., 25% of individuals over 65 ingest under two thirds of the RDA). Whether such low intakes contribute to the problem of osteoporosis is not known. Nevertheless, phosphate is just as important a component of bone mineral as is calcium. When serum phosphorus levels are low, bone mineralization will be limited by phosphate depletion in the immediate environment of the mineralizing front before calcium depletion occurs. It is probable that osteoblast function is severely compromised by low ambient phosphate concentrations even sooner.

Vitamins and Trace Minerals

Vitamins C and K and the minerals manganese, copper, and zinc are necessary cofactors for enzymes involved in the synthesis or post translational modification of various constituents of bone matrix; when these micronutrients are deficient in the diets of growing animals various bone lesions develop (15). Bone fragility has been reported with manganese deficiency in one human patient, and a bony lesion resembling osteoporosis occurs in sheep with copper deficiency. However, it is not known as to whether acquired adult deficiencies of any of these minerals in humans play a role in pathogenesis or treatment of osteoporosis. One randomized trial involving supplementation with manganese, copper, and zinc produced suggestive, but not conclusive, evidence of some benefit when these minerals were added to a calcium supplementation regimen (16).

Vitamin C is necessary for collagen crosslinking, and bony defects are well recognized as a part of the scurvy syndrome. However, apart from general nutritional considerations, there is no known role for vitamin C in osteoporotic bony fragility.

Vitamin K is necessary for the γ carboxylation of three bone matrix proteins, a step necessary for their binding to hydroxyapatite. Osteocalcin is the best studied of these. Circulating serum osteocalcin is commonly undercarboxylated in patients with osteoporosis, especially those with hip fracture, and the defect responds to modest doses of vitamin K (17). There is also suggestive evidence that vitamin K may reduce urinary calcium loss in patients with osteoporosis. What is not known is the extent to which these changes are causal or are instead simply markers for the general debility and global malnutrition common in elderly patients with osteoporosis. Vitamin K deficiency is, however, easily treatable and, if some component of the fragility of the elderly is due to inadequate intakes or colonic synthesis of vitamin K, that component of the fracture burden could be inexpensively eliminated.

REFERENCES

1. Heaney RP. Nutrition and risk for osteoporosis. In: Marcus R, Feldman D, Kelsey J (eds) *Osteoporosis*. Academic Press, San Diego, 483–505, 1996
2. NIH Consensus Conference: Optimal Calcium Intake. *JAMA* 272: 1942-1948, 1994
3. Chan GM, Hess M, Hollis J, Book LS: Bone mineral status in childhood accidental fractures. *Am J Dis Child* 138:569–570, 1984

4. Chapuy MC, Arlot ME, Duboeuf F, Brun J, Crouzet B, Arnaud S, Delmas PD, Meunier PJ: Vitamin D$_3$ and calcium to prevent hip fractures in elderly women. *N Engl J Med* 327:1637–1642, 1992

5. Chevalley T, Rizzoli R, Nydegger V, Slosman D, Rapin C-H, Michel J-P, Vasey H, Bonjour J-P: Effects of calcium supplements on femoral bone mineral density and vertebral fracture rate in vitamin D-replete elderly patients. *Osteoporosis Int* 4:245–252, 1994

6. Recker RR, Hinders S, Davies KM, Heaney RP, Stegman MR, Kimmel DB, Lappe JM: Correcting calcium nutritional deficiency prevents spine fractures in elderly women. *J Bone Min Res* 1995 (submitted)

7. Reid IR, Ames RW, Evans MC, Gamble GD, Sharpe SJ: Effect of calcium supplementation on bone loss in postmenopausal women. *N Engl J Med* 328:460–464, 1993

8. Aloia JF, Vaswani A, Yeh JK, Ross PL, Flaster E, Dilmanian FA: Calcium supplementation with and without hormone replacement therapy to prevent postmenopausal bone loss. *Ann Intern Med* 120:97–103, 1994

9. Dawson-Hughes B, Dallal GE, Krall EA, Sadowski L, Sahyoun N, Tannenbaum S: A controlled trial of the effect of calcium supplementation on bone density in postmenopausal women. *N Engl J Med* 323:878–883, 1990

10. McKane WR, Khosla S, O'Fallon WM, Robins SP, Burritt MF, Riggs BL: Role of calcium intake in modulating age-related increases in parathyroid function and bone resorption. *J Clin Endocrinol Metab* 81:1699–1703, 1996

11. Heikinheimo RJ, Inkovaara JA, Harju EJ, Haavisto MV, Kaarela RH, Kataja JM, Kokko AM-L, Kolho LA, Rajala SA: Annual injection of vitamin D and fractures of aged bones. *Calcif Tissue Int* 51:105–110, 1992

12. Rico H, Revilla M, Villa LF, Hernandez ER, Fernandez JP: Crush fracture syndrome in senile osteoporosis: a nutritional consequence. *J Bone Min Res* 7:317–319, 1992

13. Delmi M, Rapin CH, Bengoa JM, Delmas PD, Vasey H, Bonjour JP: Dietary supplementation in elderly patients with fractured neck of the femur. *Lancet* 335:1013–1016, 1990

14. Bastow MD, Rawlings J, Allison SP: Benefits of supplementary tube feeding after fractured neck of femur. *Br Med J* 287:1589–1592, 1983

15. Heaney RP: Nutritional factors in osteoporosis. *Annu Rev Nutr* 13:287–316, 1993

16. Strause L, Saltman P, Smith K, Andon M: The role of trace elements in bone metabolism. In: Burckhardt P, Heaney RP (eds) *Nutritional Aspects of Osteoporosis*. Raven Press, New York, 223–233, 1991

17. Vermeer C, Jie K-S G, Knapen MHJ: Role of vitamin K in bone metabolism. *Annu Rev Nutr* 15:1–22, 1995

14. Evaluation and Treatment of Postmenopausal Osteoporosis

Michael Kleerekoper, M.D., F.A.C.E., and *Louis V. Avioli, M.D., F.A.C.E.

*Department of Internal Medicine, Wayne State University School of Medicine, and Harper Hospital, Detroit, Michigan; and *Departments of Medicine and Orthopedic Surgery, Washington University Medical Center, Barnes-Jewish Campus, St. Louis, Missouri*

Osteoporosis is a disease characterized by low bone mass and the development of nontraumatic or atraumatic fractures as a direct result of the low bone mass. A nontraumatic fracture has been arbitrarily defined as one occurring from trauma equal to or less than that of a fall from a standing height. In the preclinical state, the disease is characterized simply by a low bone mass without fractures. This totally asymptomatic state is often termed osteopenia. Osteoporosis and osteopenia are the most common metabolic bone diseases in the developed countries of the world, whereas osteomalacia may be more prevalent in underdeveloped countries where nutrition is suboptimal. To be able to evaluate more fully the prevalence and incidence of osteoporosis worldwide, the World Health Organization (WHO) recently convened an expert panel to define osteoporosis on the basis of bone mass measurement (1). Table 1 provides the diagnostic categories for women that were established by that panel. Osteoporotic fractures may affect any part of the skeleton except the skull. Most commonly, fractures occur in the distal forearm (Colles' fracture), thoracic and lumbar vertebrae, and proximal femur (hip fracture).

The epidemiology of osteoporosis is detailed in Chapter 9 and is only briefly summarized here. The incidence of osteoporotic fractures increases with age, is higher in whites than in blacks, and is higher in women than in men. The female to male ratio is 1.5:1 for Colles' fractures, 7:1 for vertebral fractures, and 2:1 for hip fractures. Because most osteoporotic fractures do not require admission to the hospital, it is difficult to obtain precise figures on the true prevalence of this disease. Almost without exception, a hip fracture requires admission to a hospital, and current estimates indicate that there are 275,000 new osteoporotic hip fractures each year in the United States. It has been estimated that after menopause, a woman's lifetime risk of sustaining an osteoporotic fracture is one in three. Regrettably, despite improvements in surgical techniques and anesthesiology, most hip fractures require surgical intervention on a nonelective basis, and there is a 15% to 20% excess mortality after an osteoporotic hip fracture. Perhaps more important, after such fractures, less than one third of the patients are restored to their prefracture functional state within 12 months of the fracture. Most patients require some form of ambulatory support, and many require institutional care. Current estimates indicate that each new case of osteoporotic hip fracture costs $40,000, and the annual expenditure for short-term care after an osteoporotic hip fracture already exceeds $8 billion. Chapter 15 provides more details on the special problems posed by osteoporotic fractures of the hip.

PATHOGENESIS

Once peak adult bone mass has been attained in the third, possibly fourth, decade of life, bone mass at any point in time is the difference between peak adult bone mass and the loss of bone mass that has occurred since this was attained. Because age-related bone loss is a universal phenomenon in humans, any circumstance that limits an individual's ability to maximize peak adult bone mass increases the likelihood of developing osteoporosis later in life. Strategies for maximizing peak adult bone mass have been described in Chapters 11–13.

The excessive bone loss that characterizes the pathogenesis of osteoporosis results from abnormalities in the bone remodeling cycle (2,3). In brief, bone remodeling is a mechanism for keeping the skeleton "young" by a process of removal of old bone and replacement with new bone. The cycle is initiated by resorption of old bone, recruitment of osteoblasts, deposition of new matrix, and mineralization of that newly deposited matrix. It appears that with each cycle there is a slight, imperceptible deficit in bone formation. The total bone loss is, therefore, a function of the number of cycles in process at any one time. Conditions that increase the rate of activation of the bone remodeling process thus increase the proportion of the skeleton undergoing remodeling at any one time and increase the rate of bone loss. In this circumstance, which is called high-turnover osteoporosis, the deficit per unit of remodeling is apparently constant. Most of the secondary causes of osteoporosis (Table 2) are associated with this increased rate of activation of the remodeling cycle. In the normal aging process, there appears to be a progressive impairment of the signaling between bone resorption and bone formation, such that with every cycle of remodeling, there is an increase in the deficit between resorption and formation because osteoblast recruitment is inefficient. Thus, excessive bone loss can occur even when activation of the skeleton is not increased and, in fact, when activation of the skeleton might be decreased. This gives rise to the concept of low- or normal-turnover osteoporosis.

CLASSIFICATION OF OSTEOPOROSIS

In addition to describing osteoporosis as being of the high- or low-turnover type, there are several other classification systems. The first is the classification into primary and secondary, the latter being osteoporosis for which a clearly identifiable etiologic mechanism is recognized. Primary osteoporosis is further characterized into postmenopausal

TABLE 1. *Diagnostic criteria for osteoporosis[a]*

Normal	Bone mineral density (BMD) or bone mineral content (BMC) within 1 SD of young adult reference mean
Low bone mass (osteopenia)	A value for BMD or BMC between −1.0 and −2.5 SD below young adult reference mean
Osteoporosis	A value for BMD or BMC −2.5 or more SD below the young adult reference mean
Severe (established) osteoporosis	Osteoporosis with one or more fragility fractures

SD, standard deviation
[a]From ref. 1 with permission.

and senile. In postmenopausal osteoporosis, there is an apparent excess loss of cancellous bone with relative sparing of cortical bone, and the clinical syndromes involve Colles' fracture and vertebral fracture. In senile osteoporosis, there is a more concordant loss of both cortical and cancellous bone. The pathogenesis of senile osteoporosis is uncertain, but it is postulated to result from an age-related decline in renal production of 1,25-dihydroxyvitamin D and calcium malabsorption, with subsequent secondary hyperparathyroidism. It is the hyperparathyroidism that is largely responsible for the excess cortical bone loss. The fracture syndrome often seen in the patient with senile osteoporosis involves hip fracture.

CLINICAL MANIFESTATIONS OF OSTEOPOROSIS

As mentioned previously, osteoporosis without fracture is entirely without symptoms. This does not lessen its importance, because the aim of all therapies should be to prevent even the first fracture, let alone subsequent fractures. When osteoporosis is complicated by the development of an osteoporotic fracture, the symptoms and signs are those related to the fracture itself. Osteoporotic vertebral fractures may represent a unique situation, and this will be discussed separately. Primary orthopedic management of peripheral fractures should not be influenced by the fact that the fracture results from osteoporosis. Management consists of immobilization and analgesia. There does not appear to be anything about an osteoporotic fracture that results in delayed fracture union. If delayed fracture union or fracture nonunion complicates an osteoporotic fracture, one needs to look for conditions other than osteoporosis, such as osteomalacia, hyperparathyroidism, or occult forms of osteogenesis imperfecta. Immobilization should be for only a limited period of time, sufficient to ensure primary fracture healing. Longer immobilization will lead to accelerated bone loss and must be avoided. The brittleness of the osteoporotic skeleton may complicate open surgical repair of osteoporotic fractures, with limited purchase for pins, plates, screws, or nails. Restoration of the prefracture anatomic and functional state is the goal in the management of osteoporotic fractures of the appendicular skeleton. Regrettably, with respect to osteoporotic hip fractures, this is not often

TABLE 2. *Factors commonly associated with osteopenic and/or osteoporotic syndrome(s)*

Genetic
  White or Asiatic ethnicity
  Positive family history
  Small body frame
Lifestyle
  Smoking
  Inactivity
  Nulliparity
  Excessive exercise (producing amenorrhea)
  Early natural menopause
  Late menarche
Nutritional factors
  Milk intolerance
  Life long low dietary calcium intake
  Vegetarian dieting
  Excessive alcohol intake
  Consistently high protein intake
Medical disorders
  Anorexia nervosa
  Thyrotoxicosis
  Hyperparathyroidism
  Cushing syndrome
  Type I diabetes
  Alterations in gastrointestinal and hepatobiliary function
  Occult osteogenesis imperfecta
  Mastocytosis
  Rheumatoid arthritis
  "Transient" osteoporosis
  Prolonged parenteral nutrition
  Prolactinoma
  Hemolytic anemia
Drugs
  Excessive dose of thyroid hormone
  Glucocorticoid drugs
  Anticoagulants
  Chronic lithium therapy
  Chemotherapy (breast cancer or lymphoma)
  Gonadotropin-releasing hormone agonist or antagonist therapy
  Anticonvulsants
  Chronic phosphate-binding antacid use
  Extended tetracycline use[a]
  Diuretics producing calciuria[a]
  Phenothiazine derivatives[a]
  Cyclosporin A[a]

[a]Not yet associated with decreased bone mass in humans, although identified as either toxic to bone in animals or as inducing calciuria or calcium malabsorption in humans.

the outcome that is attained, given the excess morbidity and mortality already discussed. In general, this is because surgical repair of an osteoporotic hip fracture is usually a nonelective procedure. Circumstances that appear to increase mortality after a hip fracture are related to the overall medical health and nutritional status of the subject sustaining the fracture. Frail, elderly subjects taking large numbers of medications and with mental impairment have the greatest mortality, and this is particularly so in men compared with women. Of those patients who survive the early operative intervention for an osteoporotic hip fracture, less than one-third are restored to their prefracture functional state, and either require institutionalized care or some form of ambulatory support.

Osteoporotic vertebral fractures are quite different from other osteoporotic fractures. Surveys of spine radiographs in older subjects suggest that many vertebral fractures have occurred in the absence of acute symptoms. If acute symptoms do occur at the time of fracture, these will be manifest as intense pain and limitation of motion. Operative intervention is infrequently required for stabilization of these fractures. However, the principles of immobilization for a short time should still hold. The concept of placing the patient with an osteoporotic fracture in a back brace for years is to be decried. Similarly, the acute skeletal pain after an osteoporotic vertebral fracture should dissipate within 4–6 weeks. If skeletal tenderness persists much beyond this, other causes for the fracture (e.g., metastatic disease, multiple myeloma) should be considered. Osteoporotic fractures of the vertebral bodies rarely result in "referred nerve pain syndrome" or long tract symptoms or signs. Again, if a fracture is complicated by these symptoms or signs, causes other than osteoporosis should be considered.

Once a vertebral body has been fractured, restoration of normal anatomy is not possible. In fact, refracture of the same vertebra with further abnormalities of shape and size is often the outcome. Thus, even those vertebral fractures that are not associated with any acute symptoms at the time of fracture give rise to chronic pain, disability, and often obvious deformity. All vertebral fractures are associated with loss of stature; in the thoracic spine this is associated with a progressive increase in the degree of kyphosis, and in the lumbar spine this is associated with a progressive flattening of the lordotic curve and scoliosis in some individuals. As the number of vertebrae involved increases and the severity of individual vertebral deformities progresses, these anatomic changes become more pronounced. There is gradual loss of the waistline contour and protuberance of the abdomen, and in severe cases the lower ribs approximate the pelvic rim and ultimately lie within the pelvis. Each of these progressive anatomic deformities is associated with symptoms. The progressive loss of stature results in progressive "shortening" of the paraspinal musculature, that is, the paraspinal muscles are actively contracting, resulting in the pain of muscle fatigue. This is the major cause of the chronic back pain in spinal osteoporosis. Careful clinical examination reveals that the skeleton (spine) itself is not tender, and most patients indicate that the pain is paraspinal. The pain is worse with prolonged standing and is often relieved by walking. After an acute fracture, there may be associated paraspinal muscle spasm, but this dissipates with time. The loss of height and the protuberant abdomen are usually not associated with direct symptoms per se, but do give the patient the emotional discomfort of the altered body image. Many patients attempt to wear abdominal flattening girdles or go on weight-reduction diets, both of which will be of limited benefit and potential harm. It is important that the patient be advised of the irreversible nature of these anatomic changes. One common complaint of patients with advanced disease is vague gastrointestinal distress aggravated by eating. This can be alleviated somewhat by having the patient consume frequent smaller meals. This is a particularly vexing problem for patients with chronic airway disease who have osteoporosis as a result of therapy with corticosteroids. In these patients, the flattened diaphragm coupled with the shortened spinal column results in marked diminution of the size of their abdominal cavity.

There are several important approaches to the long-term management of patients with these chronic deformities from spinal osteoporosis. Of particular importance is educating the patient to understand the nature of the deformity so that he or she can have realistic expectations concerning body image and the anticipated goals of therapy (relief of pain, restoration of function, maintenance of a reasonable quality of life, and prevention of further fractures). The major focus of therapy should be rehabilitation and analgesia aimed at lessening the chronic back pain. However, caution must be used with analgesics and nonsteroidal anti-inflammatory agents, many of which cause significant constipation. Straining of the stool to relieve constipation from narcotic analgesics tends to aggravate back pain substantially. In this regard, it is worth noting that many generic calcium preparations also tend to cause vague gastrointestinal symptoms, including constipation in some patients. It is equally important to instruct the patient adequately in activities of daily living so that he or she bends, lifts, and stoops in a manner that does not increase strain on the brittle skeleton. Nurses, physical therapists, and occupational therapists become important partners in the management of the patient with spinal osteoporosis. In many respects, this nonpharmacologic approach to these patients is far more important than the pharmacologic therapy.

DIAGNOSTIC STUDIES IN OSTEOPOROSIS

The same diagnostic approach should be taken with patients suspected of having osteoporosis whether or not they have already sustained an osteoporotic fracture. These studies should only be undertaken once an appropriate history and physical examination have been completed. The history, physical examination, and studies should all be conducted with the aim of determining the extent and severity of disease, pathogenesis of the bone loss, and physiology of the skeleton at the time of presentation. Although postmenopausal and senile osteoporosis are the most prevalent forms of the disease, it must be remembered that as many as 20% of women who otherwise appear to have postmenopausal osteoporosis can be shown to have additional etiologic factors above and beyond their age, gender, and ethnic background. Many of these secondary causes of osteoporosis (Table 2) can be suggested from the history and physical examination so that appropriate investigations can be ordered.

If an osteoporotic fracture is suspected, it is imperative that radiographs be taken of the appropriate part of the skeleton. However, there is no clear indication for radiographs of the skeleton if fracture is not suspected. All patients suspected of having osteoporosis, with or without fracture, should have measurement of bone mass (see Chapter 7 for details). The one possible exception is the patient with far advanced disease clinically and radiographically. Because osteoporosis may be the only manifestation of many of the secondary causes listed earlier, it is appropriate to perform simple screening studies looking for these causes in each patient. A biochemical profile will provide information about renal and hepatic function, primary hyperparathyroidism, and possible malnutrition. A hematologic profile might also provide clues to the presence of myeloma and malnutrition. The precise role of hyperthyroidism, particularly exogenous, in the pathogenesis of accelerated bone loss and osteoporosis remains unresolved. Nonetheless, for the time being at least, it seems prudent to obtain a sensitive thyroid-stimulating hormone assay in all patients with documented bone loss. A 24-hour urine collection for measurement of calcium (which should always be accompanied by measurement of creatinine and sodium) will detect patients with hypercalciuria, which may be the end result of excess skeletal loss or may contribute to excess skeletal loss. In contrast, a very low urine calcium level (50 mg or less for 24 hours) may provide a clue to the presence of vitamin D malnutrition or malabsorption (4). It is our practice to obtain a 24-hour urine collection in all osteoporotic subjects. A 24-hour urine-free cortisol determination should be considered as the only test that can document occult Cushing's disease, which may have osteoporosis as the only presenting feature. The yield from using the urinary-free cortisol test is quite small, but it is probably the only way to detect this uncommon disorder. In general, the intensity with which one looks for occult secondary causes of accelerated bone loss should be related to any unusual features of the clinical presentation, such as bone loss in a premenopausal woman, in a woman very early in menopause, or in a man without obvious hypogonadism. One should also pay particular attention to patients whose fractures occur at unusual sites.

CALCITROPIC HORMONES AND BIOCHEMICAL MARKERS OF BONE REMODELING

In most cases of osteoporosis, there is no need to measure the calcitropic hormones (parathyroid hormone, calcitriol, or calcitonin) unless there is a specific indication for these measurements based on the history, physical examination, and biochemical screening. Although there are reports of abnormalities in some of these measurements when compared with published reference ranges, this is not the case when the reference values are appropriately adjusted for age, gender, and ethnic background.

In contrast, it is becoming increasingly important to monitor the biochemical markers of bone remodeling that are discussed in detail in Chapter 6. The control of bone remodeling is detailed in ref. 2, and the role of abnormalities in the remodeling cycle in the pathogenesis of osteoporosis has been described briefly. It may be useful to make an analogy between turnover abnormalities leading to osteoporosis and abnormalities in the red cell life cycle leading to anemia. High-turnover bone loss with increased resorption and increased, but insufficient, formation would be analogous to hemolytic anemia with increased red cell destruction and increased (but insufficient) red cell formation, characterized by the increased reticulocyte count in this type of anemia. Low-turnover bone loss with normal resorption and subnormal formation would be analogous to anemia of chronic disease.

There is increasing evidence that biochemical markers of bone formation and resorption are a useful adjunct in predicting the rate of bone loss and the response to therapy. Table 3 lists the biochemical markers of bone resorption and formation that were available through commercial diagnostic laboratories at the time of this writing (December 1995). The reader should remain aware that this is a rapidly changing field and that other markers are available in laboratories of individual investigators. Table 3 also provides details of the reference intervals for these tests in healthy premenopausal white women.

Theoretically, patients with high-turnover osteoporosis should have increased levels of resorption and formation markers, should be experiencing bone loss at an accelerated rate, and should respond best to therapy with drugs that inhibit bone resorption. In contrast, those with low- or normal-turnover osteoporosis should have normal or low levels of the markers, should not be losing bone at an accelerated rate, should respond less well to antiresorptive therapy, and should be treated preferentially with drugs that primarily enhance bone formation. To date, only a small fraction of these theoretical scenarios has been formally documented in prospective studies. This is mainly because the studies are not yet complete, and not necessarily because the theory is defective. The biggest difficulty has been demonstrating that the markers can be used to select therapy for individual patients, principally because the only therapies available are all antiresorptive. As therapeutic options broaden over the next several years, the usefulness of biochemical markers in this fashion will become more apparent.

At present, the most practical use of these markers is to monitor the response to therapy. It has been demonstrated that changes in markers after just 3 months of therapy are significantly related to changes in bone mass after 24 months of therapy (5). This is of considerable practical importance, particularly with respect to patient compliance with treatment, as changes in bone mass in response to therapy may not become apparent within 12 months of treatment. The markers may also provide confidence for dose adjustment, allowing the clinician to use a smaller than recommended dose of therapy if that proves sufficient to restore biochemical markers of remodeling to the normal premenopausal range.

In summary, the current approach to evaluation of the osteoporotic patient involves documentation of bone mass, documentation of fractures if present, a diligent search for secondary causes, and then an evaluation of the biochemistry of skeletal remodeling.

MEDICAL THERAPY

At the time of this writing, the only drugs approved by the Food and Drug Administration (FDA) for treatment of postmenopausal osteoporosis are estrogen, calcitonin, and the bisphosphonate alendronate. The FDA is evaluating a request for approval of a sustained-release sodium fluoride preparation. Although calcitriol and etidronate are both approved by the FDA for use in the United States, osteoporosis is currently not an approved indication. Oral calcium supplements are not subject to FDA regulation, and sodium

TABLE 3. *Biochemical markers of bone remodeling[a]*

Marker	Reference interval[b]
Bone resorption	
Lysylpyridinoline (LP)	24–52 nM Pyd/mM Cr
Deoxylysylpyridinoline (DPD)	2.5–6.2 nM Dpd/mM Cr
N-telopeptide of the cross-links of collagen (NTX)	5–65 nM/mM creatinine based upon 95% CI
C-telopeptide of the cross-links of collagen (PICP)	13–96 nM/mM Cr
Bone formation	
Osteocalcin (OCN) [bone Gla protein (BGP)]	1.6–9.2 ng/ml
Bone specific alkaline phosphatase (BSAP)	11.6–30.6 BAP, U/L
Carboxy-terminal extension peptide of type I procollagen (PICP)	45–190 µg/L

[a]All resorption markers are based on urine collected after an overnight fast. Usually a spot sample of the first or second voided urine is analyzed. Data are normalized for creatinine excretion. All formation markers are based on random serum samples. CI, confidence interval.

[b]Reference interval is for premenopausal women.

fluoride as a supplement is also not subject to FDA regulation. In the following sections, we will discuss what is known about each of these possible therapies for postmenopausal osteoporosis.

The primary role for estrogen in the prevention of early postmenopausal bone loss and the subsequent development of osteoporotic fractures has been discussed in detail in Chapter 12. A definitive role for the use of estrogen in established osteoporosis with fractures is much less well established. Estrogen is an "antiresorptive" agent in that it inhibits bone resorption by decreasing the frequency of activation of the bone remodeling cycle. Estrogen would be expected to be most efficient if bone remodeling or bone turnover were increased. This is why it is so effective in the early stages of menopause. If an individual patient with established osteoporosis can be shown to have increased bone remodeling, estrogen will be effective in inhibiting remodeling, no matter how long it has been since the patient had her menopause. Thus, estrogen therapy will slow down the rate of bone loss in any estrogen-deficient woman so treated. However, the ability of estrogen to result in any net gain in bone mass is limited, with the best results being a 2% to 4% annual increase for 2 years. Recent studies have suggested that older women may also receive benefit from estrogen of similar magnitude (6). There are some studies showing that estrogen reduces the rate of occurrence of new vertebral fractures in patients with established osteoporosis. The usual starting dose is 0.625 mg of conjugated equine estrogen (Premarin®) or 0.05 mg of transdermal estrogen (Estraderm®). Short-term complications of estrogen therapy in women with established osteoporosis include breast tenderness and vaginal bleeding (7). If estrogens are given without progesterone, there is an increased likelihood of endometrial hyperplasia. The relationship between estrogen therapy and breast cancer is not well established, but most studies suggest that there is little,

if any, increased risk of breast cancer during the first 10–15 years of therapy. Such long-term studies in established osteoporosis have not been conducted, and as long as therapy is tolerated, estrogen therapy, once indicated, should be continued indefinitely.

Synthetic salmon calcitonin (Calcimar® and Miacalcin®) is available in the United States as a subcutaneous injection or nasal spray formulation. Like estrogen, calcitonin inhibits bone resorption and slows down the rate of bone loss. The ability of calcitonin to increase bone mass is a function of the rate of bone remodeling at the time calcitonin therapy is initiated. The response is better in patients with increased bone turnover than in patients with low turnover (8). Again, a beneficial effect is observed as long as the medication is used, especially in intermittent-pulse regimens (8–13). There is increasing evidence that calcitonin has inherent analgesic properties, and many physicians recommend its use in the early postfracture period because of this effect (13). The major side effects of calcitonin are transient flushing of the face and nausea. These side effects are all dose dependent and virtually disappear with nasal spray formulations. The recommended dose is 100 U subcutaneously daily, but few patients tolerate this large dose initially. We have found that starting with a dose as low as 25 U subcutaneously three times per week is tolerated by most patients, and the dose can be increased gradually over a period of 2–3 months if needed. Intermittent-pulse dose regimens have also been used, with documentation of increased bone mass and decreased fracture incidence (14). Calcitonin is dispensed in a concentration of 200 U/ml. Because most patients use insulin syringes calibrated for a dose of 100 U/ml, it is important that they receive adequate instruction on the amount of solution to inject to achieve the desired dosage. Therapy should be continued for as long as the drug is tolerated (14). The recommended dose of nasal spray calcitonin is 200 U daily, with limited opportunity for dose adjustment.

As discussed earlier, use of the biochemical markers may assist in finding a suitable dose of estrogen or calcitonin for individual patients, particularly if side effects or other concerns limit the recommended starting dose. For example, breast tenderness on estrogen is less likely in older women if initiated in a dose of Premarin 0.3 mg/d. If this dose can be demonstrated to have reduced the rate of resorption, dose adjustment might not be indicated. Similarly, if the markers of resorption have not changed appropriately (arbitrarily a 40% to 50% reduction from baseline after 8–12 weeks of therapy), the patient might be more willing to consider a higher dose of therapy. This is equally appropriate when trying to minimize the gastrointestinal side effects of calcitonin.

Alendronate (Fosamax®) is an amino-bisphosphonate for which extensive clinical trials have been completed worldwide; it was recently approved by the FDA for the treatment of osteoporosis. In the clinical trials, there was a progressive increase in spine and hip bone mineral density during 3 years of daily therapy at a dose of 10 mg once a day (15–17). There were fewer and less severe spinal fractures in patients receiving therapy compared with those on placebo. The drug was well tolerated with few side effects, and more than 80% of those on therapy responded with an increase in bone mass. The major potential problem with this therapy is that, in common with other bisphosphonates, oral absorption of alendronate is very poor, with less than 1% of an orally administered dose being absorbed. This poor absorption is further impaired if the medication is taken with food, any liquid except water, or with calcium supplements. These problems can be avoided if patients are advised to take the medication first thing in the morning with water and to delay breakfast for at least 30 minutes. The major side effect is esophagitis in a small proportion of patients.

Etidronate (Didronel®), the first bisphosphonate to become clinically available, has been used in several clinical trials to stabilize or increase bone mass and also to possibly reduce the vertebral fracture rate (16,18–20). However, the effect on the vertebral fracture rate is still controversial and by no means well established. The major short-term effect of bisphosphonate is nausea (16,18–20). The treatment regimen for etidronate is 400 mg orally daily for 2 weeks followed by a 10–12-week etidronate-free period, with a repeat of this 3-month cycle for 2 years. Because this bisphosphonate is poorly absorbed orally and because its absorption is obliterated when given concurrently with calcium, it is important to advise the patient not to ingest any calcium, either as a supplement or in food, for 4 hours before or after ingestion of each tablet. Clinical trials of this therapy used 1500 mg calcium as a daily supplement during the etidronate-free periods. It is imperative that etidronate be used in this rigorous treatment cycle and that the dose not be exceeded in amount or duration. There is evidence from long-term treatment of Paget's disease that large doses or longer duration of therapy with etidronate may result in a mineralization defect and an increased risk of developing osteomalacia and hip fractures. This drug is not an FDA-approved therapy for osteoporosis. As noted earlier for calcitonin and estrogen, etidronate is an antiresorptive drug. There is very little formal evidence that its effectiveness is a function of remodeling activity at the time therapy is initiated. One can anticipate a gain of 2% to 4% annually in spinal bone mass.

Although calcitriol (Rocaltrol®) in a dose of 0.25 μg/d has been shown in one study to reduce the vertebral fracture rate compared with a group of patients taking calcium alone (21), other clinical trials have not found calcitriol to be effective in this regard. However, because calcitriol is the most potent metabolite (19) of vitamin D, it does increase intestinal calcium absorption, often resulting in hypercalciuria or hypercalcemia. Patients should be cautioned to monitor their calcium intake to avoid excessive amounts and should also be monitored every 6–8 weeks for development of hypercalciuria or hypercalcemia, because clinical symptoms and signs of these conditions may be very subtle and not evident until irreversible renal damage has occurred. It is unclear what specific effect calcitriol has on bone mass, although in some instances, increments in bone mass of 1% to 2% per annum have been recorded.

The effect of calcium supplementation on bone mass and vertebral fracture rate in established osteoporotic syndromes is not well studied. Studies that are available suggest that calcium supplementation in postmenopausal women does decrease the rate of bone loss when administered in doses of 1000–1500 mg/d, especially in individuals with histories of marginally low calcium intake (7,22–26). A combination of calcium supplements and exercise has also proven effective in stabilizing skeletal bone loss rates in postmenopausal female populations. Obviously, it is important to maintain adequate calcium supplement in addition to the active drug during estrogen, calcitonin, or alendronate therapeutic interventions, because it is difficult to mineralize newly formed matrix fully in the absence of adequate calcium. However, calcium should be taken at least 1 hour after alendronate.

Sodium fluoride is widely used as a therapy for postmenopausal osteoporosis. In doses of 50–75 mg/d, the increase in spinal bone mass achieved with sodium fluoride approximates 8% per year, twice that seen with either estrogen, calcitonin, or bisphosphonates. However, there is little evidence from properly conducted clinical trials that this increase in bone mass translates into a reduction in vertebral fractures. Moreover, sodium fluoride is associated with a significant degree of gastrointestinal distress and also a painful lower-extremity syndrome believed to represent stress fractures induced by fluoride. Recently reported studies with a lower dose of a slow-release sodium fluoride preparation administered cyclically have indicated a beneficial effect on vertebral fracture rates (27). The best results were reported in those osteoporotic patients with the highest bone mass (>65% of peak adult bone mass). Therapy was most effective in preventing fractures in previously nonfractured vertebrae; there was no significant effect on the progression of fractures in vertebra that were already fractured before initiation of treatment. It should be emphasized that these patients were also subjected to estrogen therapy. An FDA advisory panel recently recommended that a slow-release sodium fluoride preparation be approved for treatment of osteoporosis (28).

There are reports that the prevalence of osteoporotic hip fractures decreases in hypertensive patients receiving long-term therapy with hydrochlorothiazide (15,18,20). This has not been confirmed in all studies. To our knowledge, there are no formal prospective studies of thiazide diuretic therapy in osteoporotic or postmenopausal normotensive populations. Until such studies are reported and shown to be effective, thiazide diuretics should not be used as therapy for osteoporosis. However, a case could be made for selecting thiazides as the diuretic of choice in patients with osteoporosis, should diuretic therapy be otherwise indicated. Because thiazides decrease renal excretion of calcium and, uncommonly, may lead to mild hypercalcemia, extreme caution should be used when considering calcitriol therapy in a patient taking thiazides, or thiazide therapy in a patient taking calcitriol. Side effects such as hypomagnesemia, hyperglycemia, hypercholesterolemia, and hypokalemia preclude advocating this drug as potentially therapeutic for osteoporotic patients who are not hypertensive (29,30).

Newer generations of bisphosphonates, synthetic parathyroid hormone, selective estrogen receptor modulators (SERMs), and various combinations and treatment regimens of these experimental drugs, as well as the drugs listed earlier, are currently undergoing extensive clinical trials. At present, the safety and efficacy of these various drugs and their potential combinations are not well established. Consequently, their use cannot be recommended. One exception is the antiestrogen tamoxifen. This drug is widely prescribed for women with breast cancer to minimize the likelihood of recurrence. Tamoxifen inhibits bone resorption in the same manner as estrogen and is effective in preserving bone mass. However, because of reported side effects, not the least of which is endometrial carcinoma, its use should be restricted to women for whom it is prescribed as adjunctive therapy for breast cancer. Table 4 lists the several therapies that are currently under active investigation in the United States. It is anticipated that some of these therapies will become available for clinical use by the year 2000.

SELECTING A THERAPY AND MONITORING THE RESPONSE TO THERAPY

At a minimum, every patient with established osteoporosis, with or without fractures, should be given supplemental calcium at 1000–1500 mg/d. Specific therapy for osteoporosis should be restricted to estrogen, calcitonin, and alendronate, given that these drugs are approved by the FDA for an osteoporosis indication. Bone mass, which should always be measured at baseline, should be monitored at the end of 12 months of therapy. A decrease in bone mass of 2% or greater should prompt a change in therapy—either a change in dose or a change in medication. After a patient has experienced 1 full year of successful therapy, that is, 1 year of therapy with either an increase in bone mass or a 2% decrease, monitoring can be restricted to biannual measurement of bone mass. At present, there is no indication that therapy should be discontinued as long as the patient is tolerating the medication and there is no progressive decrement in bone mass. It should be noted that the antifracture efficacy of each of these drugs during the early therapeutic phase is not well established, and the occurrence of an osteoporotic fracture within the first 6–12 months of therapy should not be taken as an indication of failed therapy. The patient should be made completely aware of this before initiation of therapy. We recommend that each patient have a baseline measurement of biochemical markers of bone remodeling before initiating therapy. The patient should be seen and clinically evaluated 6–8 weeks later to ascertain compliance and possible side effects from therapy. It would also be appropriate to repeat the biochemistry at this time to determine that there is indeed a decrease in the rate of bone remodeling. If there is no satisfactory change in the biochemistry, one should consider increasing the dose. If the dose of medication is changed for whatever reason, clinical and biochemical evaluation should be repeated in 6–8 weeks until a satisfactory response is achieved. If there is no response to 3 months of therapy, one should consider a change in medication. Studies confirming the scientific rationale for monitoring biochemical markers of bone remodeling have not been fully completed. However, available data suggest that the anticipated early (3 months or less) change in several of the markers, in response to successful therapy, is greater than the precision error of the biochemical measurement. This is in contrast to serial measurement of bone mineral density, for which even a good response to therapy cannot be detected within 1 year in most patients because the anticipated change is close to the precision limits of the methods. Furthermore, there is evidence

TABLE 4. *Pharmacologic therapies for osteoporosis*

Approved by the FDA with an osteoporosis indication
  Estrogen
  Calcitonin, subcutaneous or nasal spray
  Alendronate
Approved by the FDA without an osteoporosis indication
  Calcitriol
  Etidronate
  Thiazide
Approval pending for an osteoporosis indication
  Sodium fluoride, slow-release
In clinical trial
  I. SERM
    Droloxifene
    Roloxifene
  II. Bisphosphonate
    Ibandronate
    Risedronate
    Tiludronate
  III. Parathyroid hormone

FDA, Food and Drug Administration; SERM, selective estrogen receptor modulator.

that early (3 months) changes in biochemical markers reliably predict later (24 months) changes in bone mass. Most patients and their treating physicians are reluctant to take therapy for 12 months before measurable feedback is available, and this practical consideration may dictate the frequency with which biochemical markers are monitored. As far as is known, there are no ill effects of long-term use of calcitonin or alendronate in the treatment schedules described previously. Cost and convenience become important factors in long-term patient acceptance of these drugs. Because of the potential association between long-term estrogen therapy and development of endometrial and breast cancer, appropriate monitoring for these complications must be continued. Patients must be instructed in the technique of monthly breast self-examination and must undergo an annual examination by a clinician and an annual mammogram. All episodes of unexplained vaginal bleeding must be fully evaluated by a gynecologist. In women with an intact uterus, progesterone should be given along with estrogen; most patients will soon develop either amenorrhea or a stable, recognizable bleeding pattern, which should not give rise to concern or investigation.

It is important to reemphasize that drug therapy should never be substituted for the common-sense approaches to daily living discussed in some detail in earlier sections. This includes emphasizing safety and fall prevention and avoiding drugs such as sedatives, hypnotics, and antihypertensives, which might predispose to sedation, ataxia, or postural hypotension. Patients should all be encouraged to become involved in a regular active exercise/rehabilitation program. With appropriate medical, nursing, and rehabilitation care, most patients, except for those with the most advanced disease with multiple vertebral compression fractures, can be expected to be restored to reasonable functional health with a good quality of life. Likewise, an anticipated goal of therapy should be to prevent even the first osteoporotic fracture in patients whose therapy is initiated early.

REFERENCES

1. World Health Organization: Assessment of fracture risk and its application to screening for postmenopausal osteoporosis. Report of a WHO Study Group. *World Health Organ Tech Rep Ser* 843: 1–129, 1994
2. Canalis E: Regulation of bone remodeling. In: Favus MJ, Christakos S, Goldring SR, et al. (eds) *Primer on the Metabolic Bone Diseases and Disorders of Mineral Metabolism, Third edition.* Lippincott-Raven Publishers, Philadelphia, 29–34, 1996
3. Recker RR: Bone biopsy and histomorphometry in clinical practice. In: Favus MJ, Christakos S, Goldring SR, et al. (eds) *Primer on the Metabolic Bone Diseases and Disorders of Mineral Metabolism, Third edition.* Lippincott-Raven Publishers, Philadelphia, 164–167, 1996
4. Villareal DT, Civitelli R, Chines A, Avioli LV: Subclinical vitamin D deficiency in postmenopausal women with low vertebral bone mass. *J Clin Endocrinol Metab* 72:628–634, 1991
5. Garnero P, Shih WJ, Gineyts E, Karpf DB, Delmas PD: Comparison of new biochemical markers of bone turnover in late postmenopausal women in response to alendronate treatment. *J Clin Endocrinol Metab* 79:1693–1700, 1994
6. Lufkin EG, Wahner HW, O'Fallon WM, et al: Treatment of postmenopausal osteoporosis with transdermal estrogen. *Ann Intern Med* 117:1–9, 1992
7. Prince RL, Smith M, Dick IM, et al: Prevention of postmenopausal osteoporosis. Comparative study of exercise, calcium supplementation, and hormone replacement therapy. *N Engl J Med* 325:1189–1195, 1991
8. Civitelli R, Gonnelli S, Zacchei F, et al: Bone turnover in postmenopausal osteoporosis. *J Clin Invest* 82:1268–1274, 1988
9. Avioli LV: Heterogeneity of osteoporotic syndromes and the response to calcitonin therapy. *Calcif Tissue Int* 49(Suppl 2):S16–19, 1991
10. Rico H, Hernandez ER, Diaz-Mediaville J, et al: Treatment of multiple myeloma with nasal spray calcitonin: A histomorphometric and biochemical study. *Bone Miner* 8:231–237, 1990
11. Mazzuoli GF, Passeri M, Gennari C, et al: Effects of salmon calcitonin in postmenopausal osteoporosis: A controlled double-blind clinical study. *Calcif Tissue Int* 38:3–8, 1986
12. Overgaard K, Riis BJ, Christiansen C, et al: Effect of calcitonin given intranasally on early postmenopausal bone loss. *BMJ* 299:477–479, 1989
13. Lyritis GP, Tsakalabos S, Magiasis B, et al: Analgesic effect of salmon calcitonin on osteoporotic vertebral fractures. Double-blind, placebo-controlled study. *Calcif Tissue Int* 49:369–372, 1991
14. Rico H, Hernandez ER, Revilla M, Gomez-Castresana F: Salmon calcitonin reduces vertebral fracture rate in the postmenopausal crush fracture syndrome. *Bone Miner* 16:131–138, 1992
15. Jones G, Nguyen T, Sambrook PN, Eisman JA: Thiazide diuretics and fractures: can meta-analysis help? *J Bone Miner Res* 10:106–111, 1995
16. Storm T, Thamsborg G, Steiniche T, Genant HK, Sorensen OH: Effect of intermittent cyclical etidronate therapy on bone mass and fracture rate in women with postmenopausal osteoporosis. *N Engl J Med* 322:1265–1271, 1990
17. Leiberman UA, Weiss SR, Broll J, et al: Effect of all alendronate on bone mineral density and the incidence of fracture in postmenopausal osteoporotic women. *N Engl J Med* 333:1437–1443, 1995
18. LaCroix AZ, Wienpahl J, White LR, et al: Thiazide diuretic agents and the incidence of hip fracture. *N Engl J Med* 322:286–290, 1990
19. Ott SM, Chesnut CH III: Calcitriol treatment is not effective in postmenopausal osteoporosis. *Ann Intern Med* 110:267–274, 1989
20. Watts NB, Harris ST, Genant HK, et al: Intermittent cyclical etidronate treatment of postmenopausal osteoporosis. *N Engl J Med* 323:73–79, 1990
21. Tilyard MW, Spears GFS, Thompson J, Dovey S: Treatment of postmenopausal osteoporosis with calcitriol or calcium. *N Engl J Med* 326:357–361, 1992
22. Overgaard K, Hansen MA, Nielsen V-AH, Riis BJ, Christiansen C: Discontinuous calcitonin treatment of established osteoporosis: Effects of withdrawal of treatment. *Am J Med* 89:1–6, 1990
23. Dawson-Hughes B, Dallal GE, Krall EA, Sadowski L, Sahyoun N, Tannenbau S: Controlled trial of the effect of calcium supplementation on bone density in postmenopausal women. *N Engl J Med* 323:878–883, 1990
24. Dawson-Hughes B: Calcium supplementation and bone loss: A review of controlled clinical trials. *Am J Clin Nutr* 54:274S–280S, 1991
25. Elders PJM, Netelenbos JC, Lips P, et al: Calcium supplementation reduces vertebral bone loss in perimenopausal women: A controlled trial in 248 women between 46 and 55 years of age. *J Clin Endocrinol Metab* 73:533–540, 1991
26. Licata AA, Jones-Gall DJ: Effect of supplemental calcium on serum and urinary calcium in osteoporotic patients. *J Am Coll Nutr* 11:164–167, 1992
27. Pak YC, Sakhaee K, Adams-Huet B, Piziak V, Peterson RD, Poindexter JR: Treatment of postmenopausal osteoporosis with slow-release sodium fluoride. Final report of a randomized controlled trial. *Ann Intern Med* 123:401–408, 1995
28. Hedlund LR, Gallagher JC: Increased incidences of fractures in osteoporosis patients treated with sodium fluoride. *J Bone Miner Res* 4:223–225, 1989
29. Martin BJ, Milligan K: Diuretic associated hypomagnesemia in the elderly. *Arch Intern Med* 147:1768–1771, 1987
30. Ray WA: Thiazide diuretics and osteoporosis: Time for a clinical trial? (Editorial). *Ann Intern Med* 115:64–65, 1991

15. The Special Problem of Hip Fracture

Eric S. Orwoll, M.D.

Department of Endocrinology and Metabolism, Portland Veterans Affairs Medical Center; and Department of Medicine, Oregon Health Sciences University, Portland, Oregon

Metabolic skeletal disorders are commonly generalized and may cause fracture of virtually any bone. Fractures of the proximal femur are unique. They are devastating both to the health of the affected individual as well as to society, and have been the focus of intense study. The understanding of their causation is more complete than for other complications of metabolic skeletal disease. They justifiably deserve special comment.

THE IMPORTANCE OF HIP FRACTURE

The public health impact of hip fracture is enormous. In 1990, there were more than 350,000 hip fractures in North America, more than 400,000 in Europe, and almost 600,000 in Asia (1). As the population increases and ages, these numbers will rise dramatically. The economic implications are obvious (2,3).

The effects of osteoporosis on individuals are equally impressive. In elderly women, there is a 12% to 30% reduction in expected survival after hip fracture (4), and the mortality rate is even greater in men (5). Age and prefracture condition are important indicators of outcome, as the increased mortality after hip fracture is probably the result of an interaction between preexisting conditions and the fracture itself (6,7). In addition to acute morbidity and mortality, hip fracture is commonly the precedent to prolonged or permanent dependency. Fifty percent of patients who survive the acute care of hip fracture are discharged to nursing homes, and 25% remain institutionalized 1 year later (8,9). Essentially permanent nursing home care is needed in an important fraction of patients (10). Not surprisingly, the determinants of function after recovery from hip fracture are complex, and include comorbid conditions as well as social context (11).

EPIDEMIOLOGY

Hip fracture is uncommon below the age of 50. When it occurs at younger ages, it is frequently the result of intense trauma or the presence of conditions known to affect skeletal health (12). Most hip fractures occur in the elderly, at a median age of approximately 80 years (6,13,14). In middle age, the incidence of hip fracture begins to rise rapidly, so that by age 50, the lifetime risk of hip fracture is 17% among U.S. women. The rise in the incidence of hip fracture is also dramatic in men, but it begins about a decade later, resulting in a fairly consistent male to female incidence ratio of roughly 1:2 in most developed countries (15,16). However, there is considerable geographic variation in the male to female ratio, with a complete reversal observed in some areas (14). Finally, there are pronounced racial effects on hip fracture rates, with blacks and Asians having lower fracture rates than whites (17–19).

CAUSATION

Skeletal Fragility

A convincing body of evidence links proximal femoral bone mass to the subsequent risk of hip fracture in women. An older woman with hip bone mineral density (BMD) 1 standard deviation (SD) below the mean is about seven times more likely to suffer a hip fracture than a woman with BMD 1 SD above the mean (20) (Fig. 1). Interestingly, BMD measures of the femoral neck do not predict femoral neck fracture risk in very elderly women (>80 years) (21), suggesting that in older age, factors other than bone mass become more prominent in the causation of fracture. Bone mineral density measures at other skeletal sites (spine, radius, calcaneus) also predict hip fracture risk, but with slightly less power (20) (Fig. 1).

Proximal femoral BMD is influenced by a wide variety of factors. Density increases rapidly during childhood and adolescence, and several variables have been found to influence the accumulation of peak bone mass (22), including heredity, gender, nutrition, mechanical forces, and hormonal factors. In turn, peak femoral bone mass appears to influence lifetime fracture risk. For instance, gender- and race-related differences in fracture risk can be traced in part to differences in adolescent skeletal development (22,23).

Bone mineral loss occurs from the proximal femur in adults of both sexes. There is presumed to be an accelerated phase of bone loss during the early postmenopausal period, and femoral BMD is higher in women who receive estrogen replacement (24). The rate of bone loss is similar in men and women after the age of 60 (25,26), and actually appears to accelerate in the oldest segment of the population (26,27). The determinants of femoral bone mass in adults are numerous, including body weight, gonadal status, activity and strength, nutrition (calcium, vitamin D), lifestyle (alcohol, caffeine, tobacco), and a variety of medications and medical conditions (7,21,26).

Although measures of bone mass provide valuable insight into skeletal fragility, other factors may also be important. This is an area of considerable research attention, but already it is apparent that several aspects of gross femoral structure (hip axis length, cortical thickness, trochanteric width, trabecular structure) independently influence fracture risk (28–33) (Fig. 2).

The likelihood of hip fracture appears to be related to the history of previous fragility fractures. For instance, a woman who has a prevalent vertebral fracture is about twice as likely to experience a subsequent hip fracture (34). To

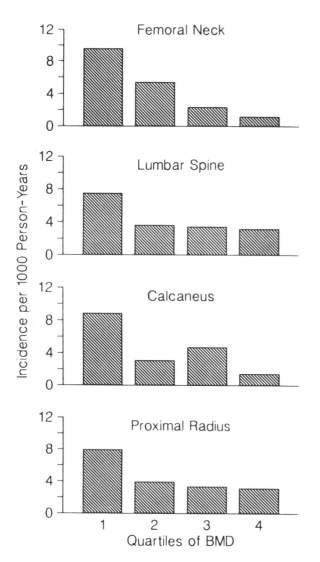

FIG. 1. Incidence of hip fracture by age-adjusted quartile of bone mineral density (BMD) (20).

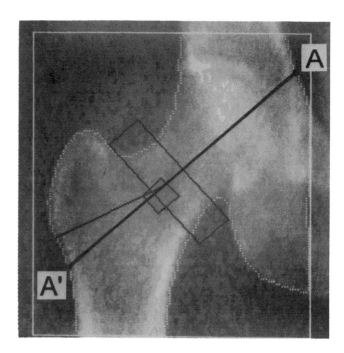

FIG. 2. Definition of the hip axis length (A-A′) from a dual-energy x-ray absorptiometry scan of the proximal femur (29).

some extent, this is the result of reduced bone mass, but there appears to be added risk independent of BMD, suggesting that other factors (skeletal structure, trauma propensity) may also be important.

The two major subtypes of hip fracture (femoral neck and trochanteric) have somewhat distinct epidemiologic patterns and clinical character (35,36), suggesting different etiologies (Table 1). In general, trochanteric fractures occur relatively more frequently in older women, are associated with lower trochanteric and higher femoral neck BMD, are less strongly associated with a maternal history of femoral fracture, and occur more frequently in patients who have experienced other osteoporotic fractures. On the other hand, fall characteristics, body habitus, and hip axis length have been found to be similar in the two kinds of fractures (35,37).

Osteoporosis is the major metabolic disorder underlying skeletal fragility, but osteomalacia also has been found in a minority of patients with hip fracture. This is particularly true in the elderly with restricted nutrition and sunlight exposure. For unclear reasons, in the last 10–15 years the prevalence of osteomalacia in patients with hip fracture appears to have declined (38).

Trauma

As opposed to vertebral fractures, the vast majority of hip fractures in the elderly occur as a direct result of falls (7). Even an uncomplicated fall from a standing height generates enough force to fracture an elderly femur (39). Factors that increase the likelihood of falls are important determinants of hip fracture risk (7,21,40), including drugs or medications (sedatives, alcohol, antidepressants), muscle weakness, disorders of gait and balance (neuromuscular impairment, visual dysfunction), cognitive impairment, and environmental hazards. The contribution of fall propensity to the risk of hip fractures is as important as that of skeletal fragility, and may be more important in the most elderly.

TABLE 1. *Fracture type*

Characteristic	Trochanteric	Femoral neck
More likely in older women	X	
Lower trochanteric bone mineral density	X	
Osteoporotic fractures common	X	
Maternal hip fracture		X
Falling increases risk	X	X
More likely in thin subjects	X	X
Greater hip axis length	X	X

In addition to the frequency of falls, the character of the fall is crucial in defining fracture risk. Whereas approximately one third of the elderly fall each year, only a small fraction experience hip fracture. A fall to the side, particularly in tall and thin individuals, is much more likely to cause a fracture (7,31). Falls associated with fractures most often occur in frail individuals, with little ability to protect themselves from direct impact on the trochanter. Women are more likely to fall on a hip than are men (41).

TREATMENT

Virtually all proximal femoral fractures require surgical fixation and an intense (and often prolonged) period of rehabilitation. During this time, there is considerable risk of additional bone loss (42) and other complications. Delayed union and femoral head avascular necrosis are notorious, especially in femoral neck fractures, and osteoporotic bone is particularly susceptible to added problems (43). During the immediate postoperative period, attention to factors that promote the rehabilitation process is important. For instance, many elderly who experience a hip fracture are not well nourished, a problem that can be exacerbated during the postoperative inpatient stay. Nutritional supplementation during this time has reduced hospital-associated complications and mortality (44). This regimen should include adequate vitamin D and calcium supplementation (45). Early restoration of mobility is preferred to preserve as much function as possible.

PREVENTION

Current efforts to prevent hip fracture have focused on maximizing proximal femoral biomechanical strength and reducing fall propensity. In both areas, there are as yet insufficient long-term data. In men, there have been no trials of strategies to prevent fracture.

In women, postmenopausal estrogen replacement has been shown reliably to reduce the risk of hip fracture (24). Other drugs are less well demonstrated as effective (46). Dietary calcium and vitamin D supplementation have reduced hip fracture risk dramatically in some frail older women (47). The effectiveness of some other potentially useful interventions (calcitonin, anabolic steroids, bisphosphonates, parathyroid hormone) has not been adequately documented (48).

The prevention of falls in the elderly is also important. Strength and balance can be improved quickly and dramatically in the elderly with appropriate exercise regimens, and successful programs for the reduction of falls in the elderly have been described (49). Such mundane apparatus as hip pads and cushioned floors in high-risk environments (e.g., nursing homes) may be quite effective (50). It is important to identify those at highest risk, to whom the most intensive preventive interventions should be directed.

REFERENCES

1. Cooper C, Campion G, Melton LJ III: Hip fractures in the elderly: A world-wide projection. *Osteoporosis Int* 2:285–289, 1992
2. Norris RJ: Medical costs of osteoporosis. *Bone* 13:S11–S16, 1992
3. Barrett-Connor E: The economic and human costs of osteoporotic fracture. *Am J Med* 98:2A-3S–7S, 1995
4. Cummings SR, Kelsey JL, Nevitt MC, O'Dowd KJ: Epidemiology of osteoporosis and osteoporotic fractures. *Epidemiol Rev* 7:178–208, 1985
5. Jacobsen SJ, Goldberg J, Miles TP, Brody JA, Stiers W, Rimm AA: Race and sex differences in mortality following fracture of the hip. *Am J Public Health* 82:1147–1150, 1992
6. Keene GS, Parker MJ, Pryor GA: Mortality and morbidity after hip fractures. *BMJ* 307:1248–1250, 1993
7. Nevitt MC: Epidemiology of osteoporosis. *Rheum Dis Clin North Am* 20:535–559, 1994
8. Ray WA, Griffin MR, Baugh DK: Mortality following hip fracture before and after implementation of the prospective payment system. *Arch Intern Med* 150:2109–2114, 1990
9. Palmer RM: The impact of the prospective payment system on the treatment of hip fractures in the elderly. *Arch Intern Med* 149:2237–2241, 1989
10. Chrischilles EA, Butler CD, Davis CS, Wallace RB: A model of lifetime osteoporosis impact. *Arch Intern Med* 151:2026–2032, 1991
11. Weatherall M: Case mix and outcome for patients with fracture of the proximal femur. *N Z Med J* 106:451–452, 1993
12. Gray AJR, Parker MJ: Intracapsular fractures of the femoral neck in young patients. *Injury* 25:667–669, 1994
13. Cummings SR: Are patients with hip fractures more osteoporotic? *Am J Med* 78:487–494, 1985
14. Elffors I, Allander E, Kanis JA, Gullberg B, Johnell O, Dequeker J, Dilsen G, Gennari C, Lopes Vaz AA, Lyritis G, Mazzuoli GF, Miravet L, Passeri M, Perez Cano R, Rapado A, Ribot C: The variable incidence of hip fracture in southern Europe: The MEDOS Study. *Osteoporosis Int* 4:253–263, 1994
15. Jones G, Nguyen T, Sambrook PN, Kelly PJ, Gilbert C, Eisman JA: Symptomatic fracture incidence in elderly men and women: The Dubbo Osteoporosis Epidemiology Study (DOES). *Osteoporosis Int* 4:277–282, 1994
16. Jacobsen SJ, Goldberg J, Miles TP, Brody JA, Stiers W, Rimm AA: Hip fracture incidence among the old and very old: A population-based study of 745,435 cases. *Am J Public Health* 80:871–873, 1990
17. Farmer ME, White LR, Brody JA, Bailey KR: Race and sex differences in hip fracture incidence. *Am J Public Health* 74:1374–1380, 1984
18. Ross PD, Norimatsu H, Davis JW, Yano K, Wasnich RD, Fujiwara S, Hosoda Y, Melton LJ III: A comparison of hip fracture incidence among native Japanese, Japanese Americans, and American Caucasians. *Am J Epidemiol* 133:801–809, 1991
19. Cummings SR, Cauley JA, Palermo L, Ross PD, Wasnich RD, Black D, Faulkner KG: Racial differences in hip axis lengths might explain racial differences in the rates of hip fracture. *Osteoporosis Int* 4:226–229, 1994
20. Cummings SR, Black DM, Nevitt MC, Browner W, Cauley J, Ensrud K, Genant HK, Palermo L, Scott J, Vogt TM, S.O.F. Research Group: Bone density at various sites for prediction of hip fractures. *Lancet* 341:72–75, 1993
21. Cummings SR, Black D: Bone mass measurements and risk of fracture in Caucasian women: A review of findings from prospective studies. *Am J Med* 98:2A-24S–28S, 1995
22. Bonjour JP, Theintz G, Law F, Slosman D, Rizzoli R: Peak bone mass. *Osteoporosis Int* 1:S7–S13, 1994
23. Gilsanz V, Roe TF, Mora S: Changes in vertebral bone density in black girls and white girls during childhood and puberty. *N Engl J Med* 325:1597–1600, 1991
24. Cauley JA, Seeley DA, Ensrud K, Ettinger B, Black D, Cummings SR: Estrogen replacement therapy and fractures in older women. *Ann Intern Med* 122:9–16, 1995
25. Hannan MT, Felson DT, Anderson JJ: Bone mineral density in elderly men and women: Results from the Framingham osteoporosis study. *J Bone Miner Res* 7:547–553, 1992
26. Jones G, Nguyen T, Sambrook P, Kelly PJ, Eisman JA: Progressive loss of bone in the femoral neck in elderly people: Longitudinal findings from the Dubbo osteoporosis epidemiology study. *BMJ* 309:691–695, 1994
27. Orwoll ES, Oviatt SK, McClung MR, Deftos LJ, Sexton G: The rate of bone mineral loss in normal men and the effects of calcium and cholecalciferol supplementation. *Ann Intern Med* 112:29–34, 1990
28. Gluer CC, Cummings SR, Pressman A, Li J, Gluer K, Faulkner

KG, Grampp S, Genant HK: Prediction of hip fractures from pelvic radiographs: The Study of Osteoporotic Fractures. *J Bone Miner Res* 9:671–677, 1994

29. Faulkner KG, McClung M, Cummings SR: Automated evaluation of hip axis length for predicting hip fracture. *J Bone Miner Res* 9:1065–1070, 1994

30. Reid IR, Chin K, Evans MC, Jones JG: Relation between increase in length of hip axis in older women between 1950s and 1990s and increase in age specific rates of hip fracture. *BMJ* 309:508–509, 1994

31. Hayes WC, Piazza SJ, Zysset PK: Biomechanics of fracture risk prediction of the hip and spine by quantitative computed tomography. *Radiol Clin North Am* 29:1–18, 1991

32. Genant HK, Gluer C-C, Lotz JC: Gender differences in bone density, skeletal geometry, and fracture biomechanics. *Radiology* 190:636–640, 1994

33. Mazess RB: Fracture risk: A role for compact bone. *Calcif Tissue Int* 47:191–193, 1990

34. Kotowicz MA, Melton LJ III, Cooper C, Atkinson EJ, O'Fallon WM, Riggs BL: Risk of hip fracture in women with vertebral fracture. *J Bone Miner Res* 9:599–605, 1994

35. Greenspan SL, Myers ER, Maitland LA, Kido TH, Krasnow MB, Hayes WC: Trochanteric bone mineral density is associated with type of hip fracture in the elderly. *J Bone Miner Res* 9:1889–1894, 1994

36. Baudoin C, Fardellone P, Sebert J-L: Effect of sex and age on the ratio of cervical to trochanteric hip fracture. *Acta Orthop Scand* 64:647–653, 1993

37. Mautalen CA, Vega EM: Different characteristics of cervical and trochanteric hip fractures. *Osteoporos Int* 3 (Suppl 1):102–105, 1993

38. Robinson CM, McQueen MM, Wheelwright EF, Gardner DL, Salter DM: Changing prevalence of osteomalacia in hip fractures in southeast Scotland over a 20-year period. *Injury* 23:300–302, 1992

39. Greenspan SL, Myers ER, Maitland LA, Resnick NM, Hayes WC: Fall severity and bone mineral density as risk factors for hip fracture in ambulatory elderly. *JAMA* 271:128–133, 1994

40. Grisso JA, Kelsey JL, Strom BL, O'Brien LA, Maislin G, LaPann K, Samelson L, Hoffman S: Risk factors for hip fracture in black women. *N Engl J Med* 330:1555–1559, 1994

41. O'Neill TW, Varlow J, Silman AJ, Reeve J, Reid DM, Todd C, Woolf AD: Age and sex influences on fall characteristics. *Ann Rheum Dis* 53:773–775, 1994

42. McCarthy CK, Steinberg GG, Agren M, Leahey D, Wyman E, Baran DT: Quantifying bone loss from the proximal femur after total hip arthroplasty. *J Bone Joint Surg* 73-B:774–778, 1991

43. Cornell CN: Management of fractures in patients with osteoporosis. *Orthop Clin North Am* 21:125–141, 1990

44. Delmi M, Rapin CH, Bengoa JM, Delmas PD, Vasey H, Bonjour JP: Clinical practice: Dietary supplementation in elderly patients with fractured neck of the femur. *Lancet* 335:1013–1016, 1990

45. Ng K, St John A, Bruce DG: Secondary hyperparathyroidism, vitamin D deficiency and hip fracture: Importance of sampling times after fracture. *Bone Miner* 25:103–109, 1994

46. Kanis JA, Johnell O, Gullberg B, Allander E, Dilsen G, Gennari C, Lopes Vaz AA, Lyritis GP, Mazzuoli G, Miravet L, Passeri M, Perez Cano R, Rapado A, Ribot C: Evidence for efficacy of drugs affecting bone metabolism in preventing hip fracture. *BMJ* 305:1124–1128, 1992

47. Chapuy MC, Arlot ME, Duboeuf F, Brun J, Crouzet B, Arnaud S, Delmas PD, Meunier PJ: Vitamin D3 and calcium to prevent hip fractures in elderly women. *N Engl J Med* 327:1637–1642, 1992

48. Kanis JA: Treatment of osteoporosis in elderly women. *Am J Med* 98:2A-60S–66S, 1995

49. Tinetti ME, Baker DI, McAvay G, Clasu EB, Garrett P, Gottschalk M: A multifactorial intervention to reduce the risk of falling among elderly people in the community. *N Engl J Med* 331:821–827, 1994

50. Lauritzen JB, Petersen MM, Lund B: Effect of external hip protectors on hip fractures. *Lancet* 341:11–13, 1993

16. Juvenile Osteoporosis

Michael E. Norman, M.D.

Department of Pediatrics, University of North Carolina School of Medicine, Chapel Hill, North Carolina

The diagnosis of osteoporosis in children is usually made when skeletal radiographs reveal a generalized decrease in mineralized bone (e.g., osteopenia) in the absence of rickets or excessive bone resorption (e.g., osteitis fibrosa). Juvenile osteoporosis occurs typically before the onset of puberty, but it may also be seen in younger children, especially when they are growing rapidly. It may be due to an inherited condition that is clinically evident from birth or early infancy, or it may be acquired during childhood. There are a primary or idiopathic form and a number of secondary forms of juvenile osteoporosis. The condition is uncommon; between 1939 and 1991, ~60 cases of idiopathic juvenile osteoporosis (IJO) were reported in the literature. However, the onset of osteoporosis just before or after the onset of puberty can have far-reaching effects, because one half of skeletal mass is acquired during the adolescent years.

PATHOPHYSIOLOGY

True osteoporosis is defined histomorphometrically by a decreased total amount of normally formed bone. During bone formation (modeling) and bone remodeling, two fundamental defects may occur, singly or in combination: (i) a defect in bone-forming cells leading to decreased or defective matrix formation; and (ii) abnormalities in the coupling of bone formation and resorption, in which an imbalance develops between matrix formation (mineralization) and bone resorption. An inherited group of disorders known as osteogenesis imperfecta usually represents defects in bone-forming cells, in which mutations in one of the two genes encoding type I procollagen produce defective matrix (1). IJO and the secondary causes of osteoporosis represent various expressions of the latter type of defect. IJO and chronic corticosteroid therapy are the most important forms of acquired juvenile osteoporosis. Early reports of calcium balance have suggested that IJO changes, with initially negative or inappropriately neutral balances (2,3), progressing to positive balance during the healing phase (3,4) and in response to vitamin D administration. Jowsey and Johnson (5) and Hoekman et al. (6) presented histologic evidence of increased bone resorption, whereas Smith (7) and Reed et al. (8) found decreased bone formation as the major pathophysiologic event in IJO. Evans et al. (9) and Marder et al. (10) suggested a role for 1,25-dihydroxyvitamin D deficiency in the pathogenesis of IJO. Several reports have also suggested a role for calcitonin deficiency in some patients (11). The bone loss noted in astronauts undergoing prolonged periods of weightlessness in space may be analogous to IJO, with rapid resorption of weight-bearing bones and suppressed bone formation. Both weightlessness and IJO appear to be reversible (7). Some have speculated that IJO, like weightlessness, consists of some fundamental disturbance in the mechanical forces that stimulate new bone formation in the growing and young adult skeleton. Finally, recent data in adult osteoporotic patients suggest impaired bone formation related in part to reduced insulin-like growth factor 1 secretion (8).

CLINICAL FEATURES

The typical child presenting with IJO is immediately prepubertal and healthy. Symptoms begin with an insidious onset of pain in the lower back, hips, and feet, and difficulty walking. Knee and ankle pain and fractures of the lower extremities may be present. IJO affects both sexes equally; family and dietary histories are negative. Physical examination may be entirely normal or reveal thoracolumbar kyphosis or kyphoscoliosis, pigeon chest deformity, crown-pubis to pubis-heel ratio of less than 1.0, loss of height, deformities of the long bones, and limp. Generally, these physical abnormalities are reversible, although several of the original patients subsequently developed crippling deformities that left them wheelchair bound with cardiorespiratory abnormalities (2).

The history and physical examination of children with secondary forms of osteoporosis reflect the primary disease more than the osteoporosis (Table 1). There is usually a family history of osteoporosis or of the primary disease, evidence of failure to thrive, immobilization, or administration of corticosteroid or anticonvulsant drugs.

BIOCHEMICAL FEATURES

There are no known biochemical abnormalities characteristic of IJO, and no known endocrine disorder has been identified. In some children (2,3,6), calcium balance is markedly negative or inappropriately neutral, and serum calcium levels are normal. Urine calcium excretion may be normal or elevated. Serum phosphorus, bicarbonate, magnesium, and alkaline phosphatase levels are also normal. The disease eventually resolves with time and the onset of puberty, and can be detected by improvement in calcium balance. Increased urinary hydroxyproline excretion, an indirect indicator of increased bone resorption, as well as hypercalcemia and suppressed parathyroid hormone secretion have been observed in some patients. Suppression of parathyroid hormone secretion reduces 1,25-dihydroxyvitamin D synthesis and decreases intestinal calcium absorption, contributing to the negative calcium balance (6).

In secondary forms of osteoporosis, biochemical and clinical clues to diagnosis depend on the underlying primary disease (3,9).

TABLE 1. *Differential diagnosis of juvenile osteoporosis*

I. Primary
   Calcium deficiency
   Idiopathic juvenile osteoporosis
   Osteogenesis imperfecta
      Multiple subtypes
II. Secondary
   Endocrine
      Cushing syndrome
      Diabetes mellitus
      Glucocorticoid therapy
      Thyrotoxicosis
   Gastrointestinal
      Biliary atresia
      Glycogen storage disease, type I
      Hepatitis
      Malabsorption
   Inborn errors of metabolism
      Homocystinuria
      Lysinuric protein intolerance
   Miscellaneous
      Acute lymphoblastic leukemia
      Anticonvulsant therapy
      Cyanotic congenital heart disease
      Immobilization

RADIOLOGIC FEATURES

Conventional radiography is a relatively insensitive method for detecting bone loss; ~30% of skeletal mineral must be lost before osteopenia can be appreciated. In the absence of fractures or rickets, osteomalacia may be difficult to distinguish from osteoporosis as the cause of osteopenia. Looser lines or changes of secondary hyperparathyroidism favor rickets or osteomalacia, whereas biconcave vertebral deformities favor osteoporosis (see Chapter 8). Children with fully expressed IJO present with generalized osteopenia, fractures of the weight-bearing bones, and collapsed or misshapen vertebrae. Disc spaces may be widened asymmetrically because of wedging of the vertebral bodies (Fig. 1). Sclerosis may be noted. Long bones are usually normal in length and cortical width, unlike the thin, gracile bones of children with osteogenesis imperfecta (1). The pathognomonic x-ray finding of IJO is neoosseous osteoporosis, an impaction-type fracture occurring at sites of newly formed weight-bearing metaphyseal bone. Typically, such fractures are seen at the distal tibiae, adjacent to the ankle joint and adjacent to the knee and hip joints (3,7). Using photon absorptiometry and computed tomography for detection of decreased bone mineral

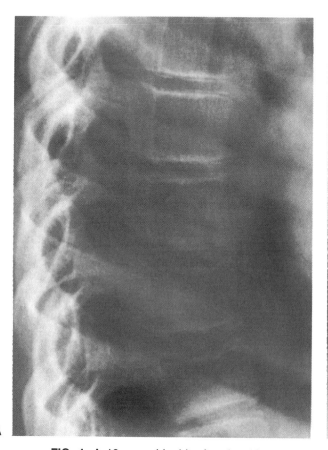
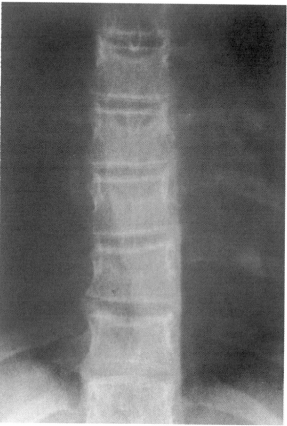

A   B

FIG. 1. A 10-year-old white female with back pain. **A:** Lateral view of thoracolumbar spine reveals wedge compression fracture of T8 and T9 with patchy sclerosis of T7. There was generalized osteopenia of the skeleton, confirmed by computed tomography. **B:** Anterior view of the same patient reveals loss of height of T8 on the right side. The vertebral bodies are osteopenic.

density, childhood osteoporosis may be diagnosed much earlier.

BONE BIOPSY

Few qualitative or quantitative studies of bone tissue have been performed in childhood osteoporosis. From microradiographs of bone, Cloutier et al. (4) and Jowsey and Johnson (5) reported increased bone resorption in IJO. They speculated that excessive dietary phosphorus intake may have stimulated parathyroid-mediated bone resorption. In contrast, Smith (7), using quantitative static histology of iliac bone, found indirect evidence of decreased bone formation. Evans et al. (9) found no abnormalities of endosteal bone formation by histomorphometry (using double tetracycline labeling) in a 12-year-old boy with severe IJO. They suggested that the major evidence for impaired periosteal new bone formation in IJO would come from careful study of skeletal radiographs and not from bone biopsy material.

DIFFERENTIAL DIAGNOSIS

Osteogenesis imperfecta is the most important entity to consider in the differential diagnosis of IJO (13). Comparisons with IJO are listed in Table 2 (1). Osteogenesis imperfecta can usually be differentiated from IJO by clinical characteristics, radiologic findings, and a positive family history. Diseases resulting in osteoporosis in childhood that must be differentiated from IJO are outlined in Table 1. Secondary causes of osteoporosis must be excluded in those children who present without the typical features of IJO. As a result, the diagnosis of IJO is reached by excluding secondary causes of osteoporosis and osteogenesis imperfecta.

THERAPY

Prompt and definitive diagnosis early in the course of the disease is important, although there is no specific medical or surgical therapy. Supportive care is instituted promptly (non-weight-bearing, crutch walking, and physical therapy) in anticipation of spontaneous recovery with the onset of puberty. There may be a role for supplemental calcitriol therapy in selected patients (9,10). Sodium fluoride increases bone mass and has been reported to reduce fracture rates in primary vertebral osteoporosis (14). Fluoride treatment has been associated with a number of toxicity symptoms and musculoskeletal complaints in adults, and it remains unclear whether the hyperosteoidosis associated with this therapy produces increased bone strength. The author has used long-term fluoride therapy with a positive clinical response in one patient with IJO (unpublished observations). Based on findings of decreased bone resorption on bone biopsy in one child, Hoekman et al. (6) reported dramatic clinical, biochemical, and radiologic responses with bisphosphonate, which inhibits bone resorption. Osteoporosis in most patients is reversible. Treatment of secondary causes of osteoporosis requires careful management of the underlying disease to minimize bone loss.

PROGNOSIS

With the exception of a few patients who develop progressive lower-extremity, spine, and chest-wall deformities and require confinement to wheelchairs or bed, the prognosis of IJO is generally excellent. Distinguishing features have been recognized that identify the subgroup of children with poor prognosis. The prognosis of osteogenesis imperfecta is dependent on the inherited subtype and is discussed in reference. 1. The most effective treatment of secondary osteoporosis is successful therapy of the underlying disease. Failing this, supportive care should be provided as with IJO.

TABLE 2. *Differential diagnosis: osteogenesis imperfecta (OI) vs. idiopathic juvenile osteoporosis (IJO)*

Characteristic	OI	IJO
Family history	Often positive	Negative
Age at onset	Birth	2–3 yr before puberty
Duration of signs/symptoms	Lifelong (intermittent)	1–4 yr
Physical findings	Thin gracile bones, short stature	Upper-lower segment ratio <1.0
	Multiple deformities and contractures	Dorsal kyphoscoliosis
	Blue sclerae[a], deafness	Pectus carinatum
	Lax joints, hernias	Abnormal gait
	Abnormal dentition	
Calcium balance	Positive	Negative in acute phase
Radiologic findings	Narrow long bones	Long bones with thin cortices
	Thin ribs	Wedge compression fractures of spine
	Pathologic fractures, rarely metaphyseal in location	Metaphyseal fractures common
	Wormian skull bones	
Molecular studies (dermal fibroblasts)	Abnormal collagen	Normal collagen

[a]Classic dominant inherited form, with associated nerve deafness.

REFERENCES

1. Whyte MP: Osteogenesis imperfecta. In: Favus MJ, Christakos S, Goldring SR, et al. (eds) *Primer on the Metabolic Bone Diseases and Disorders of Mineral Metabolism, Third edition.* Lippincott-Raven Publishers, Philadelphia, 382–385, 1996
2. Dent CE, Friedman M: Idiopathic juvenile osteoporosis. *Q J Med* 34:177–210, 1965
3. Brenton DP, Dent CE: Idiopathic juvenile osteoporosis. In: Bickel JH, Stern J (eds) *Inborn Errors of Calcium and Bone Metabolism.* Baltimore, University Park Press, 223–238, 1976
4. Cloutier MD, Hayles AB, Riggs BL, Jowsey J, Bickel WH: Juvenile osteoporosis: Report of a case including a description of some metabolic and microradiographic studies. *Pediatrics* 40:649–655, 1967
5. Jowsey J, Johnson KA: Juvenile osteoporosis: Bone findings in seven patients. *J Pediatr* 81:511–517, 1972
6. Hoekman K, Papapoulos SE, Peters ACB, Bijvoet OL: Characteristics and bisphosphonate treatment of a patient with juvenile osteoporosis. *J Clin Endocrinol Metab* 61:952–956, 1985
7. Smith R: Idiopathic osteoporosis in the young. *J Bone Joint Surg* 62-B:417–427, 1980
8. Reed BY, Zeswekh JE, Sakhaee K, Breslau N, Gottschalk F, Pak CYC: Serum IGF-I is low and correlated with osteoblastic surface in idiopathic osteoporosis. *J Bone Miner Res* 10:1218–1224, 1995
9. Evans RA, Dunstan CR, Hills E: Bone metabolism in idiopathic juvenile osteoporosis: A case report. *Calcif Tissue Int* 35:5–8, 1983
10. Marder HK, Tsang RC, Hug G, Crawford AC: Calcitriol deficiency in idiopathic juvenile osteoporosis. *Am J Dis Child* 136:914–917, 1982
11. Saggese G, Bertelloni S, Baroncelli GI, Perri G, Calderazzi A: Mineral metabolism and calcitriol therapy in idiopathic juvenile osteoporosis. *Am J Dis Child* 145:457–461, 1991
12. Jackson EC, Strife CF, Tsang RC, Marder HK: Effect of calcitonin replacement therapy in idiopathic juvenile osteoporosis. *Am J Dis Child* 142:1237–1239, 1988
13. Teotia M, Teotia SPS, Singh RK: Idiopathic juvenile osteoporosis. *Am J Dis Child* 133:894–900, 1979
14. Harrison JE: Fluoride treatment for osteoporosis. *Calcif Tissue Int* 46:287–288, 1990

17. Glucocorticoid and Drug-Induced Osteoporosis

Barbara P. Lukert, M.D., F.A.C.P.

Department of Medicine, University of Kansas Medical Center, Kansas City, Kansas

Glucocorticoid-induced bone loss has been recognized since Cushing described osteoporosis as a component of the constellation of findings in patients with hypercortisolism due to adrenocorticotropic hormone–producing pituitary tumors. The problem received little attention until cortisone was used to treat rheumatoid arthritis. These patients showed dramatic improvement in the inflammatory component of their disease, but within a year a striking percentage developed vertebral compression fractures. We are now very familiar with the rapid bone loss that occurs in patients taking glucocorticoids for the management of a number of diseases.

Glucocorticoids have a greater effect on trabecular bone than on cortical bone, hence bone loss is most rapid and fractures are most likely in vertebrae, ribs, and the ends of long bones. Bone is lost at a very rapid rate during the first year of therapy, with reports of losses as great as 20% in 1 year (1).

The true incidence of osteoporosis-related fractures in patients taking steroids for more than 6 months is unknown, but available data suggest that the incidence is between 30% and 50% (2). Even low doses of steroids, including inhaled steroids, cause bone loss, but the precise dose below which bone is not affected remains unclear. It appears that doses of prednisone exceeding 7.5 mg/day (or equivalent doses of other steroids) cause significant loss of trabecular bone in most people.

All patients—young and old, men and women, and all races—are susceptible to steroid-induced bone loss. Young people who have a high rate of bone remodeling appear to be particularly susceptible. Deceleration of growth and reduced total body calcium have been reported in children treated with glucocorticoids, even when only inhaled steroids are used. Although longitudinal studies are not available, children treated with glucocorticoids are not likely to achieve an optimum peak bone mass, thus becoming at greater risk for osteoporosis-related fractures in adulthood. Postmenopausal women are at greater risk for fractures, presumably because they have preexisting age-related and menopause-related bone loss.

EFFECTS OF GLUCOCORTICOIDS

A multitude of systemic and local effects of glucocorticoids on bone and mineral metabolism lead to a very rapid acceleration of bone loss (Fig. 1).

Histomorphometry

Bone histomorphometry shows a reduction in mean wall thickness of trabecular bone packets, low mineral apposition rate, elevation of parameters of bone resorption, suppression of osteoblastic recruitment, and depression of mature osteoblast function. The total amount of bone replaced in each remodeling cycle is reduced by 30%. There appears to be a shortening of the life span of the active osteoblast population in each basic multicellular unit (3).

Effect on Osteoblasts and Bone Formation

Physiologic concentrations of glucocorticoids enhance the function of differentiated osteoblasts and increase collagen synthesis (4). However, prolonged exposure to supraphysiologic concentrations inhibits synthetic processes (5). Cell replication is decreased after 48 hours of exposure; thus, prolonged inhibition of bone formation may be due in part to a decrease in proliferation of periosteal precursor cells (6). There is an additional direct inhibitory effect on differentiation of osteoblasts for collagen synthesis and on osteocalcin production (7,8).

Effect on Bone Resorption

Glucocorticoids have a biphasic effect on osteoclasts. Physiologic concentrations are required for the late stages of differentiation and function, whereas the generation of new osteoclasts involving cell replication is inhibited by high doses and prolonged exposure. Resorption is stimulated by glucocorticoids in fetal rat parietal bones *in vitro* (9). Glucocorticoids can enhance the attachment of macrophages to bone by altering cell surface oligosaccharides.

Glucocorticoid-induced enhanced resorption observed *in vivo* may be due in large part to secondary hyperparathyroidism. Secondary hyperparathyroidism increases the birth rate of bone-remodeling units and probably also increases the amount of bone resorbed at each site. Animal experiments have shown that the increase in resorption can be prevented by parathyroidectomy.

Effect on Sex Hormones

Glucocorticoids inhibit pituitary secretion of gonadotropins, ovarian and testicular secretion of estrogen and testosterone, and adrenal secretion of androstenedione and dehydroepiandrosterone (10,11). Because these hormones decrease bone resorption, their absence accelerates glucocorticoid-induced bone loss.

Intestinal Absorption and Renal Excretion of Calcium

Most patients taking pharmacologic doses of glucocorticoids have impaired active transcellular transport of calcium. The exact mechanisms are poorly understood, but are partially independent of vitamin D. Intestinal absorption and renal tubular reabsorption of calcium are significantly impaired in patients taking glucocorticoids, and these abnormalities may play an important role in the development of secondary hyperparathyroidism (12,13). Fasting urinary calcium excretion and parathyroid hormone (PTH) levels are elevated in normal subjects receiving glucocorticoids for only 5 days. The origin is probably twofold: increased skeletal mobilization and decreased tubular reabsorption that occurs despite elevated parathyroid hormone (PTH). The transport defect is made worse by high sodium intake and is decreased by sodium restriction and thiazide diuretics (14).

Effect on Parathyroid Hormone and Vitamin D Metabolism

The effects of glucocorticoids on serum concentrations of PTH and the vitamin D metabolites remain controversial. Both high and low levels of 25-hydroxyvitamin D (25(OH)D) have been reported. The discrepancies are probably due to variations in dietary intake and sunlight exposure rather than to steroid-induced changes in absorption or metabolism of vitamin D. Both PTH and 1,25-dihydroxyvitamin D [1,25(OH)$_2$D] levels in serum are higher in glucocorticoid-treated patients with asthma than in age-matched controls, despite higher calcium levels (15). This suggests that there may be a change in cell calcium receptors resulting in altered transport of calcium.

Glucocorticoids enhance the sensitivity of osteoblasts to PTH, and PTH-mediated inhibition of alkaline phosphatase activity, collagen synthesis, and citrate decarboxylation are all potentiated by glucocorticoids. The sensitivity to renal tubule effects of PTH are also increased by glucocorticoids.

Many of the actions of 1,25(OH)$_2$D are inhibited by glucocorticoids even though 1,25(OH)$_2$D levels are elevated. The inhibition may be mediated by both alterations in membrane response to vitamin D and receptor changes. The effect of glucocorticoids on calcitriol receptors depends on the species and growth phase of cell cultures. Glucocorticoids down-regulate the receptor in mouse osteoblasts but up-regulate the receptor in rats. The expression by osteoblasts of osteocalcin, the major noncollagenous bone protein, is stimulated by 1,25(OH)$_2$D and inhibited by glucocorticoids (16).

Effect of Glucocorticoids on Prostaglandins, Cytokines, and Growth Factors

Prostaglandins

Glucocorticoids inhibit the production of prostaglandins, particularly PGE$_2$, in bone (17). The major long-term effect of PGE$_2$ on bone in organ culture is to stimulate collagen and noncollagen protein synthesis. When PGE$_2$ is added to bones treated with glucocorticoids, the glucocorticoid-induced decrease in cell replication and collagen synthesis is partially reversed. Glucocorticoid effects cannot be explained entirely on the basis of low prostaglandin levels because the effect cannot be reproduced by inhibition of prostaglandin synthesis with nonsteroidal drugs such as indomethacin.

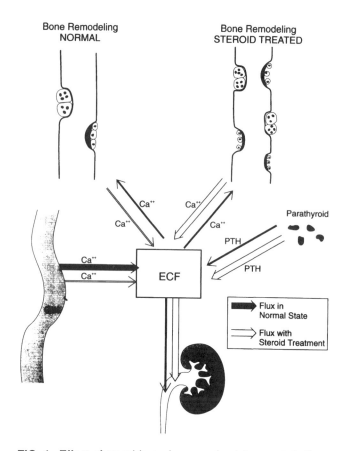

FIG. 1. Effect of steroids on bone and calcium metabolism. Glucocorticoids inhibit gastrointestinal absorption and increase renal excretion of calcium. Negative calcium balance and perhaps failure to transport calcium into the parathyroid cell cause an increase in secretion of PTH. PTH increases the number of sites undergoing bone remodeling. Glucocorticoids inhibit osteoblastic bone formation at each site. The combination of an increased number of sites undergoing remodeling and a decrease in bone formation at each site causes rapid bone loss.

Cytokines

Interleukin-1 (IL-1) and interleukin-6 (IL-6) induce bone resorption and inhibit bone formation. It is unlikely that these cytokines play a major role in glucocorticoid-induced bone loss because their production by T-lymphocytes is inhibited by glucocorticoids, and both the bone-resorbing activity and the inhibitory effect of IL-1 on collagen synthesis are partially inhibited by cortisol.

Growth Factors

The growth hormone–dependent peptide, insulin-like growth factor 1 (IGF-1) or somatomedin C, is synthesized by bone cells and stimulates bone cell replication and collagen synthesis (18). Pharmacologic doses of cortisol inhibit synthesis of IGF-1 by fetal rat calvaria. Glucocorticoids also affect IGF-binding proteins (IGFBP), which inhibit or enhance IGF activity (19). The composite effect of glucocorticoids is to decrease IGFBP-5, which enhances the anabolic effect of the IGF system, and to increase IGFBP-3 and IGFBP-4, which inhibit anabolic effects.

Transforming growth factor beta (TGF-ß) enhances osteoblast replication and bone matrix protein synthesis. Glucocorticoids decrease these anabolic effects by redistributing the binding of TGF-ß1 toward extracellular matrix storage sites and away from receptors involved in intracellular signal transduction.

Osteonecrosis

Osteonecrosis (also known as aseptic or avascular necrosis) is a serious complication of steroid therapy. It occurs in 4% to 25% of patients receiving glucocorticoid therapy. The hip, head of the humerus, and distal femur are most frequently affected. Possible mechanisms for etiology include a vascular theory, proposing that ischemia is caused by microscopic fat emboli; a mechanical theory that attributes ischemic collapse of the epiphysis to osteoporosis and the accumulation of unhealed trabecular microcracks, resulting in fatigue fractures; and the theory that increased intraosseous pressure due to fat accumulation as part of Cushing syndrome leads to mechanical impingement on the sinusoidal vascular bed and decreased blood flow.

Management of Glucocorticoid-Induced Osteoporosis

It is important to be aggressive and to maintain a positive attitude in the prevention and treatment of steroid-induced bone loss. Patients who are losing bone rapidly are unlikely to manifest any clinical or biochemical signs or symptoms of abnormalities of bone metabolism until bone loss is so severe that atraumatic fractures occur. Awareness of potential problems and prior planning can prevent and even reverse bone loss to some degree.

Patients who will be taking either high- or low-dose glucocorticoids for more than 2 months should be considered at risk. The major components of management are listed in Table 1. It is important to use a short-acting steroid in the lowest effective dose and to use topical steroids when possible, remembering, however, that even inhaled steroids cause bone loss. Secondary hyperparathyroidism should be prevented by controlling urinary loss of calcium with salt restriction and, if necessary, a thiazide diuretic, and by maintaining an oral intake of calcium of 1500 mg/day. An exercise program should be prescribed to prevent myopathy and reduce bone resorption. Estrogen/progesterone replacement in women and testosterone replacement in men should be used when there are no contraindications (20). Even mild degrees of vitamin D insufficiency should be treated and monitored with serum 25(OH)D levels. Bone density should be measured every 6 months during the first 2 years of therapy to assess adequacy of the treatment program. If rapid bone loss continues, treatment with calcitonin (21), a bisphosphonate (22), or sodium fluoride (23) should be considered.

Deflazacort, an oxazoline derivative of prednisone, may prove to have fewer adverse effects on the skeleton while maintaining approximately 80% of the anti-inflammatory effects of prednisone. Although deflazacort inhibits gas-

TABLE 1. *Management of patients taking glucocorticoids*

General measures
  Use lowest effective dose of glucocorticoid with shortest half-life.
  Encourage weight-bearing and isometric exercises.
  Maintain good nutritional status.
Prevent secondary hyperparathyroidism
  Restrict sodium intake to 3 g/d to decrease hypercalciuria and improve absorption of calcium. Add thiazide and potassium-sparing diuretic if necessary.
  Maintain a calcium intake of 1500 mg/d.
  Maintain serum 25(OH)D level at upper limits of normal.
Replace gonadal hormones
  Begin estrogen/progesterone replacement therapy in postmenopausal women and women whose menses become irregular.
  Give Depo-Testosterone to men if serum free testosterone is low.
Assess bone density every 6 months for first year.
  If bone mass continues to fall in spite of conservative measures, consider treatment with a bisphosphonate or calcitonin.

25(OH)D, 25-hydroxyvitamin D.

trointestinal absorption of calcium and bone formation, these inhibitory effects are less than those of prednisone.

CYCLOSPORINE

Cyclosporine is frequently given with prednisone to suppress the immune response, particularly in organ transplant recipients. This combination of drugs causes rapid bone loss. The effects of cyclosporine on bone and calcium metabolism are not as well understood as those of glucocorticoids, but its effects on bone differ. Serum osteocalcin levels are elevated in patients taking cyclosporine, whereas they are depressed in patients taking prednisone (24). Synthesis of $1,25(OH)_2D$ is elevated by cyclosporine, but not by glucocorticoids (25). This may explain the differences in osteocalcin levels.

EXCHANGE RESINS

Exchange resins such as cholestyramine, which are used to lower cholesterol by binding bile salts in the intestine, can decrease the absorption of fat-soluble vitamins A, D, and K and result in deficiency of these vitamins. If cholestyramine is given for long periods of time, levels of these vitamins should be monitored and supplemented when indicated.

ANTICONVULSANT-INDUCED ABNORMALITIES IN BONE METABOLISM

The anticonvulsant drugs diphenylhydantoin (DPH), phenobarbital, and carbamazepine, and combinations of these drugs, cause alterations in calcium metabolism. In patients taking these particular anticonvulsant drugs, serum levels of calcium and 25OHD are significantly lower and alkaline phosphatase levels are higher than in control subjects. Frank hypocalcemia has been reported in 3% to 30%, elevated alkaline phosphatase in 10% to 70%, and low serum 25(OH)D in 8% to 33%. Serum 1,25(OH)$_2$D may be high early in treatment and low later in treatment. Valproate has not been shown to induce any of the changes in calcitropic hormones or in other bone-related biochemical parameters.

Changes in calcium homeostatic mechanisms associated with anticonvulsant drugs have been ascribed to treatment-induced vitamin D deficiency, which leads to poor calcium absorption and secondary hyperparathyroidism. All of the commonly used anticonvulsant agents induce the liver cytochrome P 450 system. This system mediates drug oxidation reactions and enhances the hepatic conversion of steroid hormones, including vitamin D metabolites, to polar, biologically inactive products, which are excreted in urine and bile (26). These changes increase the requirement for vitamin D, and a state of vitamin D insufficiency or deficiency ensues unless the supply of vitamin D is increased. The dose of vitamin D required to maintain serum 25(OH)D in the normal range is between 400 and 4000 IU/day. The majority of patients appear to maintain normal levels on 2400 IU/day (27).

Susceptibility to the adverse effects of anticonvulsant drugs on calcium and vitamin D metabolism is increased by poor dietary intake of vitamin D, limited ultraviolet light exposure, multidrug therapy, prolonged therapy, and combination with other drugs that induce the hepatic P 450 enzyme system (28).

Anticonvulsant drugs also have direct effects on cellular metabolism unrelated to vitamin D. Diphenylhydantoin inhibits calcium transport in the gut and suppresses osteoblastic and osteoclastic activity in bone in vitro (29), and both phenobarbital and DPH inhibit the resorptive response to PTH and vitamin D metabolites. Paradoxically, elevated serum levels of osteocalcin, bone-specific alkaline phosphatase, and C-terminal extension peptide of type I procollagen, all markers of bone formation; and cross-linked carboxyl-terminal telopeptide of type I collagen, a marker of bone matrix resorption, reflect high rates of remodeling in patients taking anticonvulsant drugs (30). This apparent paradox is most likely due to a composite of opposing effects of anticonvulsants on cellular metabolism and the effect of an anticonvulsant-induced decrease in vitamin D metabolites and increase of PTH secretion. The ultimate effect of anticonvulsants on bone is quite variable, as is the frequency of anticonvulsant-related bone disease. The bone disease may present as full-blown osteomalacia; however, the patient is more often asymptomatic but has low serum 25(OH)D levels, mild hypocalcemia, and slightly elevated alkaline phosphatase and PTH.

Early measurements of bone density of the mid-radius using single-photon absorptiometry demonstrated a 10% to 30% decrease when compared with normal age-matched controls (31). A more recent study using dual-photon absorptiometry failed to show significant bone loss in the femoral neck in a group aged 5–20 years who were taking anticonvulsants but were otherwise healthy (32). Adult women taking DPH were found to have decreased bone density in the femoral neck. Bone densities were normal for men even though biochemical markers of bone remodeling showed increased turnover (30).

TABLE 2. *Management of patients taking anticonvulsant drugs*

Beginning of therapy
Maintain good nutritional status and level of physical activity.
Assure intake of 1500 mg of calcium and 800 IU vitamin D daily.
After 6 or more months of therapy
1. Measure serum calcium, alkaline phosphatase, 25(OH)D
2. If 25(OH)D is low, begin vitamin D 50,000 IU once a week.
3. Measure 25(OH)D 3 months after beginning high dose of vitamin D.
4. Adjust dose to maintain 25(OH)D in normal range.
5. Measure 24-hr urine calcium. If low, increase calcium intake.
6. Assess serum 25(OH)D yearly once it is normal.

25(OH)D, 25-hydroxyvitamin D.

Diagnosis and Treatment

Alterations in calcium and bone metabolism should be suspected in all patients who are taking DPH, phenobarbital, or carbamazepine. All patients should be encouraged to remain physically active and to consume 800 IU of vitamin D and 1500 mg of calcium daily (Table 2). Serum calcium, phosphorous, and 25(OH)D levels should be measured. If the 25(OH)D level is below normal, vitamin D 50,000 IU once weekly should be prescribed. The serum 25(OH)D level should then be assessed 3 months after starting this dose, and the dose should be adjusted as needed to maintain a level in the normal range. Assessment should be repeated yearly. When the 25(OH)D level is normal, 24-hour excretion of calcium should be measured, and if this is low, calcium supplementation should be increased, as a low level is indicative of impaired intestinal absorption.

REFERENCES

1. Gennari C, Imbimbo B, Montagnani M, Bernini M, Nardi P, Avioli LV: Effects of prednisone and deflazacort on mineral metabolism and parathyroid hormone activity in humans. *Calcif Tissue Int* 36:245–252, 1984
2. Adinoff AD, Hollister JR: Steroid-induced fractures and bone loss in patients with asthma. *N Engl J Med* 309:265–268, 1983
3. Dempster DW: Bone histomorphometry in glucocorticoid-induced osteoporosis. *J Bone Miner Res* 4:137–141, 1989
4. Wong GL: Basal activities and hormone responsiveness of osteoblastic activity. *J Biol Chem* 254:6337–6340, 1979
5. Dietrich JW, Canalis EM, Maina DM, Raisz LG: Effect of glucocorticoids on fetal rat bone collagen synthesis in vitro. *Endocrinology* 104:715–721, 1979
6. Canalis EM: Effect of cortisol on periosteal and nonperiosteal collagen and DNA synthesis in cultured rat calvariae. *Calcif Tissue Int* 36:158–166, 1984
7. Lukert B, Mador A, Raisz LG, Kream BE: The role of DNA synthesis in the responses of fetal rat calvariae to cortisol. *J Bone Miner Res* 6:453–460, 1991
8. Morrison N, Eisman J: Role of the negative glucocorticoid regulatory element in glucocorticoid repression of the human osteocalcin promoter. *J Bone Miner Res* 8:969–975, 1993
9. Gronowicz G, McCarthy MB, Raisz LG: Glucocorticoids stimulate resorption in fetal rat parietal bones in vitro. *J Bone Miner Res* 5:1223–1230, 1990

10. Crilly RG, Cawood M, Marshall DH, Nordin BE: Hormonal status in normal, osteoporotic and corticosteroid-treated postmenopausal women. *J R Soc Med* 71:733–736, 1978
11. MacAdams MR, White RH, Chipps BE: Reduction of serum testosterone levels during chronic glucocorticoid therapy. *Ann Intern Med* 104:648–651, 1986
12. Suzuki Y, Ichikawa Y, Saito E, Homma M: Importance of increased urinary calcium excretion in the development of secondary hyperparathyroidism of patients under glucocorticoid therapy. *Metabolism* 32:151–156, 1983
13. Lukert BP, Stanbury SW, Mawer EB: Vitamin D and intestinal transport of calcium: Effects of prednisolone. *Endocrinology* 93:718–722, 1973
14. Adams JS, Wahl TO, Lukert BP: Effects of hydrochlorothiazide and dietary sodium restriction on calcium metabolism in corticosteroid treated patients. *Metabolism* 30:217–221, 1981
15. Bikle DD, Halloran B, Fong L, Steinbach L, Shellito J: Elevated 1,25-dihydroxyvitamin D levels in patients with chronic obstructive pulmonary disease treated with prednisone. *J Clin Endocrinol Metab* 76:456–461, 1993
16. Price PA, Otsuka AA, Poser JW, Kristaponis J, Raman N: Characterization of gamma-carboxyglutamic acid containing protein form bone. *Proc Natl Acad Sci USA* 73:1447–1451, 1976
17. Raisz LG, Pilbeam CC, Fall PM: Prostaglandins: Mechanisms of action and regulation of production in bone. *Osteoporosis Int* 3(Suppl 1):136–140, 1993
18. Canalis E, McCarthy T, Centrella M: Isolation of growth factors from adult bovine bone. *Calcif Tissue Int* 43:346–351, 1988
19. Kream BE, LaFrancis PM, Fall PM, Feyen JHM, Raisz LG: Insulin-like growth factor binding protein-2 blocks the stimulatory effect of glucocorticoids on bone collagen synthesis. *J Bone Miner Res* 7(Suppl 1):5100, 1992
20. Lukert BP, Johnson BE, Robinson RG: Estrogen and progesterone replacement therapy reduces glucocorticoid-induced bone loss. *J Bone Miner Res* 7:1063–1069, 1992
21. Luengo M, Picado C, Del Rio L, Guanabens N, Monserrat JM, Setoain J: Treatment of steroid-induced osteopenia with calcitonin in corticosteroid-dependent asthma: A one-year follow-up study. *Am Rev Respir Dis* 142:104–107, 1990
22. Mulder H, Smelder HAA: Effect of cyclical etidronate regimen on prophylaxis of bone loss of glucocorticoid (prednisone) therapy in postmenopausal women. *J Bone Miner Res* 7:S331, 1992
23. Meunier PJ, Birancon D, Chavassieux P, et al: Treatment with fluoride: Bone histomorphometric findings. In: Christiansen C, Johansen JS, Riis BJ (eds) *Osteoporosis 1987.* Copenhagen, Osteopress, 824–828, 1987
24. Shane E, Rivas MDC, Silverberg SJ, Kim TS, Staron RB, Bliezikian JP: Osteoporosis after cardiac transplantation. *Am J Med* 94:257–264, 1993
25. Stein B, Halloran BP, Reinhardt T, et al: Cyclosporin-A increases synthesis of 1,25-dihydroxyvitamin D_3 in the rat and mouse. *Endocrinology* 128:1369–1373, 1991
26. Hahn TJ, Hendin BA, Scharp CR, Haddad JG Jr: Effect of chronic anticonvulsant therapy on serum 25-hydroxycalciferol levels in adults. *N Engl J Med* 287:900–904, 1972
27. Collins N, Maher J, Cole M, Baker M, Callaghan N: A prospective study to evaluate the dose of vitamin D required to correct low 25-hydroxyvitamin D levels, calcium, and alkaline phosphatase in patients at risk of developing antiepileptic drug-induced osteomalacia. *Q J Med* 78:113–122, 1991
28. Gough H, Goggin T, Bissessar A, Baker M, Crowley M, Callaghan N: A comparative study of the relative influence of different anticonvulsant drugs, UV exposure and diet on vitamin D and calcium metabolism in out-patients with epilepsy. *Q J Med* 59:569–577, 1986
29. Dietrich JW, Duffield R: Effects of diphenylhydantoin on synthesis of collagen and non-collagen protein in tissue culture. *Endocrinology* 106:606–610, 1990
30. Valimiaki MJ, Tiihonen M, Laitinen K, Tahtela R, Karkkainen M, Lamberg-Allardt C, Makela P, Tunninen R: Bone mineral density measured by dual-energy x-ray absportiometry and novel markers of bone formation and resorption in patients on antiepileptic drugs. *J Bone Miner Res* 9:631–367, 1994
31. Barden HS, Mazess RB, Chesney RW, Rose PG, Chun R: Bone status in children receiving anticonvulsant therapy. *Metab Bone Dis Relat Res* 4:43–47, 1982
32. Timperlake RW, Cook SD, Thomas KA, Harding AF, Bennett JT, Haller JS, Anderson RM: Effects of anticonvulsant drug therapy on bone mineral density in a pediatric population. *J Pediatr Orthop* 8:467–470, 1988

18. Osteoporosis in Men

Jeffrey A. Jackson, M.D.

Division of Endocrinology, Scott & White Clinic, Texas A & M University Health Science Center, Temple, Texas

Osteoporosis in men has received much less attention and study than its counterpart in women. Recent studies suggest that vertebral fractures in men occur more commonly than previously appreciated, with an incidence in men up to one half of that in women (1,2). The greatest morbidity, mortality (actually greater in men than women), and societal expense, however, are caused by hip fractures in men, which account for 25% to 30% of all hip fractures. This constitutes a significant public health problem, predicted to increase considerably in the next 30 years. The lower incidence of osteoporosis in men is due to higher peak bone cross-sectional area and size; lower rate of age-related cortical bone loss; a different pattern of trabecular bone loss with age, with predominant thinning rather than perforation; the absence of a distinct menopause equivalent with associated acceleration of bone loss; shorter life expectancy; and reduced propensity to fall.

The differential diagnosis of osteopenia, or moderately reduced bone mass (not strictly defined yet in men) without fractures, and osteoporosis in men is shown in Table 1. This list also applies to other groups of patients, such as black and premenopausal women. Detailed discussions of bone loss associated with endocrinopathies other than hypogonadism, osteomalacia, neoplastic diseases, glucocorticoids and other drugs, and other disorders such as osteogenesis imperfecta, immobilization, and rheumatoid arthritis are presented elsewhere in this book.

HYPOGONADISM

Long-standing testosterone deficiency is typical of up to 30% of men presenting with spinal osteoporosis (3). These men most commonly present in the sixth decade and in retrospect, most have had hypogonadal symptoms of impotence and decreased libido in excess of 20–30 years. Virtually any cause of hypogonadism (primary or secondary) may be associated with osteoporosis in men, including Klinefelter syndrome, hypogonadotropic hypogonadism, hyperprolactinemia, hemochromatosis, mumps orchitis, and castration (4). Testosterone deficiency may be a significant risk factor for hip fracture in elderly men (5) and may contribute to bone loss associated with aging in general, malignancy and other systemic diseases (see Chapters 20 and 22), malnutrition, ethanol abuse, and glucocorticoid excess (see Chapter 17).

Detection of hypogonadism in osteoporotic men may be quite challenging. Pitfalls include lack of palpably abnormal testes (not uncommon in secondary hypogonadism occurring after puberty), denial of hypogonadal symptoms (testosterone-deficient men may be capable of adequate sexual function), and presence of "normal" serum total testosterone levels despite clear elevations in serum luteinizing hormone (sometimes due to associated increases in sex hormone-binding globulin). Every osteopenic or osteoporotic man should have routine measurement of serum testosterone (total or free) and of luteinizing hormone.

Histomorphometric heterogeneity in hypogonadal osteoporotic men (similar to that of postmenopausal osteoporosis, except for lack of subnormal bone formation rates) (3) may reflect a gradual transition from osteoclast- to osteoblast-dependent bone loss over time. The increased remodeling activation and bone turnover in such men appear to be correctable by testosterone replacement (3) or calcitonin (4). Testosterone deficiency may reduce calcitonin secretion, and synthesis of calcitriol may be impaired, particularly when substrate (calcidiol) is deficient (3,6). Parallels between the bone effects of gonadal hormone deficiency in men and women may be due to similar direct effects on bone; both estrogen and androgen receptors have been demonstrated *in vitro* in human osteoblasts and osteoblast-like cells as well as in bone

TABLE 1. *Differential diagnosis of osteopenia and osteoporosis in men[a]*

Endocrinopathies	Hypogonadism, Cushing syndrome, hyperthyroidism, primary hyperparathyroidism, hyperprolactinemia, acromegaly, and idiopathic hypercalciuria
Osteomalacia	Vitamin D deficiency, phosphate-wasting syndromes, metabolic acidosis, and inhibitors of mineralization
Neoplastic disease	Multiple myeloma, systemic mastocytosis, diffuse bony metastases, vertebral metastases, myelo- and lymphoproliferative disorders
Drug-induced	Glucocorticoids, ethanol, excessive thyroid hormone, heparin, anticonvulsants, and tobacco smoking
Hereditary disorders	Osteogenesis imperfecta, Ehlers-Danlos and Marfan syndromes, and homocystinuria
Other disorders	Immobilization, chronic disease (rheumatoid arthritis, liver/kidney failure), malnutrition, skeletal sarcoidosis, Gaucher's disease, hypophosphatasia, and hemoglobinopathies
Idiopathic	Juvenile and adult
Age-related	

[a]Adapted from: Jackson JA, Kleerekoper M: *Medicine* 69:139–152, 1990.

marrow stromal cells and osteoclast-like multinucleated cells (7). The recent finding of markedly reduced bone mineral density in a man with severe estrogen resistance (8) suggests that local aromatization of testosterone to estradiol may be necessary for normal bone homeostasis.

Study of the effects of testosterone replacement therapy on bone mineral density has been quite limited. Significant increases in radial and spinal bone mineral densities have been reported in patients with hypogonadotropic hypogonadism and initially open epiphyses after testosterone treatment for up to 2 years, but those with initially closed epiphyses showed minimal improvement (9). Restoration of gonadal function after successful treatment of hyperprolactinemic hypogonadal men resulted in significant increases in only cortical bone density (10). Spine and forearm bone mineral densities increased in hypogonadal men with hemochromatosis treated by testosterone replacement and venesection (11).

IDIOPATHIC OSTEOPOROSIS

The diagnosis of idiopathic osteoporosis should be made only after all other causes have been excluded (1,12). Idiopathic juvenile osteoporosis is discussed in Chapter 16. In adults, men predominate by a 10:1 ratio, although some investigators have reported more equal representation by women (13). Idiopathic osteoporosis accounts for at least 30% to 40% of osteoporosis in adult men. These men usually present with vertebral compression fractures in the third to sixth decades. The trend toward early recognition of radiographic osteopenia and measurement of bone mineral density will likely detect more of these patients in the future before fracture occurrence. This would be vastly preferable to the current practice of delayed diagnosis until after three or four vertebral fractures have occurred, followed by a lengthy (although necessary) workup for secondary causes before therapeutic decisions are made.

Performance of dynamic bone histomorphometry on these patients is generally unnecessary with the clinical availability of improved biochemical markers of bone turnover (14). However, bone histomorphometry has been useful in exploring the pathophysiology of bone homeostasis in idiopathic osteoporosis. Most studies have shown defective osteoblast function with low bone-formation rates (3,13), correlated with reduced levels of insulin-like growth factor 1 in one study (13). There appears to be considerable heterogeneity, however, with at least one subgroup of men having hypercalciuria and increased bone turnover (15), perhaps related to excessive interleukin-1 or other humoral growth factors. Alterations in calcitriol synthesis may also contribute to bone loss in some of these patients.

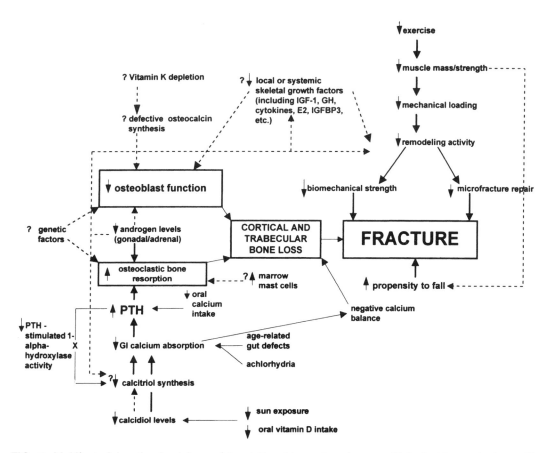

FIG. 1. Multifactorial pathophysiology of involutional bone loss in men. (Adapted from: Jackson JA, Kleerekoper M: *Medicine* 69:139–152, 1990.)

The utility of bone-turnover assessment in selection of treatment modalities (i.e., therapies stimulating bone formation in patients with low bone-turnover and antiresorptive agents for those with increased bone turnover), though intuitively gratifying, has not yet been confirmed in clinical studies of osteoporosis. At present, because there is a void in approved pro-osteoblastic agents, it appears reasonable to use antiresorptive agents (bisphosphonates or calcitonin) combined with oral calcium and low-dose vitamin D (for patients with low urinary calcium) or thiazides (for those with urinary calcium >200 mg/d) and to follow biochemical markers of turnover and serial bone densitometry. Physical therapy and counseling on osteoporotic precautions and safe exercises also are essential, as in all osteoporotic patients.

INVOLUTIONAL BONE LOSS IN MEN

Cross-sectional studies of bone mass and density in aging men have shown a gradual decline in bone mineral content at cortical sites (3% to 4% loss per decade after age 40), although recent longitudinal studies suggested a higher rate of loss (5% to 10% per decade). There may be a more rapid decline in men after age 50 (much less than menopausal losses in women). Periosteal bone formation in men appears to compensate for endosteal resorption, with no reduction in bending strength with age (16). Cancellous bone loss appears similar in both sexes (7% to 12% loss per decade), with only a slightly greater rate of loss in women. Quantitative computed tomography shows greater trabecular decline, as bone densitometric techniques measure integral bone density including cortical shell, posterior processes, and extravertebral calcifications. Qualitative differences in trabecular microarchitecture between the sexes may be quite distinct: men appear to have more reduction in trabecular width with age, whereas women have a greater fall in trabecular number (17), which may disproportionately reduce biomechanical strength in women.

Figure 1 summarizes the current understanding of the multifactorial pathophysiology of involutional bone loss in men (1,2,12). The major factor appears to be reduction in osteoblast function with age, possibly due to decreased osteoblast longevity or impaired regulation of osteoblast activity and recruitment or formation-resorption coupling by systemic or local skeletal growth factors. Decreased mechanical loading, exercise, and muscle mass in the elderly may impair remodeling activity. Negative calcium balance in aging men is due to insufficient oral calcium intake and decreased gastrointestinal calcium absorptive efficiency, which may partly relate to subnormal calcitriol levels reported by some investigators. An age-related increase in bone resorption appears less prominent and may relate to several hormonal factors. Increases in serum parathyroid hormone with age have been reported by most investigators. Calcitonin levels measured by monomeric assays do not fall with age in either sex. A fall in gonadal function with age (18) may contribute significantly to involutional bone loss in men. Increased propensity to fall

TABLE 2. *Prevention of osteoporosis in men: general measures*[a]

Routine maintenance of adequate calcium intake throughout life
1000 mg/d elemental calcium in younger men and preadolescent boys
1500 mg/d in adolescent boys and men > ages 60–65
Routine maintenance of adequate vitamin D intake throughout life
Low-dose vitamin D supplementation to push total intake to 600–800 IU/d in men > ages 60–65
Lifelong regular physical exercise
Recognize and treat testosterone deficiency early
Limit ethanol use and avoid tobacco smoking
Recognize other high-risk men (Table 3); consider specific prophylactic treatment regimens
Postgastric surgery (oral calcium ± vitamin D)
Chronic glucocorticoid therapy (oral calcium ± vitamin D and thiazides)
Avoidance of falls

[a]Adapted from: Jackson JA, Kleerekoper M: *Medicine* 69:139–152, 1990.

also plays a major role in involutional fractures; elderly women fall two to four times more often than men.

PREVENTION

Because current therapy of established osteoporosis is inadequate and no therapeutic agent has yet been convincingly proven effective in preventing osteoporotic fractures in men, emphasis must be placed on prevention of bone loss (Table 2). Specific measures may include routine calcium and vitamin D supplementation in men after ages 60–65, lifelong regular exercise, prompt recognition and treatment of testosterone deficiency, moderation of ethanol intake, and avoidance of tobacco smoking. Recognition of risk factors for osteoporosis in men (19) (listed roughly in order of importance in Table 3) is also important. In the future, specific programs for prevention of falls (and selective use of hip padding) will likely yield beneficial results for the elderly.

TABLE 3. *Risk factors for osteoporosis in men*[a]

Caucasian (? Asiatic) ancestry
Impaired gonadal function
Significant ethanol use
Cigarette smoking
Drugs, particularly glucocorticoids
Chronic illness/immobilization
Inactive lifestyle
Postgastric surgery or intestinal resection
Low dietary calcium intake
Lean body build
? Family history of osteoporotic fractures
? Chronic excess sodium, caffeine, protein, and phosphorus intake

[a]Adapted from: Jackson JA, Kleerekoper M: *Medicine* 69:139–152, 1990.

REFERENCES

1. Orwoll ES, Klein RF: Osteoporosis in men. *Endocr Rev* 16:87–116, 1995
2. Seeman E: The dilemma of osteoporosis in men. *Am J Med* 98(Suppl 2A):76S–88S, 1995
3. Jackson JA, Kleerekoper M, Parfitt AM, Rao DS, Villanueva AR, Frame B: Bone histomorphometry in hypogonadal and eugonadal men with spinal osteoporosis. *J Clin Endocrinol Metab* 65:53–58, 1987
4. Stepan JJ, Lachman M, Zverina J, Pacovsky V, Baylink DJ: Castrated men exhibit bone loss: Effect of calcitonin treatment on biochemical indices of bone remodeling. *J Clin Endocrinol Metab* 69:523–527, 1989
5. Jackson JA, Riggs MW, Spiekerman AM: Testosterone deficiency as a risk factor for hip fractures in men: A case-control study. *Am J Med Sci* 304:4–8, 1992
6. Francis RM, Peacock M, Aaron JE, et al.: Osteoporosis in hypogonadal men: Role of decreased plasma 1,25-dihydroxyvitamin D, calcium malabsorption and low bone formation. *Bone* 7:261–268, 1986
7. Vanderscheueren D, Bouillon R: Androgens and bone. *Calcif Tissue Int* 56:341–346, 1995
8. Smith EP, Boyd J, Frank GR, et al.: Estrogen resistance caused by a mutation in the estrogen-receptor gene in a man. *N Engl J Med* 331:1056–1061, 1994
9. Finkelstein JS, Klibanski A, Neer RM, et al.: Increases in bone density during treatment of men with idiopathic hypogonadotropic hypogonadism. *J Clin Endocrinol Metab* 69:776–783, 1989
10. Greenspan SL, Oppenheim DS, Klibanski A: Importance of gonadal steroids to bone mass in men with hyperprolactinemic hypogonadism. *Ann Intern Med* 110:526–531, 1989
11. Diamond T, Stiel D, Posen S: Effects of testosterone and venesection on spinal and peripheral bone mineral in six hypogonadal men with hemochromatosis. *J Bone Miner Res* 6:39–43, 1991
12. Jackson JA, Kleerekoper M: Osteoporosis in men: Diagnosis, pathophysiology, and prevention. *Medicine* 69:139–152, 1990
13. Reed BY, Zerwekh JE, Sakhaee K, Breslau NA, Gottschalk F, Pak CYC: Serum IGF 1 is low and correlated with osteoblastic surface in idiopathic osteoporosis. *J Bone Miner Res* 10:1218–1224, 1995
14. Garner P, Shih WJ, Gineyts E, Karpf DB, Delmas PD: Comparison of new biochemical markers of bone turnover in late postmenopausal osteoporotic women in response to alendronate treatment. *J Clin Endocrinol Metab* 79:1693–1700, 1994
15. Perry HM, Fallon MD, Bergfield M, Teitelbaum SL, Avioli LV: Osteoporosis in young men: A syndrome of hypercalciuria and accelerated bone turnover. *Arch Intern Med* 142:1295–1298, 1982
16. Ruff CB, Hayes WC: Sex differences in age-related remodeling of the femur and tibia. *J Orthop Res* 6:886–896, 1988
17. Aaron JE, Makins NB, Sagreiya K: The microanatomy of trabecular bone loss in normal aging men and women. *Clin Orthop* 215:260–271, 1987
18. Vermeulen A: Clinical review 24: Androgens in the aging male. *J Clin Endocrinol Metab* 73:221–224, 1991
19. Seeman E, Melton LJ III, O Fallon WM, Riggs BL: Risk factors for spinal osteoporosis in men. *Am J Med* 75:977–983, 1983

19. Hyperthyroidism, Thyroid Hormone Replacement, and Osteoporosis

Daniel T. Baran, M.D.

Departments of Medicine, Orthopedics, and Cell Biology, University of Massachusetts Medical Center, Worcester, Massachusetts

Thyroid hormone increases bone remodeling (1). Although both osteoblast and osteoclast activities are increased by elevated levels of thyroid hormone, osteoclast activity predominates, with a resultant loss of bone mass. It appears that thyroid hormones stimulate osteoclastic bone resorption by an indirect effect mediated by osteoblasts. The presence of osteoblasts is required for thyroid hormones to increase bone resorption (2,3). Osteoblasts possess thyroid hormone receptors, based on biochemical binding studies and detectable messenger ribonucleic acid (mRNA) levels for thyroid hormone receptor (4). Bone cell–specific triiodothyronine responses appear to be associated with differing patterns of receptor gene expression and stages of osteoblast phenotype expression.

Thyroid hormone directly stimulates osteoblast production of alkaline phosphatase (5), osteocalcin (6), and insulin-like growth factor (7). Thyrotoxicosis is associated with increased serum levels of osteocalcin (8) and alkaline phosphatase (9). Despite increased osteoblastic activity, the enhanced bone formation cannot compensate for thyroid hormone–induced increments in bone resorption. The increased bone resorption is detected by increased urinary levels of hydroxyproline and collagen cross-links in thyrotoxic patients (1,10,11). The levels of these biochemical markers of bone turnover appear to correlate with circulating levels of thyroid hormone.

Abnormalities in serum calcium concentrations are also observed in patients with hyperthyroidism. Mild hypercalcemia has been reported in 20% of patients with thyrotoxicosis (12), but the modest degree of hypercalcemia rarely causes symptoms. Serum parathyroid hormone (PTH) levels and bioactivity (13), serum 1,25-dihydroxyvitamin D_3 [$1,25(OH)_2D_3$] (14), and intestinal calcium absorption (15) are decreased in patients with thyrotoxicosis, suggesting that thyroid hormone–induced increases in bone resorption explain the occurrence of hypercalcemia.

Hypercalciuria also is common in patients with thyrotoxicosis. The increased calcium excretion normalizes after treatment of thyrotoxicosis (12).

In thyrotoxicosis, the surface area of unmineralized matrix (osteoid) is increased. In contrast to osteomalacia, mineralization rates are increased. The increased bone turnover in the presence of excessive levels of thyroid hormone is characterized by an increase in the number of osteoclasts, the number of resorption sites, and the ratio of resorptive to formative surfaces. In contrast to the normal bone-remodeling cycle, which lasts about 200 days, in hyperthyroid patients the cycle is shortened, primarily because of a decrease in the length of the formation period, with failure to replace resorbed bone completely (1) (Fig. 1). The histologic changes in cortical bone in hyperthyroidism are characterized by increased porosity (1). In hyperthyroidism, there are also changes in the gene expression markers in cortical bone.

In summary, thyroid hormone effects on osteoblasts and osteoclasts result in alterations in mineral metabolism and in the remodeling cycle, manifested by histologic and molecular changes in bone. These changes appear to be reflected in altered bone mineral density.

BONE MASS AND FRACTURE RISK IN THYROID DISEASE

Bone mass is reduced in patients with thyrotoxicosis (16,17). The detrimental effects of thyroid hormone on the skeleton appear to occur more frequently in female patients. As a result of the decrease in bone density, individuals with a history of thyrotoxicosis have an increased risk of fracture (18) and sustain fractures at an earlier age than individuals who have never been thyrotoxic (19).

The decreased bone density noted in thyrotoxic patients is reversible after effective treatment. Normalization of the thyroid function tests results in significant increases in axial and appendicular bone density compared with pretreatment values (16,17). If the detrimental skeletal effects of supraphysiologic levels of thyroid hormone were restricted to individuals with thyrotoxicosis, therapy would be expected to prevent any further skeletal damage and in fact restore at least a portion of the bone mass that was lost before effective treatment.

Administration of high doses of thyroid hormone to suppress thyroid-stimulating hormone (TSH) secretion in patients with differentiated thyroid carcinoma and nontoxic goiter is considered appropriate therapy for those conditions. In patients prone to osteoporosis, however, this therapy may aggravate fracture risk. TSH-suppressive doses of thyroid hormone have been reported to decrease or to have no effect on bone mineral density (BMD) in women. A metanalysis of the reports in which BMD was assessed in women receiving TSH-suppressive doses of thyroxine concluded that treatment led to a 1% increase in annual bone loss in postmenopausal women (20). In contrast, thyroid hormone replacement therapy in the absence of TSH suppression does not appear to be associated with detrimental effects on BMD (21).

PREVENTION OF THYROID HORMONE–INDUCED BONE LOSS

Treatment of thyrotoxic patients increases bone density compared with pretreatment values (16,17). A more difficult situation is presented by the patient who requires

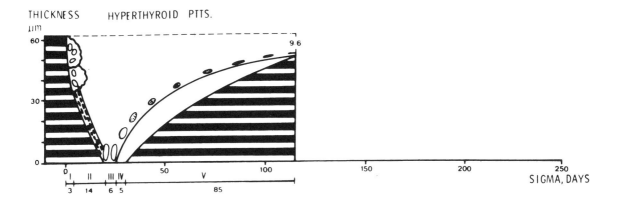

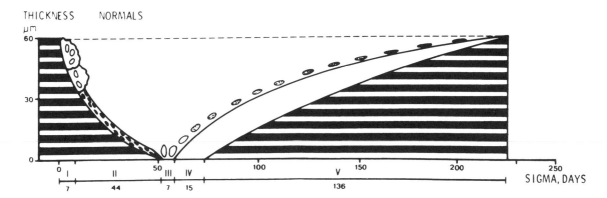

FIG. 1. Smoothed resorption and formation curves in hyperthyroid patients and their controls. The durations of the different resorption and formation periods are given below the curves. I, osteoclastic function period; II, mononuclear function period; III, preosteoblast-like cell function period; IV, initial mineralization lag time; V, mineralization period. For the hyperthyroid group, the negative balance between resorption depth and formation thickness is indicated (-9.6 µM). (Reprinted from: Eriksen EF, Mosekilde L, Melsen F. *Bone* 6:421–428, 1985, with kind permission from Elsevier Science, Ltd, The Boulevard, Langford Lane, Kidlington OX5 1GB, UK.)

TSH-suppressive doses of thyroid hormone. Bone mass measurements at 1- to 2-year intervals will detect those patients with accelerated rates of bone loss. In animal models of thyroid hormone–induced TSH suppression, bisphosphonates appear to prevent the detrimental effects of thyroid hormone on the skeleton (22), whereas calcitonin does not inhibit thyroid hormone–induced bone loss in these animal models (23). Bisphosphonates also prevent the increases in the biochemical markers of osteoblast and osteoclast activity that occur after thyroid hormone administration in humans (24). In a cross-sectional study, estrogen appeared to negate the thyroid hormone–associated loss of bone density in postmenopausal women taking replacement doses of thyroid hormone (25). Women taking suppressive doses of thyroid hormone who were also taking estrogen had significantly higher BMD values than women who were taking suppressive doses of thyroid hormone alone, and similar values to those women taking neither thyroid hormone nor estrogen. Bone density values did not differ by estrogen status in women taking replacement doses of thyroid hormone (25). Thus, current evidence suggests that estrogen or bisphosphonate therapy should be considered for those individuals requiring TSH-suppressive doses of thyroid hormone who demonstrate accelerated rates of bone loss or who already manifest decreased bone mass.

REFERENCES

1. Mosekilde L, Eriksen EF, Charles P: Effects of thyroid hormone on bone and mineral metabolism. *Endocrinol Metab Clin North Am* 19:35–63, 1990
2. Allain TJ, Chambers TJ, Flanagan AM, McGregor AM: Triiodothyronine stimulates rat osteoclastic bone resorption by an indirect effect. *J Endocrinol* 133:327–331, 1992
3. Britto JM, Fenton AJ, Holloway WR, Nicholson GC: Osteoblasts mediate thyroid hormone stimulation of osteoclastic bone resorption. *Endocrinology* 134:169–176, 1994
4. Williams GR, Bland R, Sheppard MC: Characterization of thyroid hormone (T_3) receptors in three osteosarcoma cell lines of distinct osteoblast phenotype: Interactions among T_3, vitamin D_3, and retinoid signaling. *Endocrinology* 135:2375–2385, 1994
5. Sato K, Han DC, Fujii Y, Tsushima T, Shizume K: Thyroid hormone stimulates alkaline phosphatase activity in cultured rat osteoblastic cells (ROS 17/2.8) through 3,5,3′-triiodo-L-thyronine nuclear receptors. *Endocrinology* 120:1873–1881, 1987
6. Rizzoli R, Poser J, Burgi U: Nuclear thyroid hormone receptors in cultured bone cells. *Metabolism* 35:71–74, 1986

7. Schmid C, Schlapfer I, Futo E, et al.: Triiodothyronine (T₃) stimulates insulin-like growth factor (IGF)-1 and IGF binding protein (IGFBP)-2 production by rat osteoblasts *in vitro*. *Acta Endocrinol (Copenh)* 126:467–473, 1992

8. Garrel DR, Delmas PD, Malaval L, Tourniaire J: Serum bone Gla protein: A marker of bone turnover in hyperthyroidism. *J Clin Endocrinol Metab* 62:1052–1055, 1986

9. Cooper DS, Kaplan MM, Ridgway EC, Maloof F, Daniels GH: Alkaline phosphatase isoenzyme patterns in hyperthyroidism. *Ann Intern Med* 90:164–168, 1979

10. Harvey RD, McHardy KC, Reid IW, et al.: Measurement of bone collagen degradation in hyperthyroidism and during thyroxine replacement therapy using pyridinium cross-links as specific urinary markers. *J Clin Endocrinol Metab* 72:1189–1194, 1991

11. Krakerauer JC, Kleerekoper M: Borderline low serum thyrotropin level is correlated with increased fasting urinary hydroxyproline excretion. *Arch Intern Med* 152:360–364, 1992

12. Baxter JD, Bondy PK: Hypercalcemia of thyrotoxicosis. *Ann Intern Med* 65:429–442, 1966

13. Mosekilde L, Christensen MS: Decreased parathyroid function in hyperthyroidism: Interrelationships between serum parathyroid hormone, calcium-phosphorus metabolism and thyroid function. *Acta Endocrinol (Copenh)* 84:566–575, 1977

14. Bouillon R, Muls E, DeMoor P: Influence of thyroid function on the serum concentration of 1,25-dihydroxyvitamin D₃. *J Clin Endocrinol Metab* 51:793–797, 1980

15. Haldimann B, Kaptein EM, Singer FR, Nicoloff JT, Massry SG: Intestinal calcium absorption in patients with hyperthyroidism. *J Clin Endocrinol Metab* 51:995–997, 1980

16. Rosen CJ, Alder RA: Longitudinal changes in lumbar bone density among thyrotoxic patients after attainment of euthyroidism. *J Clin Endocrinol Metab* 75:1531–1534, 1992

17. Diamond T, Vine J, Smart R, Butler P: Thyrotoxic bone disease in women: A potentially reversible disorder. *Ann Intern Med* 120:8–11, 1994

18. Cummings SR, Nevitt MC, Browner WS, Stone K, Fox KM, Ensrud KE, Cauley J, Black D, Vogt TM: Risk factors for hip fracture in white women. Study of Osteoporotic Fractures Research Group. *N Engl J Med* 332:767–773, 1995

19. Solomon BL, Wartofsky L, Burman KD: Prevalence of fractures in postmenopausal women with thyroid disease. *Thyroid* 3:17–23, 1993

20. Faber J, Galloe AM: Changes in bone mass during prolonged subclinical hyperthyroidism due to L-thyroxine treatment: A meta-analysis. *Eur J Endocrinol* 130:350–356, 1994

21. Duncan WE, Chung A, Solomon B, Wartofsky L: Influence of clinical characteristics and parameters associated with thyroid hormone therapy on the bone mineral density of women treated with thyroid hormone. *Thyroid* 4:183–190, 1994

22. Ongphiphadhanakul B, Jenis LG, Braverman LE, et al.: Etidronate inhibits the thyroid hormone-induced bone loss in rats assessed by bone mineral density and messenger ribonucleic acid markers of osteoblast and osteoclast function. *Endocrinology* 133:2502–2507, 1993

23. Ongphiphadhanakul B, Alex S, Braverman LE, Baran DT: TSH-suppressive L-thyroxine therapy decreases bone density in the rat: Effect of hypogonadism and calcitonin. *J Bone Miner Res* 7:1227–1231, 1992

24. Rosen HN, Moses AC, Gundberg C: Therapy with parenteral pamidronate prevents thyroid hormone-induced bone turnover in humans. *J Clin Endocrinol Metab* 77:664–669, 1993

25. Schneider DL, Barrett-Connor EL, Morton DJ: Thyroid hormone use and bone mineral density in elderly women: Effects of estrogen. *JAMA* 271:1245–1249, 1994

20. Miscellaneous Causes of Osteoporosis

Socrates E. Papapoulos, M.D.

Department of Endocrinology and Metabolic Diseases, University Hospital, Leiden, The Netherlands

The title of this chapter encompasses a collection of heterogeneous conditions that can be associated with increased bone loss, low bone mass, and fractures. In some of these conditions a causal relation to osteoporosis is established; in others there may be more than one link to osteoporosis, and in some the etiology is unknown. The first category includes endocrinopathies such as Cushing's disease; thyrotoxicosis; severe primary hyperparathyroidism and hypogonadism of varying etiologies (e.g., hypothalamic amenorrhea, prolacting secreting pituitary adenomas, treatment of endometriosis with synthetic luteinizing hormone-releasing hormone analogs), drugs such as glucocorticosteroids, anticonvulsants, and cyclosporin A; or genetic disorders such as osteogenesis imperfecta. These subjects are discussed elsewhere in this volume. In the second category belong conditions thought to adversely affect bone metabolism and/or structure through multiple disease- and therapy-related mechanisms such as rheumatoid arthritis (see Chapter 22), gastrointestinal diseases (1), organ transplantation (see Chapter 17), and prolonged immobilization (see Chapter 11). Finally, in the third category belong conditions the pathogeneses of which are still ill defined such as, for example, pregnancy-associated osteoporosis. This chapter focuses on this third category and on disorders that have as common pathogenetic mechanism the definite or possible interaction between the bone tissue and its bone marrow microenvironment.

In recent years the role of the bone marrow microenvironment in the regulation of bone metabolism has attracted considerable attention. It becomes increasingly clear that these two compartments cannot be considered separately, and better understanding of the bone marrow physiology and pathology may enhance our knowledge of bone pathology. Although examination of bone tissue by sophisticated morphometric techniques provides invaluable information about bone remodeling and its disturbances, for the elucidation of the driving forces for the observed changes, concurrent examination of the bone marrow may be essential. This approach is gaining popularity but we currently lack the necessary knowledge and tools to interpret or recognize all important pathology that may be related to osteoporosis. Identification of such relations not only is essential for understanding the mechanisms of bone loss and the pathogenesis of bone destruction but may also lead to more rational therapeutic interventions. For some bone marrow disorders, however, the link to bone pathology is clear. These include mainly disorders in which the bone marrow is infiltrated by malignant cells.

MULTIPLE MYELOMA

Multiple myeloma is typically associated with bone pathology. Nearly 80% of patients have bone pain at presentation and pathologic fractures have been reported in up to 60% of patients. Bone lesions are usually focal and lytic but diffuse osteopenia can also be present. In rare cases osteosclerotic lesions may also be seen. The prevalence of vertebral fractures, assessed morphometrically in x-rays of the spine of 250 patients with multiple myeloma was 56%, and there was a relation between the presence of vertebral fractures and the severity and prevalence of bone pain (2). This high prevalence together with the fact that the incidence of multiple myeloma is highest in the seventh decade of life, a period when the incidence of fractures due to primary osteoporosis is also high, makes this disease an important cause of secondary osteoporosis, which may not be recognized unless appropriate investigations are performed.

In our unit last year we encountered three women with vertebral fractures and multiple myeloma who had been diagnosed with primary osteoporosis and were treated accordingly by their physicians. With the greater awareness of osteoporosis and the wider availability of means to diagnose and treat it, we may be confronted with more cases like these unless major efforts are taken to inform the medical profession about the need to carefully assess patients presenting with vertebral fractures.

Bone destruction in multiple myeloma is due to increased osteoclastic activity induced by bone-acting cytokines, which are produced by the malignant cells. These have been named in the past, collectively, osteoclast-activating factor (OAF) and probably include interleukin-6, tumor necrosis factor, interleukin-1β, and macrophage colony stimulating factor (M-CSF). In multiple myeloma there is an uncoupling between bone resorption and bone formation and this is reflected in the generally normal serum alkaline phosphatase activity, normal to low serum osteocalcin concentrations, and in the increased urinary excretion of biochemical indices of bone resorption. In addition, bone scans show usually no abnormalities, which contrasts the findings in patients with metastatic bone disease from solid tumors. In patients with multiple myeloma bone complaints respond generally well to chemotherapy but bone destruction may progress. Because this is due to increased bone resorption bisphosphonates have not only been used in the treatment of hypercalcemia, which occurs in about one third of the patients, but also for the prevention of the other skeletal complications.

Evidence is accumulating that newer bisphosphonates can reduce significantly, skeletal morbidity in patients with multiple myeloma, especially those on second-line chemotherapy (2). The doses of bisphosphonates used are, however, substantially higher than those used in the treatment of primary osteoporosis. Positive results have been obtained in large clinical trials with oral clodronate and intravenous pamidronate leading to registration of these compounds for this indication in various countries.

Apart from multiple myeloma, leukemia may also be associated with diffuse osteopenia and vertebral fractures especially in children (adolescents) with acute lymphoblastic leukemia (3) and may be due to local release of osteotropic factors by the malignant cells. Convincing evidence for that is, however, lacking. Development of osteopenia and fractures after treatment of the leukemia is most probably multifactorial and therapeutic interventions appear to play a major role in that (4). With improving survival of patients with this common childhood malignancy, osteoporosis may become an important clinical issue in such patients.

BREAST CANCER

Breast cancer is the most frequent malignant tumor and the most common cause of death due to cancer among women in industrialized countries. Breast cancer metastasizes frequently to the skeleton and about 70% of patients with advanced cancer develop symptomatic skeletal disease (5). Metastases are usually localized in bone that is rich in red marrow, particularly at sites of active hematopoiesis, and the axial skeleton (spine, ribs, pelvis) is most frequently affected.

In a placebo-controlled trial to evaluate the effect of the bisphosphonate clodronate on skeletal complications in patients with breast cancer and bone metastases, the rate of new vertebral fractures in the placebo group was 124 per 100 patient-years (6). This incidence exceeds by far published incidences of vertebral fractures in patients with primary osteoporosis.

Skeletal complications in patients with breast cancer are a major cause of morbidity and deterioration of the quality of life. Furthermore, patients with first metastasis to the skeleton live longer and if the disease remains confined to the skeleton survival may be even longer, but requires efficient preventive and/or palliative interventions.

The reason for the strong preference of breast cancer cells (and of other osteotropic tumors) for the skeleton is not known. There is, however, general agreement that bone destruction involves mainly the activation of the normal osteoclastic pathway (7). Breast cancer cells in the direct vicinity of bone release factors which stimulate the formation and/or the activity of osteoclasts leading to increased bone resorption.

Current evidence suggests that bone resorption may also be systemically stimulated by parathyroid hormone-related protein (PTHrP). Bone components (e.g., growth factors, cytokines, collagen fragments) that are released during bone resorption may in turn stimulate the chemotaxis and attachment of new cancer cells to bone, thus amplifying the process. Inhibition of bone resorption may therefore not only decrease bone destruction but may also disrupt this cycle.

Ample evidence in support of the first notion has been obtained in human studies with the use of bisphosphonates. Clodronate and pamidronate were shown in controlled studies to significantly decrease skeletal morbidity in patients with breast cancer and bone metastases and to decrease the frequency of new vertebral fractures (clodronate) (6,8). Evidence for the second notion was recently obtained in an ani-

mal model of metastatic breast cancer. It was shown that inhibition of cancer-induced bone resorption by the bisphosphonate risedronate induced a significant reduction in the tumor burden in the bone marrow (9). Thus, although the differential diagnosis of vertebral fractures in patients with breast cancer presents usually no difficulties, their pathogenesis as well as their management are a challenge to physicians involved in the care of patients with skeletal disorders.

For completeness, it should also be mentioned that anticancer treatment of premenopausal women can lead to early menopause and bone loss. As estrogen therapy is contraindicated in these but also in postmenopausal patients with breast cancer, other therapeutic options need to be considered. Compounds antagonizing the effects of estrogens on breast (and uterus) while acting agonistically on bone and lipid metabolism are gaining popularity. Such compounds are currently named SERMs (selective estrogen receptor modulators). Up until now results have been obtained with the use of tamoxifen, which is used in the treatment of patients with breast cancer but may increase the risk of uterine carcinoma. Tamoxifen has been also shown to reduce bone loss in women with breast cancer (10). However, in a recent study of healthy late postmenopausal women given tamoxifen (20 mg/day) there was only a small protective effect on bone mineral density of the axial skeleton. This was comparable in magnitude to that of calcium supplements and less than that of estrogens or bisphosphonates (11). Other SERMs are currently under clinical development but it is too early to derive any conclusions about their effectiveness.

CHRONIC ANEMIAS

Homozygous β-thalassemia is usually described as an example of chronic anemia predisposing to osteoporosis. Evidence for that has been obtained by skeletal radiographs, by bone density measurements, and by bone histology (12,13). In patients with thalassemia there is expansion of the bone marrow space, due to hyperplasia of the marrow, with thinning of the adjacent trabeculae. In addition, iron deposits have been described in the bone marrow, the bone marrow–bone interface at the mineralization front, but also in osteoblasts due to frequent blood transfusions as in patients with hemochromatosis. Apart from these potential mechanisms for the development of osteoporosis, patients with thalassemia have also a multiplicity of other metabolic disturbances that may predispose to osteoporosis such as, for example, hepatic and gonadal dysfunction. Hypogonadism appears to be a major contributing factor as suggested recently in cross-sectional as well as in longitudinal studies of thalassemic patients on different transfusion and iron chelation regimens with or without hormonal replacement (14). Thus, all the evidence collected so far suggests multiple causes for the low bone mass with hypogonadism perhaps being the predominant cause. However, Greep et al. (15) reported reduced bone mass in patients with thalassemia trait (thalassemia minor). These patients have a mild hemolytic anemia, do not need blood transfusions, have no endocrine or hepatic dysfunction, and have a normal life expectancy. These clearly preliminary observations, if confirmed, can have a significant impact on our understanding of the role of the bone marrow microenvironment in the regulation of bone metabolism and further studies in this area are certainly worth undertaking.

MASTOCYTOSIS

Mastocytosis, a multiorgan disease of unknown etiology, is characterized by abnormal mast cell proliferation limited to the skin (urticaria pigmentosa) or involving, in addition, lymph nodes, the bone marrow, the liver, the spleen, and the gastrointestinal tract. Because of the multiorgan involvement and the biologic potential of the mast cells, the disease has heterogeneous manifestations and variable prognosis.

Skeletal symptoms are present in about 60% to 75% of the patients with systemic mast cell disease, being the presenting clinical manifestation in about 5% (16). Skeletal changes are usually confined to the axial skeleton and include, among others, generalized osteopenia and vertebral fractures. Bone biopsies from patients with mast cell infiltration of the bone marrow and osteoporosis show increased bone turnover but imbalance in the remodeling activity in favor of resorption has also been reported (17,18).

The mechanism of bone destruction in mastocytosis is not known and is thought to be due to increased heparin production by the mast cells (see further) and/or to bone-acting cytokines that are produced in excess by these cells. Of particular interest are reports of patients with vertebral osteoporosis and bone marrow mast cell lesions without any other manifestation of mast cell disease (17). These patients would have been classified as primary osteoporosis if a bone biopsy had not been taken.

The prevalence of mast cell lesions in the bone marrow of patients with symptomatic spinal osteoporosis is about 3% to 4%. This is admittedly low but such patients tend to have more severe and progressive osteoporosis. At present the diagnosis of mast cell lesions can only be established by bone marrow histology but the diagnostic value of measurements of products of the mast cells, such as histamine metabolites, in biological fluids needs to be properly assessed. The relevant question is whether the increase in mast cells in the bone marrow of these patients is causally related to osteoporosis. Mast cells may be increased in the bone marrow of patients with primary osteoporosis (19) but their number is less than that observed in mast cell disease. In addition, the pattern of mast cell infiltration of the bone marrow as well as cell morphology in patients with osteoporosis as the sole manifestation of mastocytosis appears to differ from those seen in the marrow of patients with systemic mast cell disease. The condition may thus represent part of the spectrum of primary osteoporosis or, alternatively, a variant of mast cell disease. There is no specific treatment for osteoporosis associated with mast cell disease and only case studies have reported variable success with the use of histamine antagonists or bisphosphonates (20–22).

HEPARIN TREATMENT

Heparin is an effective treatment for thromboembolic disorders. It is usually given for a few days and if long-term treatment with antithrombotic agents is indicated this is done with the use of oral anticoagulants, mainly coumarin derivatives. There are, however, instances when heparin therapy may be prolonged and these include, first, contraindications to oral anticoagulant therapy and, second, prevention and treatment of thromboembolic episodes during pregnancy as vitamin K antagonists may carry increased risks for the fetus.

Early studies have already reported increased incidence of osteoporotic fractures in heparin-treated patients (23). A number of subsequent reports supported this observation and it was suggested that development of osteoporosis during heparin therapy depends on the dose of the drug and the duration of treatment.

Recently, two relatively large studies examined the relation between heparin therapy and osteoporosis in clinically relevant groups of patients. In the first study occurrence of symptomatic vertebral fractures was assessed in 184 pregnant women who received a mean dose of 19,000 IU/day of heparin for an average period of 25 weeks (24). Spinal fractures occurred in 4 (2.2%) women postpartum and there was a suggestion of a relation to the amount of heparin given. This is a low incidence but it should be noted that it occurred in young women and that x-rays were made only in women with sudden severe back pain, which may have underestimated the number of incident vertebral fractures. In addition, this study provided no information about a possible effect of heparin on bone mass that may be of significance later in life.

The second study assessed the skeletal effects of heparin treatment given subcutaneously to 80 patients with venous thromboembolic episodes and contraindications to oral coumarin therapy (25). Half of the patients received unfractionated heparin 10,000 IU twice daily whereas the other half received low-molecular-weight heparin 5000 IU twice daily for a period of 3–6 months. Both treatments had similar antithrombotic effects. In total, 7 of the 80 patients (8.8%) developed symptomatic vertebral fractures and 6 of them were treated with unfractionated heparin. Patients with fractures were older (mean 79 ± 6 years vs. 67 ± 15 years in the nonfracture group) and had significantly lower baseline bone mineral density of the femur but not of the lumbar spine. Bone mineral density decreased with treatment, on average by 4% at the spine and 2% at the femur. This study suggested, in addition, that the osteopenic effects of heparin therapy may be less pronounced with the use of low-molecular-weight heparin preparations, a conclusion that was also supported by animal studies (26).

The mechanism responsible for the skeletal effects of heparin is unknown and may involve the same pathway as in mast cell disease. Various hypotheses have been proposed to explain the action of heparin on bone including stimulation of osteoclastic activity by enhancement of parathyroid hormone (PTH)–dependent bone resorption or stimulation of collagenase synthesis, suppression of osteoblastic activity, and/or interference with the parathyroid–vitamin D axis.

A recent study with bone cultures from rat fetuses showed stimulation of osteoclastic resorption by unfractionated heparin to a level similar to that induced by PTH or calcitriol; low-molecular-weight heparin appeared to be less effective in stimulating resorption (27). The authors concluded that heparin promotes bone resorption and that the size and the sulfation of the molecule are major determinants of this action. On the other hand, van der Wiel et al. (28) failed to detect any changes in biochemical indices of bone resorption in healthy volunteers given heparin 5000 IU twice daily subcutaneously for 10 days. Thus, although the pathogenesis of heparin-induced osteoporosis remains to be resolved and its true clinical significance to be determined, caution is needed when treating older patients with heparin for long, as this may predispose to symptomatic spinal osteoporosis.

PREGNANCY-ASSOCIATED OSTEOPOROSIS

Osteoporosis occurring during pregnancy is an intriguing syndrome first described about 40 years ago (29). In the following years reports of sporadic cases supported the view that this is a rare condition, but recent evidence suggests that it may not be that uncommon (30). Pregnancy-associated osteoporosis presents during the third trimester or postpartum usually with back pain, loss of height, and vertebral fractures, but pain in the hips and femoral fractures have also been described in a few patients. The primary involvement of the axial skeleton is further supported by bone densitometry measurements. In bone biopsies taken from patients 2 weeks to 5 years after the affected pregnancy, histologic features of osteoblast failure have been reported (31). In two thirds of the cases the disease occurs during the first pregnancy and does not generally recur in subsequent pregnancies. Isolated cases of recurrence, however, have also been described. Clinical recovery is rapid and the long-term prognosis is usually good.

During pregnancy there is a stress on maternal calcium stores to meet the needs of the fetus that is compensated by alterations in maternal calcium and bone metabolism, particularly by the marked increases in estrogen production. This has led to the hypothesis that pregnancy-associated osteoporosis occurs at an already pathologic background rather than being a separate entity. However, analysis of published cases reveals possible risk factors for osteoporosis in a minority of patients. For example, Smith et al. (31) reported that in only 4 of 24 patients a preexisting disorder known to decrease bone mass was present; this was also the case in 6 of 35 patients with pregnancy-associated osteoporosis evaluated by postal questionnaire (30). In these two studies preexisting conditions included heparin therapy (4), glucocorticoid treatment (3), mild osteogenesis imperfecta (2), history of anorexia nervosa and of thyroid disease (3), celiac disease (2), and antiepileptic treatment (2). In an analysis of 72 cases (mainly from the literature but also own), Saraux et al. (32) reported the use of heparin as a potential risk factor in 6 patients. It is also of interest that in the above-mentioned postal survey it was found that the mothers of patients with pregnancy-associated osteoporosis had a significantly higher prevalence of fractures compared

with controls (30), suggesting that genetic factors may also be involved in the pathogenesis of the disease. On the other hand, the rapid clinical improvement, the densitometric evidence of recovery, and the nonoccurrence in subsequent pregnancies led to the suggestion that the disease may be related to a particular pregnancy (or to a particular fetus) for reasons not yet clear (31).

Elucidating the pathogenesis of pregnancy-associated osteoporosis is not easy. Apart from the rarity of the disease, its delayed recognition, when alterations in bone metabolism have already occurred, contribute to this difficulty. The inability of radiologic investigations during pregnancy and the difficulty in interpreting changes in biochemical indices of bone metabolism, especially during the third trimester, complicate the evaluation of such patients further. Finally, back complaints are common in pregnant women and it has been hypothesized that some of them may in fact have unrecognized milder forms of pregnancy-associated osteoporosis (33). Designing strategies to approach this intriguing syndrome may provide some clues of its real prevalence and its possible consequences for the skeletal integrity of such patients later in life.

REFERENCES

1. Rao DS, Honasoge M. Metabolic bone disease in gastrointestinal, hepatobiliary, and pancreatic disorders. In: Favus MJ, Christakos S, Goldring SR, et al. (eds) *Primer on the Metabolic Bone Diseases and Disorders of Mineral Metabolism, Third edition.* Philadelphia, Lippincott-Raven Publishers, 306–311, 1996
2. McCloskey E. Bisphosphonates in multiple myeloma. In: Bijvoet OLM, Fleisch HA, Canfield RE, Russell RGG (eds) *Bisphosphonate on Bons.* Amsterdam, Elsevier Science, 391–402, 1995
3. Newman AJ, Melhorn DK. Vertebral compression in childhood leukemia. *Am J Dis Child* 125:863–865, 1973
4. Atkinson SA, Fraher L, Gundberg CM, Andrew M, Pai M, Barr RD. Mineral homeostasis and bone mass in children treated for acute lymphoblastic leukemia. *J Pediatr* 114:793–800, 1989
5. Rubens RD. Bone involvement in solid tumours. In: Bijvoet OLM, Fleisch HA, Kanfield RE, Russell RGG (eds) *Bisphosphonate on Bons.* Amsterdam, Elsevier Science, 337–347, 1995
6. Paterson AHG, Powels TJ, Kanis JA, McCloskey E, Hanson J, Ashley S. Double-blind controlled trial of oral clodronate in patients with bone metastases from breast cancer. *J Clin Oncol* 11:59–65, 1993
7. Guise TA, Mundy GR. Breast cancer and bone. *Cur Opin Endocrinol Diab* 2:548–555, 1995
8. van Holten-Verzantvoort ATM, Kroon HM, Bijvoet OLM, et al. Palliative pamidronate treatment in patients with bone metastases from breast cancer. *J Clin Oncol* 11:491–498, 1993
9. Sasaki A, Boyce BF, Story B, et al. Bisphosphonate risedronate reduces metastatic human breast cancer burden in bone in nude mice. *Cancer Res* 55:3551–3557, 1995
10. Love RR, Mazess RB, Barden HS, et al. Effects of tamoxifen on bone mineral content in postmenopausal women with breast cancer. *N Engl J Med* 326:852–856, 1991
11. Grey AB, Stapleton JP, Evans MC, Tatnell MA, Ames RW, Reid IR. The effect of the antiestrogen tamoxifen on bone mineral density in normal late postmenopausal women. *Am J Med* 99:636–641, 1995
12. Orvietto R, Leichter I, Rachmilewitz EA, Margulies JY. Bone density, mineral content and cortical index in patients with thalassemia major and the correlation to their bone fractures, blood transfusion and treatment with desferioxamine. *Calcif Tissue Int* 50:397–399, 1992

13. Vernejoul MC de, Girot R, Geuris J et al. calcium phosphate metabolism and bone disease in patients with homozygous thalassemia. *J Clin Endocrinol Metab* 54:276–281, 1982
14. Anapliotou MLG, Kastanias IT, Psara P, Evangelou EA, Liparaki M, Dimitriou P. The contribution of hypogonadism to the development of osteoporosis in thalassaemia major: new therapeutic approaches. *Clin Endocrinol* 42:279–287, 1994
15. Greep N, Anderson AL, Gallaher JCh. Thalassemia minor: a risk factor for osteoporosis? *Bone Miner* 16:63–72, 1992
16. Travis WD, Li C, Bergstrahl EJ, Yam LT, Swee RG. Systemic mast cell disease: analysis of 58 cases and literature review. *Medicine* 67:345–368, 1988
17. Chines A, Pacifici R, Avioli LV, Teitelbaum SC, Korenblat PE. Systemic mastocytosis presenting as osteoporosis. A clinical and histomorphometric study. *J Clin Endocrinol Metab* 72:140–144, 1991
18. de Gennes C, Kuntz D, de Vernejoul MC. Bone mastocytosis. *Clin Orth Rel Res* 279:281–291, 1992
19. Frame B, Nixon R. Bone marrow mast cells in osteoporosis and aging. *N Engl J Med* 279:626–630, 1968
20. Cundy T, Beneton MHC, Darby AJ, Marshall WJ, Kanis JA. Osteopenia in systemic mastocytosis: natural history and response to treatment with inhibitors of bone resorption. *Bone* 8:149–155, 1987
21. Graves L, Stechschulte DJ, Morris DC, Lukert BP. Inhibition of mediator release in systemic mastocytosis is associated with reversal of bone changes. *J Bone Miner Res* 5:1113–1119, 1990
22. Watts RA, Scott DGI, Crisp AJ. Mastocytosis and osteoporosis. *Br J Rheum* 31:715, 1992
23. Griffith GC, Nichols G, Asher JD, Flanagan B. Heparin osteoporosis. *J Am Med Assoc* 193:85–88, 1965
24. Dahlman TC. Osteoporotic fractures and the recurrence of thromboembolism during pregnancy and the purperium in 184 women undergoing thromboprophylaxis with heparin. *Am J Obst Gynecol* 168:1265–1270, 1993
25. Monreal M, Lafoz E, Olive A, del Rio L, Vedia C. Comparison of subcutaneous unfractionated heparin with low molecular weight heparin (Fragmin) in patients with venous thromboembolism and contraindications to coumarin. *Thromb Haem* 71:7–11, 1994
26. Monreal M, Vinas L, Monreal L, Lavin S, Lafoz E, Angles AM. Heparin-related osteoporosis in rats. A comparative study between unfractonated heparin and low molecular weight heparin. *Haemostasis* 20:204–207, 1990
27. Shaughnessy SG, Young E, Deschamps P, Hirsh J. The effects of low molecular weight and standard heparin on calcium loss from fetal rat calvaria. *Blood* 86:1368–1373, 1995
28. van der Wiel HE, Lips P, Huijgens PC, Netelenbos JC. Effects of short-term low-dose heparin administration on biochemical parameters of bone turnover. *Bone Miner* 22:27–32, 1993
29. Nordin BEC, Roper A. Postpregnancy osteoporosis - a syndrome. *Lancet* 1:431–434, 1995
30. Dunne F, Walters B, Marshall T, Heath DA. Pregnancy associated osteoporosis. *Clin Endocrinol* 39:487–490, 1993
31. Smith R, Athanasou NA, Ostlere SJ, Vipond SE. Pregnancy-associated osteoporosis. *Q J Med* 88:865–878, 1995
32. Saraux A, Bourgeais F, Ehrhart A, Baron D, Le Goff P. Osteoporose de la grossesse: Quatre observation. *Rev Rhum Ed Fr* 60:596–600, 1993
33. Khastgir G, Studd J. Pregnancy-associated osteoporosis. *Br J Obst Gynecol* 101:836–838, 1994

21. Orthopedic Complications of Osteoporosis

Thomas A. Einhorn, M.D.

Department of Orthopedics, Mount Sinai School of Medicine, New York, New York

Most osteoporosis-related complications in orthopedics relate to problems associated with fractures and fracture management, and how the osteoporotic skeleton responds to joint reconstructive procedures. Specific attention to the quality of fracture fixation and the use of implants in weak bone is required. Control of the metabolic condition, including treatment of the underlying cause of the osteoporosis (if known), and pharmaceutical management of the condition may improve surgical results. It may be necessary to alter the surgeon's usual preference for specific fixation devices to meet the anatomic and physiologic needs of the deformed or qualitatively impaired bone. In certain osteoporotic conditions in which bone remodeling is affected, a prolonged period of fracture healing may be anticipated and this period of healing may exceed the rate of healing in normal nonosteoporotic bone.

The orthopedist must be aware that the osteoporotic skeleton may suffer unusual types of injuries because of the fragile quality of the bone. For example, patients with osteoporosis who are engaged in athletic events may experience injuries in which their soft tissue structures have a greater ability to withstand mechanical loads than the bones that support them. As an example, a common skiing injury, rupture of the anterior cruciate of the knee, usually occurs when an anterior displacement force is applied to the knee and the ligament becomes stretched rupturing in its midsubstance. However, since the ligament is anchored in the joint to the bone of the femur and tibial plateau, if the cross-sectional area and strength of the ligament exceeds the bone's resistance to tensile loading, an avulsion fracture may occur in osteoporotic bone instead of a failure (tear) occurring in the ligament. Not only must the orthopedist be aware of the possibility of this type of problem, but the method of operative repair and the rehabilitation program must take into consideration the limited capacity of the bone to support a tensile force in the ligament. Other complications of osteoporosis relate to the reconstruction of the diseased or deformed skeleton during treatments such as osteotomy, arthrodesis, and arthroplasty. In each case, the ability of the osteoporotic skeleton to respond to mechanical conditions, implant devices, or cementation techniques must be recognized and addressed. This chapter will review some of these situations.

MANAGEMENT OF FRACTURES IN PATIENTS WITH OSTEOPOROSIS

Skeletal fractures are the most common orthopedic condition associated with osteoporosis. The goals of treatment are rapid mobilization and a return to normal activities; prolonged immobilization through the use of conservative fracture management is generally discouraged because it places the patient at risk of pulmonary decompensation, thromboembolic disease, decubitus formation, and further skeletal deterioration from disuse. Although the treatment of each fracture must be addressed individually, the following are general guidelines for the management of osteoporotic fractures:

1. Elderly patients are best treated by rapid, definitive fracture management aimed at early restoration of mobility and function. In general, these patients are considered to be at their healthiest on the initial day of injury and thus are in the best condition to undergo an operation at that time (1,2). In some cases, survival is benefited by judicious preoperative management to reverse medical decompensation causing or resulting from the injury. In addition, the extent and scope of the operative intervention should be minimized in order to reduce operative time, blood loss, and physiologic stress to the patient.

2. The goal of operative intervention is to achieve stable fracture fixation and permit early return of function. For the lower extremity, this is dictated by the ability of the patient to return to a weight bearing status early in the treatment period. Although anatomic restoration is important for intraarticular fractures, metaphyseal and diaphyseal fractures require early stabilization and perfect anatomic reduction is less important.

3. The primary mode of failure of internal fixation is due to the inability of the osteoporotic bone to support fixation devices. Since the strength of bone is directly related to the square of its mineral density (3), osteoporotic bone may lack the strength to support rigid fixation devices such as plates and screws. Moreover, comminution is generally more extensive in osteoporotic fractures and fixation devices should be chosen to allow compaction and settling of fracture fragments into stable patterns that minimize stresses at the bone–implant interface. Finally, implants should be chosen that minimize stress shielding in order to avoid further regional bone loss. For these reasons, sliding nail-plate devices, intramedullary systems, and tension band wiring constructs that allow load sharing and compaction are generally preferred over rigid systems.

4. Although the events of fracture healing proceed normally in almost all osteoporotic patients, an inadequate calcium intake could result in deficits in callus mineralization or remodeling (4). Since it has been shown that many elderly patients are malnourished, fracture healing may be enhanced when nutritional deficiencies are corrected (4,5). Therefore, for optimal results, nutritional assessment should be included in patient evaluation and in certain cases protein supplementation, physiologic doses of vitamin D (400–800 IU/day) and calcium (1.5 g elemental calcium/day) should be administered in the perioperative and postoperative periods.

Hip Fractures

A number of factors influence the occurrence of hip fractures. The medical and epidemiologic issues relating to hip fracture incidence are reviewed in Chapter 15. Although hip fractures have been classified according to several systems, patients with osteoporosis generally sustain one of two types of hip fractures, intracapsular or intertrochanteric. In intracapsular fractures, the fracture occurs within the hip capsule and frequently results in an interruption of the blood supply to the femoral head. These fractures are also known as cervical fractures, transcervical fractures, or femoral neck fractures (Fig. 1). Intertrochanteric fractures are extracapsular fractures that occur in an area in which biomechanical forces are only moderately high. The name "intertrochanteric" is derived from the fact that the fracture is anatomically propagated between the greater and lesser trochanters of the femur (Fig. 2).

Intracapsular fractures are problematic because of the high incidence of nonunion and avascular necrosis that occurs in spite of adequate treatment. These complications are related to the retrograde blood supply to the femoral head and the fact that the branches of the medial femoral circumflex artery, which nourish the femoral head within the hip capsule, are apposed to the femoral neck and are usually interrupted when intracapsular fractures are displaced. Closed reduction and pin and screw fixation using a variety of implants are consistently associated with a 14% incidence of nonunion and a 15% incidence of avascular necrosis (Fig. 3) (2).

The treatment options for intracapsular fractures are reduction and internal fixation vs. hemiarthroplasty. Since the degree of displacement of an intracapsular fracture may predict its prognosis, the decision of operative treatment is dictated by the extent of displacement of the fracture. The classification system used to help make these assessments is known as the Garden classification (Fig. 4). This is a four-stage classification system in which stage I fractures are those that are incomplete, nondisplaced, and frequently angled into a valgus position; stage II fractures are those that are complete, nondisplaced, but potentially unstable; stage III fractures are completely displaced, but a portion of the capsule remains intact; and in stage IV fractures, the fracture is completely displaced and the capsule is completely disrupted. Studies have shown that stage III and IV fractures have the highest rates of nonunion. Therefore, reduction and fixation with pins is generally preferred in stage I and II fractures while hemiarthroplasty is often used in the treatment of stage III and IV injuries (Fig. 5). The advantages of internal fixation are that the anatomy is restored, the patient undergoes a normal period of fracture healing, and if the joint has not been injured, the patient can expect normal service from the hip after the fracture has healed. The advantage of hemiarthroplasty is the immediate return to function because the replaced joint does not need to undergo a period of healing. However, hemiarthroplasty is associated with its own set of complications including loosening and breakage of implants, and the risk of infection. Most authors agree that treatment by hemiarthroplasty is associated with a higher perioperative morbidity.

Intertrochanteric fractures have received less attention than femoral neck fractures because nonunion and avascular necrosis are uncommon in intertrochanteric fractures. However, the prevalence of malunion with resulting varus, short-

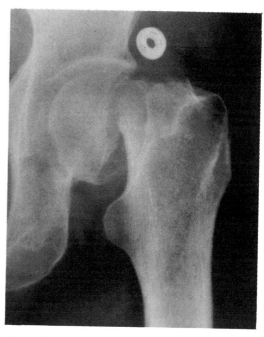

FIG. 1. Anteroposterior view of a typical intracapsular (femoral neck) fracture. Since the hip capsule inserts just above the greater and lesser trochanters of the femur, this fracture is anatomically located within the hip joint. As such, it is referred to as an intracapsular fracture.

ening, and external rotational deformity is significant and can be disabling. In addition, when bone quality is particularly poor, the use of fixation devices may be beset with problems such as loss of fixation and screw penetration into the hip joint (2). Telescoping or sliding hip screw devices are an improvement over fixed nail devices in that they allow controlled compaction of the fracture until a stable fracture pattern is achieved. However, it is still necessary for the surgeon to obtain an adequate reduction before using such a device. When used properly, a load-sharing device will result in a decrease in the stresses between the implant and the bone and a more favorable biomechanical situation (Fig. 2B).

In some situations, the bone in the trochanteric region of the femur is so osteoporotic that any type of fixation system is at risk of failure. In these situations, orthopedists have resorted to the use of methyl methacrylate cement to enhance the purchase of implant devices in the bone and prevent penetration or cutting out of the device. More recently, a calcium phosphate-based material has been developed that may prove effective when injected into the site of a fracture or used with a fixation device at the time of fracture management. This material is presently experimental but current investigations on its use in the treatment of hip fractures have yielded encouraging results (6).

Fractures About the Knee

Osteoporotic bone that supports the knee joint is susceptible to supracondylar fractures of the distal femur and fractures of the tibial plateau. Because both of these fractures may be associated with comminution and intraarticular

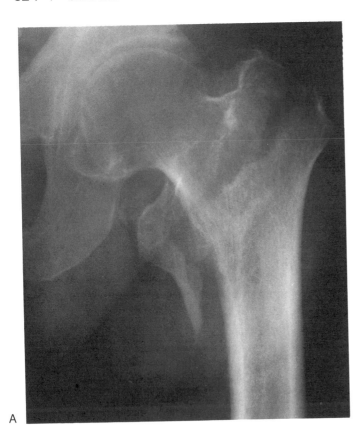

A

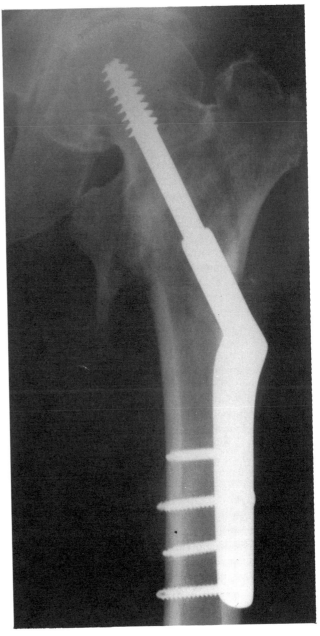

B

FIG. 2. A: Anteroposterior view of a typical intertrochanteric fracture. Note that the fracture line is propagated between the greater and lesser trochanters, and the lesser trochanter is actually displaced from the femur being pulled medially by the iliopsoas muscle insertion. **B:** Anteroposterior view of the same fracture 2 months after operative treatment. Note that with the use of a sliding hip screw the fracture fragments have settled or compacted into a stable configuration.

extension, they carry a high risk for postoperative degenerative joint disease and arthrofibrosis. Treatment protocols are therefore aimed at early knee rehabilitation and strengthening of the quadriceps mechanism.

Management of fractures about the knee in patients with osteoporosis can be difficult. Frequently, the degree of comminution is so extensive that choices of internal fixation are limited. Occasionally, special imaging techniques such as computed tomography (CT) scanning and plain tomography can help delineate the size and position of the fracture fragments. Because these fractures can be immobilized in a well-padded long leg cast or brace, the urgency for operative treatment is usually not as great as for the hip or the femoral shaft. However, long-term immobilization of these fracture not only limits a patient's activity but can lead to joint stiffness particularly in the elderly population.

In supracondylar fractures, the objectives of operative treatment are anatomic restoration and rigid fixation to allow immediate rehabilitation. Although good results have been obtained with one-piece blade plates and 90° telescoping screw plates, the recent advent of short locked intramedullary nails (GSH Nail®, Richards Manufacturing Company, Memphis, Tennessee) has aided in the management of these injuries. The advantage of this rigid type of fixation is that the patient's knee can be immediately moved in rehabilitation protocols.

Tibial plateau fractures generally result from a valgus stress to the knee in conjunction with falling and twisting. The degree of compromise that occurs as a result of tibial plateau fractures depends on the degree of instability and angular deformity. Minimally displaced fractures, i.e., those with less than 5 mm of depression, can be treated with

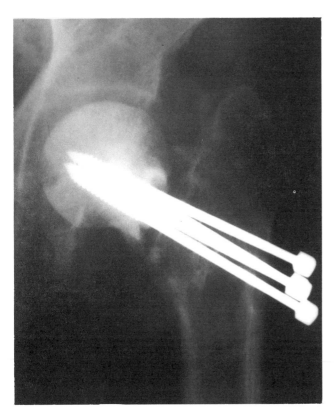

FIG. 3. Anteroposterior view of the proximal femur of a patient 3 months after open reduction and internal fixation of a displaced intracapsular fracture. Note that there is a diastasis at the fracture site, the pins have begun to migrate laterally, and the femoral head is radiodense, suggesting osteonecrosis.

immobilization of the knee followed by active motion. Non-weightbearing of the injured limb should be maintained until fracture healing has occurred at approximately 6–8 weeks. The use of continuous passive motion (CPM) has been found to be extremely helpful and the use of a hinge knee brace between CPM sessions enhances recovery. Fractures displaced by more than 8 mm, or those with associated varus or valgus instability of 5–10° or greater, require open reduction and internal fixation. Postoperatively, a varus molded cast brace followed by CPM is used. Weight bearing is delayed for a period of 8–10 weeks posttreatment.

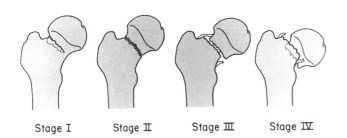

FIG. 4. Schematic of the Garden classification of intracapsular hip fractures.

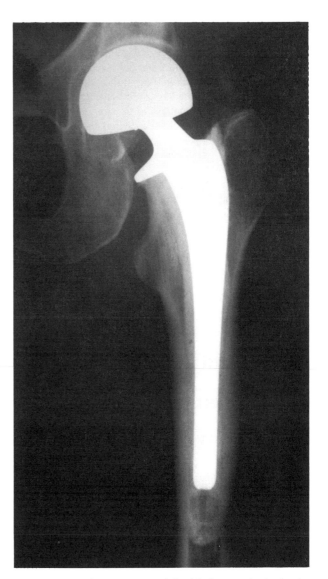

FIG. 5. Anteroposterior view of the hip in a patient who has undergone a hemiarthroplasty for the treatment of a displaced (stage IV) intracapsular hip fracture.

Fractures of the Humerus

Three types of humeral fractures occur in osteoporotic patients: fractures of the proximal humerus, the humeral diaphysis, and the supracondylar region of the elbow. Generally, these fractures result from minor falls and usually occur with minimal displacement.

Fractures of the proximal humerus are common and account for approximately 5% of fractures in this patient population. Eighty percent of these fractures occur through the cancellous bone of the surgical neck and are impacted without significant displacement (2). These fractures are considered stable and can be treated by immobilization in a sling or sling like system. Range of motion activities including pendulum exercises can be started to avoid shoulder stiffness. Generally, 3–4 weeks is sufficient to allow for early healing prior to full passive range of motion with active range of motion taking place by 5–6 weeks. Unimpacted fractures can be treated with a sling or sling like device. Occasionally, closed reduction and percutaneous pin fixation are required to achieve stable reduction. Comminuted fractures involving three- or four-part displacement are best treated by prosthetic replacement followed by early vigorous physical therapy. Open reduction and internal fixation can be used when the fragments are sufficiently large and there is less than extensive comminution. Open reduction and internal fixation using screws and tension band wires have been shown to work well. However, if difficulty is encountered in obtaining adequate purchase of screws, pins, or wires in bone, hemiarthroplasty is recommended.

Humeral shaft fractures in most cases are treated by nonoperative means. Occasionally, intramedullary nailing is needed to control angulation; however, because of the large amount of soft tissue in the arm, more angulation is acceptable with humeral shaft fractures than with fractures of other long bones.

Fractures of the distal humerus, especially those with an intraarticular component, present a particular challenge to orthopedic treatment. The potential for chronic disability is high and hence anatomic reduction and stable fixation is required. These fractures are associated with a high degree of morbidity and elbow stiffness is not uncommon. Early operative intervention followed by carefully planned physical therapy is needed.

Fractures of the Distal Radius

Fractures of the distal radius, most notably Colles' fractures, are a common complication of osteoporosis. Although it is generally held that substantial deformity of the distal radius can be acceptable when associated with relatively normal function, complications arise from this injury including loss of reduction, radial shortening, and painful prominence of the ulna (2). Many of these complications can be avoided by accurate reduction that restores the normal length and orientation of the distal radioulnar joint followed by early mobilization of the hand and upper extremity. Closed reduction and casting under local or regional anesthesia are generally successful in restoring the length of the distal radius. Healing is usually rapid and return to function occurs in about 6 weeks. Adequate reduction implies no radial shortening and at least a neutral angulation of the distal radial articular surface in the anterior–posterior plane. Unstable and severely comminuted fractures are best treated with internal or external fixation. External fixation is frequently difficult in osteopenic bone due to loosening of the pins in bone of poor quality. Therefore, the goal of treatment in these types of injuries is to obtain adequate reduction and control over the fracture fragments and immobilization long enough for early healing to take place. Once this has occurred, conversion to a cast or a splint is recommended. Current investigations using a calcium phosphate-based bone paste suggest that this material may enhance the fixation of these fragments and allowing for early conversion from a full-length arm cast to a short arm volar splint (6).

Spinal Fractures

Fractures of the spinal column are common in patients with osteoporotic bone. Vertebral fractures are grouped according to fracture type (wedge, biconcavity, or compression) and by degree of deformity (7). However, the vast majority of fractures of the osteoporotic spine are considered stable because the posterior spinal elements remain intact. Therefore, operative intervention is rarely required in spinal osteoporosis.

Symptomatic relief of spinal pain is often difficult to achieve because the causes are related not only to microcracks or fractures within the bone but also to stresses placed on the interspinous ligaments, facet joint capsules, and paraspinal muscles. Although narcotic medications are sometimes effective, their use should be discouraged or at least limited because the abuse potential is high. In many instances, significant symptomatic relief can be achieved through physical therapy, rehabilitation, and bracing. External support in the form of a bivalved custom polypropylene body jacket is useful during the acute painful phase of a fracture but should be discontinued when symptoms subside. These devices may cause paraspinal muscles to undergo atrophy with prolonged use, and it is those paraspinal muscles that are ultimately needed for support in maintaining the integrity of the spinal column complex. In those patients who upon careful evaluation are deemed able to withstand some low-level spinal stresses, a program of back extension and deep breathing exercises should be prescribed (8). In addition, counseling and instruction should be provided to all patients on the subjects of correct posture and body mechanics to prevent further pathologic fractures and the propensity to fall.

Operative management of osteoporotic spinal fractures is rarely indicated and should be reserved for the patient who has a fracture that is causing gross deformity resulting in pulmonary or neurologic impairment. The ability of the surgeon to obtain adequate purchase in bone is the main problem affecting any type of spinal fixation system. The recent development of the calcium phosphate-based materials may lead to the availability of new, fast-setting cements that could be effective in this application.

PROBLEMS ASSOCIATED WITH RECONSTRUCTIVE OPERATIVE PROCEDURES

Patients with osteoporosis are more prone to develop skeletal deformities as a result of physiologic bowing of qualitatively impaired bone or malunions of previous fractures. Correction of these deformities involves osteotomy, fixation, and bone healing. Planning of the osteotomy site and the placement of the bone cuts follow the same principles used in reconstructive surgery of the normal skeleton. Fixation, however, follows the principles outlined above for fracture management. In general, load-sharing devices such as intramedullary nails are preferred to rigid fixation systems. In addition, a very popular and effective method of osteotomy correction, small pin external fixation, is not suitable for patients with severe osteoporosis because of the propensity of small pins to cut out of qualitatively impaired bone.

Patients with diseased joints such as degenerative osteoarthritis are candidates for arthrodeses or total joint arthroplasties. While there are no special problems associated with arthrodeses in patients with osteoporosis, the types of fixation systems used in conjunction with these procedures follow the same principles described for fractures. With respect to total joint arthroplasty, surgeons should follow the same principles used in the management of joints supported by normal bone; however, special care should be taken during reaming and component insertion. When reaming the acetabular socket, reamers should be used at lower speeds and the results of the reaming should be checked more frequently so that penetration of the acetabulum does not occur. This is particularly relevant in patients who use corticosteroids. When reaming the femoral canal, special attention should be paid to the positioning of all reamers and guide wire systems because it is easy to penetrate the cortex.

Insertion of cement under pressure in patients with osteoporotic bone can lead to unusual complications. For example, even when there are no breaks in the cortices of the femoral canal, highly pressurized cement and implant insertion can result in a blow out of the cortical wall. Similarly, once an implant has been seated in the joint and the cement cured, settling or subsidence of the implant–cement composite may occur leading to increased joint laxity.

Fractures occur more frequently around total joint prostheses in osteoporotic bone and the surgeon must be prepared to handle these complications. A common example occurs in the patient who has a total knee replacement and subsequent supracondylar fracture. Although controversy exists concerning the management of these injuries in patients with normal bone, the prolonged period of healing associated with osteoporotic bone and the limited amount of trabecular bone in this area dictates that the best method of management is fixation. The use of a short intramedullary nail can be very useful in this setting. Finally, although most fractures occur from traumatic events, the surgeon must be aware that resistance encountered intraoperatively in the process of reduction or dislocation of the joint can lead to an increased risk of iatrogenic fracture. For this reason, particular care must be taken in the gentle intraoperative manipulation of the limbs of osteoporotic patients who are undergoing total joint arthroplasty.

SUMMARY

Patients with osteoporosis present a special challenge to the orthopedist. While most issues relate to the management of fractures sustained in fragile bone, special problems associated with reconstructive orthopedic procedures must also be addressed. The goal of any treatment is the rapid restoration of mobility and function and a return of the patient to a level of activity which supports their general health. Long-term immobilization should be avoided. In situations where it is possible to reduce the effects of an offending agent, such as corticosteroids, all efforts should be made to do so. Recently, several new pharmacologic agents have been approved by the U.S. Food and Drug Administration for the treatment of osteoporosis. These agents carry the hope of reducing the morbidity of this disease. Hopefully, they will also lead to an improvement in bone quality such that the response of the skeleton to operative interventions will also be improved. The combined approach of general health maintenance, the judicious use of pharmacologic agents, and a program of regular exercise should reduce the orthopedic complications associated with this disease.

REFERENCES

1. Villar RN, Allen SM, Barnes SJ: Hip fractures in healthy patients: operative delay vs. prognosis. *BMJ* 293:1203–1204, 1986
2. Cornell CN: Management of fractures in patients with osteoporosis. *Orthop Clin N Am* 21:125–141, 1990
3. Carter DR, Hayes WC: The compressive behavior of bone as a two-phase porous structure. *J Bone Joint Surg* 59:954–962, 1977
4. Einhorn TA, Bonnarens F, Burstein AH: The contributions of dietary protein and mineral to the healing of experimental fractures: A biomechanical Study. *J Bone Joint Surg* 68A:1389–1395, 1986
5. Jensen JE, Jensen TG, Smith TK, Johnston DA, Dudrick SJ: Nutrition in orthopaedic surgery. *J Bone Joint Surg* 64A:1263–1272, 1982
6. Constantz BR, Ison IC, Fulmer MT, Poser RD, Smith ST, Van Wagoner M, Ross J, Goldstein SA, Jupiter JB: Skeletal repair by in situ formation of the mineral phase of bone. *Science* 267:1796–1799, 1995
7. Eastell R, Cedel SI, Wahner HW, Riggs BL, Melton LJ III: Classification of vertebral fractures. *J Bone Min Res* 6:207–214, 1991
8. Sinaki M, Mikkelesen BA: Postmenopausal spinal osteoporosis: flexion versus extension exercises. *Arch Phys Med Rehabil* 65:593–596, 1984

22. Osteoporosis and Rheumatic Diseases

Steven R. Goldring, M.D.

Department of Medicine, Harvard Medical School; and Division of Rheumatology, Deaconess and New England Baptist Hospitals, Boston, Massachusetts

The rheumatic diseases include a diverse group of disorders that have in common their propensity to affect articular structures. The most commonly involved joints are the so-called diarthrodial joints, which consist of two articulating surfaces lined by hyaline cartilage. Arthritic processes most often affect the cartilage surfaces and the synovial lining but may also involve the subchondral bone and joint capsule. Amphiarthroses that are characterized by fibrocartilaginous union, e.g., the intervertebral disks, are also frequently affected in rheumatic disorders.

Osteoarthritis is a prototypical example of a rheumatic disease in which the pathologic events are restricted almost entirely to the joint structures. Many of the rheumatic diseases, however, may affect extraarticular organ systems and these conditions are often accompanied by significant systemic symptoms that may dominate the clinical picture. These illnesses, which include, for example, conditions such as rheumatoid arthritis (RA), systemic lupus erythematosus (SLE), and the spondyloarthropathies, are believed to be initiated by disturbances in immune regulation that involve complex interactions between unique host genetic susceptibility and specific environmental factor(s). In these disorders, not only may skeletal tissues be involved at juxtaarticular and subchondral sites, but in addition there is evidence that many of these conditions may produce generalized effects on bone remodeling that affect the entire skeleton.

Among the rheumatic disorders, RA represents an excellent model for gaining insights into the effects of local as well as systemic consequences of inflammatory processes on skeletal tissue remodeling. Three principal forms of bone disease have been described in RA. The first is that characterized by a focal process that affects the immediate subchondral and juxtaarticular bone. The synovial lesion of RA is characterized by the proliferation of the synovial lining cells and infiltration of the tissue by inflammatory cells, including lymphocytes, plasma cells, and activated macrophages (1,2). The proliferative synovial tissue (pannus) invades the immediately adjacent bone resulting in progressive focal osteolysis that gives rise to the characteristic cystic bone "erosions" that can be detected radiographically. Analysis of the immediate bone–pannus interface reveals the frequent presence of multinucleated cells with phenotypic features of osteoclasts (3,4), suggesting that the focal osteolytic lesions of RA are mediated at least in part by authentic osteoclasts. The origin of these cells is not clear, but some authors have speculated that they are derived from mononuclear cell precursors present within the inflamed synovium and that they are induced to differentiate into osteoclasts by the cytokines that are produced locally within the inflamed synovial tissue (5–7). There is also evidence that the macrophages and macrophage

polykaryons associated with this lesion can also contribute to the bone resorption (6).

A second form of bone disease observed in patients with RA is the presence of juxtaarticular osteopenia adjacent to inflamed joints. Histologic examination of this bone tissue reveals the presence of frequent osteoclasts and increased osteoid and resorptive surfaces consistent with increased bone turnover (3,8). Local aggregates of inflammatory cells, including macrophages and lymphocytes, are often detected in the marrow space. It has been suggested that these cells are derived from the synovial lining and that they migrate into the marrow where they release local products that affect bone remodeling (3). Decreased joint motion and immobilization in response to the joint inflammation likely represent additional contributing factors to this local bone loss.

The third form of bone disease associated with RA is the presence of generalized axial and appendicular osteopenia at sites that are distant from inflamed joints (9–11). Although there are conflicting data concerning the effects of RA on skeletal mass, the presence of a generalized reduction in bone mass has been confirmed using multiple different techniques and there is compelling evidence that this reduction is associated with an increased risk of hip and vertebral fracture (12–15). The conflicting data are in part related to the fact that most observations have been based on cross-sectional studies and have focused on patients late in the evolution of their disease when factors such as disability, or corticosteroid and other treatments, may confound the analyses. Histomorphometric analysis of bone biopsies from patients with RA indicate that in the absence of corticosteroid use the cellular basis of the generalized reduction in bone mass is related to a decrease in bone formation rather than an increase in bone resorption (16–18). More recently, biochemical markers of bone turnover have been used to study patients with RA and the results of these studies indicate that in patients receiving corticosteroids there is an increase in bone resorption (19,20).

Several factors have emerged as important determinants of bone mass in patients with RA. These include age and menopausal status, reduced mobility, disease activity, influence of antirheumatic therapy (especially corticosteroids), and disease duration (21–28). A recent study by Gough and coworkers (21) in a large longitudinal prospective study concluded that significant amounts of generalized skeletal bone was lost early in RA and that this loss was associated with disease activity. These findings support the previous observations of Als et al. (29), who also noted a significant decrease in bone mass during the early phases of RA.

There is still considerable controversy regarding the effects of corticosteroids in affecting the progression of bone loss in RA. In part this is related to the tendency to use these medications in patients with more severe disease. Some authors suggest that if steroids satisfactorily suppress inflammation and maintain mobility, the deleterious effects of corticosteroids may be outweighed (21,22). It is premature, however, to generally advocate the use of corticosteroids in patients with RA since there is considerable evidence that their chronic use is associated with many potentially serious extraskeletal complications (30). This cautionary note is supported by the recent findings of Saag and coworkers who noted that low-dose long-term prednisone use, ≥ 5 g/day, was correlated in a dose-dependent fashion with the development of several different adverse reactions, including fracture (31).

Although not associated with focal bone erosions, generalized bone loss is also a significant clinical problem in patients with SLE. Reductions in both cortical as well as trabecular bone mass have been reported, even in the absence of corticosteroid treatment (32–34). As in patients with RA, the effects of systemic inflammation, decreased physical activity, nutritional factors, sex steroid influences, and drug treatments all likely contribute to the adverse effects on generalized bone mass. Similar factors contribute to the reduced bone mass and increased incidence of fractures in patients with a history of juvenile chronic (rheumatoid) arthritis (35,36). In addition, there is evidence of delayed skeletal linear growth.

Ankylosing spondylitis is characterized by inflammation at the entheses in the spine and peripheral skeleton. Although local bone erosions may be detected early in the course of the disease, new bone formation and ankylosis of the spine eventually develop in many patients. Several studies have documented an increased incidence of spinal compression fractures in patients with this disorder (37–39). Because of the chronic back pain experienced by many patients with ankylosing spondylitis and the high incidence of paraspinal calcifications and syndesmophytes, many of these fractures are not detected. Although not well studied, the decrease in axial bone density has been attributed to the effects of immobilization of the spine associated with the progressive ankylosis. It is interesting that appendicular bone appears to be normal in these individuals.

In contrast to the observations in individuals with inflammatory arthropathies, several authors have suggested that there is a reduced frequency of osteoporosis in patients with osteoarthritis (40–43). In a recent study, Hart et al. (44) examined the relationship between osteoarthritis of the hand, knee, and spine and bone density using dual x-ray absorptiometry of the spine and femoral neck. Their results suggest that the two conditions are inversely related. Adjustments for age, physical activity, and obesity as well as smoking and hormone replacement therapy did not affect results. The mechanisms that account for this observed relationship are not clearly defined.

REFERENCES

1. Harris ED Jr.: Rheumatoid arthritis. Pathophysiology and implications for therapy. *N Engl J Med* 322:1277–1289, 1990
2. Krane SM, Conca W, Stephenson ML, Amento EP, Goldring MB: Mechanisms of matrix degradation in rheumatoid arthritis. *Ann NY Acad Sci* 580:340–354, 1990
3. Bromley M, Woolley DE: Chondroclasts and osteoclasts at subchondral sites of erosion in the rheumatoid joint. *Arthritis Rheum* 27:968–975, 1984
4. Harada Y, Wang JT, Gorn AH, Gravallese EM, Thornhill TS, Jasty M, Harris WH, Juppner H, Goldring SR: Identification of the cell types responsible for bone resorption in rheumatoid arthritis. *Arthritis Rheum* 37:1994
5. Ashton BA, Ashton IK, Marshall MJ, Butler RC: Localization of vitronectin receptor immunoreactivity and tartrate resistant acid phosphatase activity in synovium from patients with inflammatory and degenerative arthritis. *Ann Rheum Dis* 52:133–137, 1993
6. Chang JS, Quinn JM, Demaziere A, Bulstrode CJ, Francis MJ, Duthie RB, Athanasou NA: Bone resorption by cells isolated from rheumatoid synovium. *Ann Rheum Dis* 51:1223–1229, 1992
7. Firestein GS, Alvaro-Garcia JM, Maki R: Quantitative analysis of cytokine gene expression in rheumatoid arthritis. *J Immunol* 144:3347–3353, 1990
8. Shimizo S, Shiozawa S, Shiozawa K, Imura S, Fujita T: Quantitative histological studies on the pathogenesis of peri-articular osteoporosis in rheumatoid arthritis. *Arthritis Rheum* 28:25–31, 1985
9. Joffe I, Epstein S: Osteoporosis associated with rheumatoid arthritis: pathogenesis and management. *Semin Arthritis Rheum* 20:256–272, 1991
10. Peel NF, Eastell R, Russell RG: Osteoporosis in rheumatoid arthritis—the laboratory perspective. *Br J Rheum* 30:84–85, 1991
11. Woolf AD: Osteoporosis in rheumatoid arthritis—the clinical viewpoint. *Br J Rheum* 30:82–84, 1991
12. Spector TD, Hall GM, McCloskey EV, Kanis JA: Risk of vertebral fracture in women with rheumatoid arthritis. *BMJ* 306:558, 1993
13. Hooyman JR, Melton LJ, Nelson AM, O'Fallon WM, Riggs BL: Fractures after rheumatoid arthritis. *Arthritis Rheum* 27:1353–1361, 1984
14. Beat AM, Bloch DA, Fries JF: Predictors of fractures in early rheumatoid arthritis. *J Rheumatol* 18:804–808, 1991
15. Verstraeten A, Dequeker J: Vertebral and peripheral bone mineral content and fracture incidence in postmenopausal patients with rheumatoid arthritis: effect of low dose corticosteroids. *Ann Rheum Dis* 45:852–857, 1986
16. Kroger H, Arnala I, Alhava EM: Bone remodeling in osteoporosis associated with rheumatoid arthritis. *Calcif Tissue Int* 49:S90, 1991
17. Compston JE, Vedi S, Croucher PI, Garrahan NJ, O'Sullivan MM: Bone turnover in non-steroid treated rheumatoid arthritis. *Ann Rheum Dis* 53:163–166, 1994
18. Mellish RWE, O'Sullivan MM, Garrahan NJ, Compston JE: Iliac crest trabecular bone mass and structure in patients with non-steroid treated rheumatoid arthritis. *Ann Rheum Dis* 46:830–836, 1987
19. Hall GM, Spector TD, Delmas PD: Markers of bone metabolism in postmenopausal women with rheumatoid arthritis. Effects of corticosteroids and hormone replacement therapy. *Arthritis Rheum* 38:902–906, 1995
20. Gough AK, Peel NF, Eastell R, Holder RL, Lilley J, Emery P: Excretion of pyridinium crosslinks correlates with disease activity and appendicular bone loss in early rheumatiod arthritis. *Ann Rheum Dis* 53:14–17, 1994
21. Gough AK, Lilley J, Eyre S, Holder RL, Emergy P: Generalized bone loss in patients with early rheumatoid arthritis. *Lancet* 344:23–27, 1994
22. Kirwan JR: The effect of glucocorticoids on joint destruction in rheumatoid arthritis. *N Engl J Med* 333:142–146, 1995
23. Kroger H, Honkanen R, Saarikoski S, Alhava E: Decreased axial bone mineral density in perimenopausal women with rheumatoid arthritis —a population based study. *Ann Rheum Dis* 53:18–23, 1994
24. Laan RF, van Riel PL, van de Putte LB: Bone mass in patients with rheumatoid arthritis. *Ann Rheum Dis* 51:826–832, 1992
25. Laan RF, van Riel PL, van Erning LJ, Lemmens JA, Ruijs SH, van de Putte LB: Vertebral osteoporosis in rheumatoid arthritis patients: effect of low dose prednisone therapy. *Br J Rheumatol* 31:91–96, 1992
26. Sambrook PN, Eisman JA, Champion D, Yeates MG, Pocock

NA, Eberl S: Determinants of axial bone loss in rheumatoid arthritis. *Arthritis Rheum* 30:721–728, 1987

27. Sambrook P, Birmingham J, Champion D, Kelly P, Kempler S, Freund J, Eisman J: Postmenopausal bone loss in rheumatoid arthritis: effect of estrogens and androgens. *J Rheumatol* 19:357–361, 1992

28. Sambrook P, Nguyen T: Vertebral osteoporosis in rheumatoid arthritis patients: effect of low dose prednisone therapy. *Br J Rheumatol* 31:573–574, 1992

29. Als OS, Gotfredsen A, Riis BJ, Christiansen C: Are disease duration and degree of functional impairment determinants of bone loss in rheumatoid arthritis? *Ann Rheum Dis* 44:406–411, 1985

30. Fries JF, Williams CA, Ramsey DR, Bloch DA: The relative toxicity of disease-modifying antirheumatic drugs. *Arthritis Rheum* 36:297–306, 1993

31. Saag KG, Koehnke R, Caldwell JR, Brasington R, Burmeister LF, Zimmerman B, Kohler JA, Durst DE: Low dose long-term corticosteroid therapy in rheumatoid arthritis: an analysis of serious adverse events. *Am J Med* 6:115–123, 1994

32. Dykman TR, Gluck OS, Murphy WA, Hahn TJ, Hahn BH: Evaluation of factors associated with glucocorticoid-induced osteopenia in patients with rheumatic diseases. *Arthritis Rheum* 28:361–368, 1985

33. Kalla AA, Fataar A, Jessop SJ, Bewerunge L: Loss of trabecular bone mineral density in systemic lupus erythematosus. *Arthritis Rheum* 36:1726–1734, 1993

34. Dhillon VB, Davies MC, Hall ML, Round JM, Ell PJ, Jacobs HS, Snaith ML, Isenberg DA: Assessment of the effect of oral corticosteroids on bone mineral density in systemic lupus erythematosus: a preliminary study with dual energy x-ray absorptiometry. *Ann Rheum Dis* 49:624–626, 1990

35. Loftus J, Allen R, Hesp R, David J, Reid DM, Wright DJ, Green JR, Reeve J, Ansell BM, Woo PM: Randomized, double-blind trial of deflazacort versus prednisone in juvenile chronic (or rheumatoid) arthritis: a relatively bone-sparing effect of deflazacort. *Pediatrics* 88:428–436, 1991

36. Varonos S, Ansell BM, Reeve J: Vertebral collapse in juvenile chronic arthritis: its relationship with glucocorticoid therapy. *Calcif Tissue Int* 41:75–78, 1987

37. Hanson CA, Shagrim JW, Duncan H: Vertebral osteoporosis in ankylosing spondylitis. *Clin Orthop* 74:59–64, 1971

38. Will R, Palmer R, Bhalla AK, Ring F, Calin A: Osteoporosis in early ankylosing spondylitis: a primary pathological event? *Lancet* 2:1483–1485, 1989

39. Ralston SH, Urquhart GD, Brzeski M, Sturrock RD: Prevalence of vertebral compression fractures due to osteoporosis in ankylosing spondylitis. *BMJ* 300:563–565, 1990

40. Dequeker J: The relationship between osteoporosis and osteoarthritis. *Clin Rheum Dis* 11:271–296, 1985

41. Cooper C, Cook PL, Osmond C, Fisher L, Cawley MID: Osteoarthritis of the hip and osteoporosis of the proximal femur. *Ann Rheum Dis* 50:540–542, 1991

42. Price T, Hesp R, Mitchell R: Bone density in generalized osteoarthritis. *J Rheumatol* 14:560–562, 1987

43. Nevitt MC, Lane NE, Scott JC, Hochberg MC, Pressman AR, Genant HK, Cummings SR: Radiographic osteoarthritis of the hip and bone mineral density. *Arthritis Rheum* 38:907–916, 1995

44. Hart DJ, Mootoosamy I, Doyle DV, Spector TD: The relationship between osteoarthritis and osteoporosis in the general population: the Clingford study. *Ann Rheum Dis* 53:158–162, 1994

SECTION V

Appendix

i. Laboratory Values of Importance for Calcium Metabolism and Metabolic Bone Disease

Laboratory values of importance for calcium metabolism and metabolic bone disease[a]

Test	Source of specimen	Reference range		Reference range (SI units)
Calcium, ionized	Serum or plasma		mg/dl	mmol/L
		Cord:	5.5 ± 0.3	1.37 ± 0.07
		Newborn		
		3–24 h:	4.3–5.1	1.07–1.27
		24–48 h:	4.0–4.7	1.00–1.17
		Adult:	4.48–4.92	1.12–1.23
		>60 yr		1.13–1.30
Calcium, total	Serum[b]		mg/dl	mmol/L
		Child:	8.8–10.8	2.2–2.7
		Adult:	8.4–10.2	2.1–2.55
	Urine	Ca^{2+} in diet	mg/dl	mmol/d
		Free Ca^{2+}:	5–40	0.13–1.0
		Low to average:	50–150	1.25–3.8
		Average (20 mmol/d):	100–300	2.5–7.5
	Feces	Average: 0.64 g/d		16 mmol/d
Magnesium	Serum	1.3–2.1 mEq/L (higher in females during menses)		0.65–1.05 mmol/L
	Urine, 24-h	6.0–100 mEq/d		3.0–5.0 mmol/d
Phosphatase, acid	Serum	<3.0 ng/ml		<3.0 µg/L
Prostatic (RIA)		0.11–0.60 U/L		0.11–0.60 U/L
Roy, Brower, and				
Hayden, 37 C				
Phosphatase, alkaline	Serum			U/L
p-nitrophenyl phosphate,		Infant:		50–165
carbonate buffer, 30 C		Child:		20–150
		Adult:		20–70
		>60 yr:		30–75
Bowers and McComb, 30 C				25–90
IFFC, 30 C		Male:		30–90
		Female:		20–80
Phosphorus, inorganic	Serum		mg/dl	nmol/L
		Cord:	3.7–8.1	1.2–2.6
		Child:	4.5–5.5	1.45–1.78
		Thereafter	2.7–4.5	0.87–1.45
		>60 yr		
		Male:	2.3–3.7	0.74–1.2
		Female:	2.8–4.1	0.9–1.3
	Urine	Adult on diet containing 0.9–1.5 g P and 10 mg Ca/kg: <1.0 g/d		On diet containing 29–48 mmol P and 0.25 mmol Ca/kg: <32 mmol/d
		Unrestricted diet: 0.4–1.3 g/d		Unrestricted diet: 13–42 mmol/d
Tubular reabsorption of phosphate	Urine, 4 h (0800–1200 h), and serum	82%–95%		Fraction reabsorbed: 0.82–0.95
Vitamin A	Serum	30–65 µg/dl		1.05–2.27 mmol/L
Vitamin D_3, 25 hydroxy	Plasma	Summer: 15–80 ng/ml		37–200 nmol/L
		Winter: 14–42 ng/ml		35–105 nmol/L
Vitamin D_3, 1,25 dihydroxy	Serum	25–45 pg/ml		12–46 µmol/L

Laboratory values of importance for calcium metabolism and metabolic bone disease[a] Continued.

Test	Source of specimen	Reference range		Reference range (SI units)
Calcitonin[d]	Serum (Nichols RIA)	Basal	pg/ml	
		Male	<36	
		Female	<17	
		Pentagastrin		
		Male	<106	
		Female	<29	
	Serum (CIS 2-site IRMA)	Basal	pg/ml	
		Male	<10	
		Female	<10	
		Pentagastrin		
		Male	<30	
		Female	<30	
	Serum (Mayo Medical Lab)	Basal		
		Male	<19	
		Female	<14	
		Pentagastrin		
		Male	<110	
		Female	<30	
Parathyroid hormone[d]	Serum (intact, Mayo Lab)	Basal	1.0–5.0 pmol/L	
	Serum (intact, Nichols Institute)	Basal	10–65 pg/ml	
	Serum (mid-molecule, Nichols Institute)	Basal	50–330 pg/ml	
	Serum (N-terminal, Nichols Institute)	Basal	8–24 pg/ml	
Osteocalcin[d]	Serum (Nichols Institute)	Basal	1.6–9.2 ng/ml	
PTHrP[d]	Serum (intact, Nichols Institute)	Basal	<0.5 pmol/L	
Procollagen (PICP)	Plasma (Osteometer A/S)	Basal		
		Male	128 ng/ml	
		Female	115 ng/ml	
Pyridinium (PYD) crosslinks	Urine (Metra Biosystems)	Basal		
		Male	8–24 nM PYD/mM creatinine	
		Female	10–28 nM PYD/mM creatinine	
Type 1 collagen peptides	Urine (Osteometer A/S)	Basal		
		Female		
		(Premenopausal)	0.293 ± 0.155 µg/µmol creatinine (mean ± SD)	
		(Postmenopausal)	0.532 ± 0.229 µg/µmol creatinine	

[a]Laboratory values in this table were extracted from: Tietz NW. Reference ranges and laboratory values of clinical importance. In: Wyngaarden JB, Smith LH Jr (eds): *Cecil Textbook of Medicine,* 17th ed. Philadelphia: Saunders, 1985. This reference provides more detailed discussion of source material and units used in this table.

[b]Divide by 2 to get mEq/L.

[c]The total serum calcium can be corrected for alterations in the serum protein concentration by the following formula: Corrected total serum calcium (mg/dl) = observed total serum calcium + [(the normal mean albumin concentration - the observed albumin concentration) × 0.8]. In most situations, the normal mean albumin concentration equals 4 g/dl.

[d]The normal values listed include commercial assays. These are listed not to provide an endorsement for these assays, but because they are representative of values available for daily clinical use. It is likely that normal values in other research or commercial assays will vary to some extent.

ii. Formulary of Drugs Commonly Used in Treatment of Mineral Disorders

Formulary of drugs commonly used in treatment of mineral disorders[a]

Drug	Application in treatment of bone and mineral disorders	Dosage (adult)[b]	Rx Cat[c]	Notes[d]
Hormones and analogs				
1. Calcitonin				
Human (Cibacalcin) im or sc (0.5 mg vials)	Paget's disease	0.25–0.5 mg im or sc; q24h	Rx	
Salmon (Calcimar, Miacalcin) im or sc (100, 200 IU/ml) (sc preferred)	Paget's disease, osteoporosis, hypercalcemia	50–100 IU, im or sc; qod or qd for Paget's or osteoporosis; 4–6 IU/kg im or sc; qid for hypercalcemia	Rx	Modestly effective and short-lived in treatment of hypercalcemia
Nasal spray (200 IU/spray)		200 IU nasal qd for osteoporosis	Rx	
2. Estrogens				
Estinyl estradiol (Estinyl, Seminone), po (0.02, 0.05, 0.5 mg)	Postmenopausal osteoporosis	0.02–0.05 mg; qd 3/4 weeks	Rx	To reduce risk of . endometrial cancer, estrogens can be cycled with a progesterone during last 7–10 days or given concurrently with a progestin throughout the cycle (less break-through bleeding)
17B estradiol (Estrace), po (1, 2 mg)		1–2 mg; qd 3/4 weeks	Rx	
Transderm patch (Estraderm)		0.05–0.1 mg 2x/wk	Rx	
Conjugated equine estrogens (Premarin), po (0.3, 0.625, 0.9, 1.25, 2.5 mg)		0.625–1.25 mg qd 3/4 weeks	Rx	0.3 mg conjugated equine estrogens (CEE) with calcium may also be effective.
3. Glucocorticoids				
Prednisone (Deltasone), po (2.5, 5, 10, 20, 50 mg)	Hypercalcemia due to sarcoidosis, vitamin D intoxication, and certain malignancies such as multiple myeloma and related lymphoproliferative disorders	10–60 mg; qd	Rx	Long-term use results in osteoporosis and adrenal suppression. Other glucocorticoids with minimal mineralcorticoid activity can be used.
4. Parathyroid hormone				
Human 1–34 (Parathor), iv (200 U/vial)	Diagnosis of pseudo-hypoparathyroidism	200 U; over 10 min infusion	Rx	The use of PTH to treat osteoporosis is being evaluated.
5. Progesterone				
Medroxyprogesterone (Provera), po (2.5, 5, 10 mg)	Osteoporosis in conjunction with estrogens	10 mg; qd for final 7 to 10 days of cycle	Rx	The concurrent use of progesterone does not appear to reduce the protective cardiovascular effects of estrogen or diminish the potential risk for breast cancer.
Norethindrone (Micronor, Nor-QD, Norlutin), po (5 mg)		5 mg; qd for final 7 to 10 days of cycle 2.5 mg continuously with estrogen	Rx	

135

Formulary of drugs commonly used in treatment of mineral disorders[a] Continued.

Drug	Application in treatment of bone and mineral disorders	Dosage (adult)[b]	Rx Cat[c]	Notes[d]
6. Vitamin D preparations				
Cholecalciferol or D_3, po (125, 250, 400 U, often in combination with calcium)	Nutritional vitamin D deficiency, osteoporosis, malabsorption, hypoparathyroidism, refractory rickets	400–1000 U; as dietary supplement	OTC	
Ergocalciferol or D_2 (Calciferol), po (8000 U/ml drops; 25,000, 50,000 U tabs)		25,000–100,000 U; 3×/wk to qd	Rx, OTC	D_2 (or D_3) has been shown to reduce fractures and increase BMD in elderly women at 400–1000 U doses.
Calcifediol or 25(OH)D_3 (Calderol), (20, 50 mg)	Malabsorption, renal osteodystrophy	20–50 µg; 3×/wk to qd	Rx	25(OH)D_3 may be useful in treatment for steroid-induced osteoporosis.
Calcitriol or 1,25(OH)$_2D_3$ (Rocaltrol), po (0.25, 0.5 µg); (Calcijex), iv (1 or 2 µg/ml)	Renal osteodystrophy, hypoparathyroidism, refractory rickets	0.25–1.0 µg; qd to bid	Rx	Role of calcitriol in treatment of osteoporosis, psoriasis, and certain malignancies is being evaluated, primarily with new analogs.
Dihydrotachysterol (DHT), po (0.125, 0.2, 0.4 mg)	Renal osteodystrophy, hypoparathyroidism	0.2–1.0 mg; qd	Rx	
Bisphosphonates				
1. **Etidronate** (Didronel), po (200, 400 mg); iv (300 mg/6 ml vial)	Paget's disease, heterotopic ossification, hypercalcemia of malignancy	po: 5 mg/kg, qd for 6/12 mo for Paget's disease; 20 mg/kg, qd 1 mo before to 3 mo after total hip replacement; 10–20 mg/kg, qd for 3 mo after spinal cord injury for heterotopic ossification. iv: 7.5 mg/kg, qd for 3 d, given in 250–500 ml normal saline for hypercalcemia of malignancy.	Rx	Etidronate is the first-generation bisphosphonate. High doses may cause a mineralization disorder not seen with newer bisphosphonates.
2. **Alendronate** (Fosamax), po (10 mg)	Osteoporosis, Paget's disease	10 mg qd for osteoporosis; 40 mg qd for Paget's disease	Rx	
3. **Pamidronate** (Aredia), iv (30–90 mg/10 ml)	Hypercalcemia of malignancy, Paget's disease	60–90 mg given as a single intravenous infusion over 24 h for hypercalcemia of malignancy; 4-h infusions also effective for 30- or 60-mg doses. 30-mg doses over 4 h on 3 consecutive days for a total of 90 mg for Paget's disease	Rx	
Minerals				
1. **Bicarbonate, sodium,** po (325, 527, 650 mg)	Chronic metabolic acidosis leading to bone disease	Must be titrated for each patient	Rx, OTC	

Formulary of drugs commonly used in treatment of mineral disorders[a] Continued.

Drug	Application in treatment of bone and mineral disorders	Dosage (adult)[b]	Rx Cat[c]	Notes[d]
2. Calcium preparations				
Calcium carbonate (40% Ca), po (500, 650 mg)	Hypocalcemia (if symptomatic should be treated iv), osteoporosis, rickets, osteomalacia, chronic renal failure, hypoparathyroidism, malabsorption, enteric oxaluria	po: 400–2000 mg elemental Ca in divided doses; qd	OTC	Calcium carbonate is the preferred form because it has the highest percentage of calcium and is the least expensive, although calcium citrate may be somewhat better absorbed. In normal subjects, the solubility of the calcium salt has not been shown to affect its absorption from the intestine. In achlorhydric subjects, $CaCO_3$ should be given with meals.
Calcium citrate (Citracal) (21% Ca), po (950–1500 mg)				
Calcium chloride (36% Ca), iv (100% solution)				
Calcium bionate (6.5% Ca) (Neo-glucon), po (1.8 g in 5 ml)				
Calcium gluconate (9% Ca), po (500, 600, 1000 mg), iv (10% solution, 0.465 mEq/ml)		iv, 2–20 ml 10% calcium gluconate over several hours	Rx	Calcium gluconate is the preferred iv form because, unlike calcium chloride, it does not burn.
Calcium lactate (13% Ca), po (325, 650 mg)				
Calcium phosphate, dibasic (23% Ca), po (486 mg)				
Tricalcium phosphate (39% Ca) po (300, 600 mg)				
3. Fluoride preparations				
Fluoride, sodium (Luride, Fluoritab), po (2.25 mg/ml drops; 0.25, 0.5, 1.0 mg F tabs)	Dental prophylaxis in regions with non-fluoridated water	0.25–1 mg F, depending on age of child and fluoride content of water supply	Rx	Currently being investgated for treatment of osteoporosis at much higher doses. Also available combined with vitamins and other minerals or for topical application to teeth.
Florical (8.3 mg sodium fluoride and 364 mg calcium carbonate)	Osteoporosis	3–6 tablets/day		Fluoride is not FDA approved for treatment of osteoporosis
4. Magnesium preparations				
Magnesium oxide (Mag-Ox, Uro-Mag), po (84.5, 241.3 mg Mg)	Hypomagnesemia	240–480 mg elemental Mg; qd	OTC	Low magnesium often coexists with low calcium in alcoholics and malabsorbers. Also found in many antacids and vitamin formulations.
5. Phosphate preparations				
Neutra-Phos, po (250 mg P, 278 mg K, 164 mg Na)	Hypophosphatemia, vitamin-D-resistant rickets, hypercalcemia, hypercalciuria	po: 1–3 g in divided doses; qd	Rx, OTC	
Neutra-Phos-K, po (250 mg P, 556 mg K)				

Formulary of drugs commonly used in treatment of mineral disorders[a] Continued.

Drug	Application in treatment of bone and mineral disorders	Dosage (adult)[b]	Rx Cat[c]	Notes[d]
Fleet Phospha-Soda, po (815 mg P, 760 mg Na in 5 ml)				
In-Phos, iv (1 g P in 40 ml)		iv: 1.5 g over 6–8 h		iv phosphorus is seldom necessary and can be toxic if infusion is too rapid.
Hyper-Phos-K, iv (1 g P in 15 ml)				
Diuretics				
1. **Thiazides**				
Hydrochlorothiazide (Esidrix, Hydro-Diuril), po (25, 50, 100 mg)	Hypercalciuria, nephrolithiasis	25–50 mg; qd or bid	Rx	Other thiazides may also be effective but are less commonly used for this purpose. These uses are not FDA approved.
Chlorthalidone, po (25, 50 mg)				
2. **Loop diuretics**				
Furosemide (Lasix), po (20, 40, 80 mg), iv (10 mg/ml)	Hypercalcemia; if symptomatic, use iv	po: 20–80 mg, q6h as necessary; iv: 20–80 mg over several minutes, repeat as necessary	Rx	Ethacrynic acid may also be effective but is less commonly used for this purpose. These uses are not FDA approved.
Miscellaneous				
1. **Mitramycin or plicamycin** (Mithracin), iv (2.5 mg/vial)	Hypercalcemia of malignancy	25 µg/kg in 1 liter D5W or normal saline over 4–6 hr	Rx	Has been used in treatment of severe Paget's disease, but toxicity makes it treatment of last resort for this purpose and it has not been approved by the FDA for this purpose.
2. **Gallium nitrate** (Genite)	Hypercalcemia of malignancy	200 mg/m² qd in D5W for continuous infusion over 5 d	Rx	

[a]This table is not intended to be an official guideline.

[b]qd, every day; qod, every other day; bid, twice a day; tid, three times a day; qid, four times a day; sc, subcutaneously; im, intramuscularly; po, orally; iv, intravenously; IU, International Units.

[c]Rx Cat, prescription category: Rx, prescriptions required; OTC, over-the-counter preparations available.

[d]Where comments are not specifically aligned with preparations or their dosages, they apply to all preparations listed in that column.

iii. **Bone Density Reference Data**

The reference data displayed below were provided by the manufacturer for Hologic QDR Systems. All data, unless otherwise noted, were obtained from Caucasian sample populations. They are listed in 5-year age increments with mean ±2 standard deviations (95% confidence interval).

TABLE 1. *Normal bone mineral density (BMD) values of the AP Spine (L2 to L4) in females*

Age	BMD	DEV
20	1.051	0.110
25	1.072	0.110
30	1.079	0.110
35	1.073	0.110
40	1.056	0.110
45	1.030	0.110
50	0.997	0.110
55	0.960	0.110
60	0.920	0.110
65	0.878	0.110
70	0.840	0.110
75	0.805	0.110
80	0.775	0.110
85	0.754	0.110

TABLE 3. *Normal BMD values of the hip/femoral neck in females*

Age	BMD	DEV
20	0.895	0.100
25	0.894	0.100
30	0.886	0.100
35	0.871	0.100
40	0.850	0.100
45	0.826	0.100
50	0.797	0.100
55	0.766	0.100
60	0.733	0.100
65	0.700	0.100
70	0.667	0.100
75	0.636	0.100
80	0.607	0.100
85	0.581	0.100

TABLE 2. *Normal BMD values of the AP Spine (L2 to L4) in males*

Age	BMD	DEV
20	1.115	0.110
25	1.115	0.110
30	1.115	0.110
35	1.115	0.110
40	1.115	0.110
45	1.091	0.110
50	1.076	0.110
55	1.061	0.110
60	1.045	0.110
65	1.030	0.110
70	1.015	0.110
75	0.999	0.110
80	0.984	0.110
85	0.968	0.110

TABLE 4. *Normal BMD values of the hip/femoral neck in males*

Age	BMD	DEV
20	0.979	0.110
25	0.958	0.110
30	0.936	0.110
35	0.915	0.110
40	0.894	0.110
45	0.873	0.110
50	0.851	0.110
55	0.830	0.110
60	0.809	0.110
65	0.788	0.110
70	0.766	0.110
75	0.745	0.110
80	0.724	0.110
85	0.703	0.110

For additional information, please contact HOLOGIC, INC., 590 Lincoln Street, Waltham, MA 02154.

The following reference data were supplied by the manufacturer for HOLOGIC scanners. All data were based on ambulatory subjects free from chronic bone diseases and not currently taking medications that may affect bone.

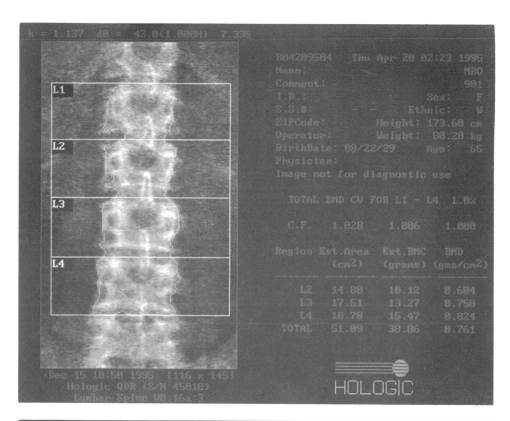

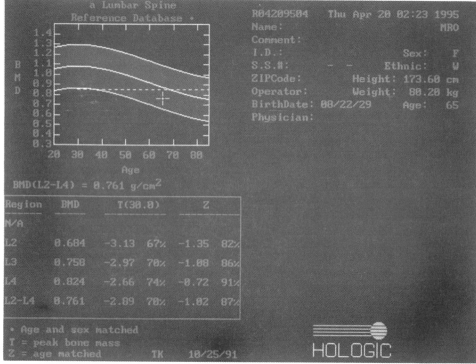

FIG. 1. Sample report obtained for lumbar spine of a 65-year-old female patient.

TABLE 5. *Mean BMD values for spine L2 to L4 (SD = 0.12 g/cm2) for reference US/Europe population*

Age	Female		Male	
	n	Mean	n	Mean
20–29	467	1.188	85	1.255
30–39	499	1.207	106	1.215
40–49	716	1.170	73	1.174
50–59	969	1.081	67	1.161
60–69	476	0.995	63	1.183
70–79	105	0.960	51	1.178

TABLE 6. *Mean female BMD values for femur regions (SD = 0.12 g/cm2)*

Age	n	Neck	Ward's	Trochanter
20–29	479	0.994	0.947	0.798
30–39	499	0.958	0.886	0.787
40–49	704	0.950	0.847	0.792
50–59	882	0.881	0.751	0.745
60–69	415	0.811	0.660	0.714
70–79	121	0.773	0.630	0.668

TABLE 7. *Mean male BMD values for femur regions (SD = 0.12 g/cm2)*

Age	n	Neck	Ward's	Trochanter
20–29	84	1.107	1.022	0.948
30–39	95	1.038	0.922	0.900
40–49	74	1.001	0.852	0.898
50–59	73	0.985	0.809	0.920
60–69	66	0.953	0.770	0.904
70–79	46	0.872	0.685	0.841

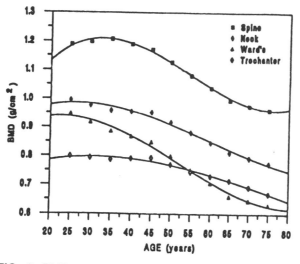

FIG. 2. BMD values of the AP spine and femur (neck, Ward's triangle, and trochanter) in Caucasian female reference subjects.

AP SPINE RESULTS
LUNAR CORPORATION
313 W. BELTLINE HWY., MADISON, WI 53713

Patient, Rkp   AP SPINE BONE DENSITY

Facility: Acquired: 09/15/95 (4.00)
42 years 12/01/52   Analyzed: 09/15/95 (4.00)
191.0cm 79.6kg White Male   Printed: 12/06/95 (4.00)
Physician: payner11.s01

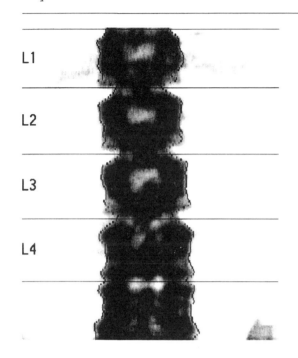

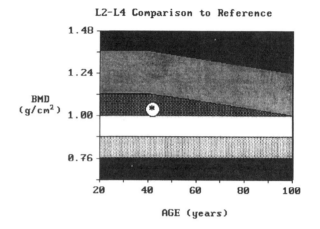

Region	BMD[1] g/cm²	Young-Adult[2] %	T	Age-Matched[3] %	Z
L2-L4	1.039	84	-1.7	84	-1.7

Image not for diagnosis
3.00:Medium DPX 0.6x1.2 1.68
813099:452773 1.385:5.0 263.79:195.56:142.67

FIG. 3. Sample report obtained for AP spine of a 42-year-old male patient.
[1]Statistically, 68% of repeat scans fall within 1 SD.
[2]USA AP spine reference population, ages 20–40.
[3]Matched for age, weight (males 25–100 kg; females 25–100 kg), ethnic background.

For additional information please contact LUNAR Corporation, 313 W. Beltline Highway, Madison, WI 53713.

Subject Index

Subject Index